P9-BID-217

Therapeutic Alternatives in the Management of Benign Prostatic Hyperplasia

Edited by

Flavio Castañeda, M.D.
Clinical Assistant Professor of Radiology
College of Medicine at Peoria
University of Illinois
Peoria, Illinois

Arthur D. Smith, M.D.
Chairman, Department of Urology
Long Island Jewish Medical Center
New Hyde Park, New York

Wilfrido R. Castañeda-Zúñiga, M.D.
Professor of Radiology
University of Minnesota
Minneapolis, Minnesota

1993
Thieme Medical Publishers, Inc., New York
Georg Thieme Verlag, Stuttgart · New York

Thieme Medical Publishers, Inc.
381 Park Avenue South
New York, New York 10016

THERAPEUTIC ALTERNATIVES IN THE MANAGEMENT
OF BENIGN PROSTATIC HYPERPLASIA
Flavio Castañeda, Arthur D. Smith, Wilfrido R. Castañeda-Zúñiga

Library of Congress Cataloging-in-Publication Data

Therapeutic alternatives in the management of benign prostatic hyperplasia
  / edited by Flavio Castañeda, Arthur D. Smith, Wilfrido R. Castañeda
  -Zúñiga.
      p.   cm.
    Includes bibliographical references and index.
    ISBN 0-86577-440-4 (Thieme Medical Publishers).—ISBN
3-13-783201-2 (Georg Thieme Verlag)
    1. Prostate—Hypertrophy—Alternative treatment.
2. Urethroplasty. I. Castañeda, Flavio. II. Smith, Arthur D.
III. Castañeda-Zúñiga, Wilfrido R.
    [DNLM: 1. Prostatic Hypertrophy—therapy.   WJ 752 T3975]
RC899.T48   1992
616.5′5—dc20
DNLM/DLC
for Library of Congress   92-49924
                                                    CIP

Important note: Medicine is an ever-changing science. Research and clinical experience are continually broadening our knowledge, in particular our knowledge of proper treatment and drug therapy. Insofar as this book mentions any dosage or application, readers may rest assured that the authors, editors, and publishers have made every effort to ensure that such references are strictly in accordance with the state of knowledge at the time of production of the book. Nevertheless, every user is requested to carefully examine the manufacturers' leaflets accompanying each drug to check on his own responsibility whether the dosage schedules recommended therein or the contraindications stated by the manufacturers differ from the statements made in the present book. Such examination is particulary important with drugs that are either rarely used or have been newly released on the market.

Some of the product names, patents, and registered designs referred to in this book are in fact registered trademarks or proprietary names even though specific reference to this fact is not always made in the text. Therefore, the appearance of a name without designation as proprietary is not to be construed as a representation by the publisher that it is in the public domain.

Printed in the United States of America.

5 4 3 2 1

(TMP) ISBN 0-86577-440-4
(GTV) ISBN 3-13-783201-2

This book is dedicated to my wife Yvonne and daughters Yvonne Jr. and Denysse for their sacrifices and continuous support that allowed me to undertake this endeavor.

To my mentors, Drs. Kurt Amplatz, Wilfrido R. Castañeda-Zúñiga, and David Hunter with deep appreciation and gratitude for their teaching and encouragement.

And finally to my partners of Peoria Radiology Associates for allowing me to continue my research and academic activities.

Flavio Castañeda, M.D.

Contents

Preface

Throughout the centuries medicine has been characterized by continuous evolution brought on by new knowledge and technological advancements that have resulted from both the need for better, safer therapies and the curiosity and genius of many pioneers in the field. Today's cost-conscious society and rising medical costs have added further pressure to the continuing need for these better and safer therapies by placing cost-efficiency as one of the main goals in the pursuit of better quality of life.

Benign prostatic hyperplasia is currently the number one cause of obstructive uropathy in the elder male population, a condition that will continue to rise due to longer life expectancies. If current trends continue, it is estimated that about 20–25% of males will require some procedure for the relief of bladder outlet obstruction at some point in their lives.

This has placed transurethral resection of the prostate, the current standard treatment modality for this ailment, as the second most costly major operation under medicare, taking approximately 1.4% of its total allowance. This reflects approximately 38% of all major surgical and 24% of all urological workloads in an average urological practice.

This book attempts to provide concise, state-of-the-art assessment and screening criteria and modalities used for the diagnosis of benign prostatic hyperplasia; to provide an in-depth historic and current overview of the different experiences with balloon dilatation of the prostatic urethra as well as its mechanism of action, which although a relatively new procedure, has now been utilized experimentally by many investigators; and lastly, a detailed review of the newest trends in the non-surgical attempts to manage or alternatively treat benign prostatic hyperplasia.

All of the contributors in this book have been pioneers in their respective specialties, in which they have gathered worldwide recognition. They all share their experiences with us by exploring new possible applications or by presenting new research on fascinating and innovative methods for the treatment of this complex but common medical problem for which the pathophysiology is still poorly understood.

Flavio Castañeda M.D.
Peoria, Illinois

Contributors

Jorn Aagaard, M.D.
Urology Research Fellow
Department of Surgery
University of Wisconsin
Madison, Wisconsin

Kurt Amplatz, M.D.
Professor of Radiology
Director, Cardiovascular and Interventional Radiology
University of Minnesota
Minneapolis, Minnesota

Dean G. Assimos, M.D.
Associate Professor of Urology
Bowman Gray School of Medicine
Wake Forest University
Winston-Salem, North Carolina

Joseph J. Banno, M.D.
Clinical Assistant Professor of Urology
University of Illinois
College of Medicine at Peoria
Peoria, Illinois

Edgardo F. Becher, M.D.
Staff Urologist
University of Buenos Aires Hospital
Buenos Aires, Argentina

J. A. Belon, M.D.
Staff of Urology Department
N. S. del Pino Hospital
Canary Islands, Spain

Ben C. Berg, M.D.
Clinical Assistant Professor of Radiology
University of Illinois
College of Medicine at Peoria
Peoria, Illinois

Terry M. Brady, M.D.
Clinical Assistant Professor of Radiology
University of Illinois
College of Medicine at Peoria
Peoria, Illinois

Reginald Bruskewitz, M.D.
Associate Professor of Surgery
University of Wisconsin-Madison Medical School
Madison, Wisconsin

Simon St. Clair Carter, M.S., F.R.C.S.
Consultant Urologist
Charing Cross Hospital
London, England, United Kingdom

Flavio Castañeda, M.D.
Director of Research
Department of Radiology
Clinical Assistant Professor of Radiology
University of Illinois
College of Medicine at Peoria
Peoria, Illinois

Wilfrido R. Castañeda-Zúñiga, M.D.
Professor of Radiology
University of Minnesota
Minneapolis, Minnesota

B.L. Davies, M.Phil.
Centre for Robotics
Imperial College London
London, England, United Kingdom

Laurel E. Emerson, R.N.
Research Assistant
Department of Urology
Queen's University
Kingston General Hospital
Kingston, Ontario, Canada

Richard M. Evans, M.D.
Assistant Professor
Department of Urologic Surgery
University of Minnesota
Minneapolis, Minnesota

S. Larry Goldenberg, M.D., F.R.C.S. (C)
Associate Professor of Urology
University of British Columbia
Vancouver, British Columbia, Canada

Lloyd H. Harrison, M.D.
Department of Urology
Bowman Gray School of Medicine
Wake Forest University
Winston-Salem, North Carolina

Lois J. Hart, M.D.
Department of Urology
Bowman Gray School of Medicine
Wake Forest University
Winston-Salem, North Carolina

Maj. José M. Hernandez-Graulau, MD USAR MC
Assistant Professor
New York Medical College
Director of Urology
Lincoln Hospital
New York, New York

R.D. Hibberd, Ph.D.
Centre for Robotics
Imperial College London
London, England, United Kingdom

David Hunter, M.D.
Professor of Radiology
University of Minnesota
Minneapolis, Minnesota

Santiago Isorna, M.D.
Director of Urology Department
Passo de Madrid #12
Canary Islands, Spain

F. Izquierdo, M.D.
Head of the Radiodiagnostic Service
Instituto de Urologia, Nefrologia y Andrologia
Hospital de la Santa Cruz y San Pablo
Escuela de Post-Graduados-Universidad
   Autonoma de Barcelona
Barcelona, Spain

Deepak A. Kapoor, M.D.
Assistant Professor of Urologic Surgery
University of Minnesota
Minneapolis, Minnesota

Fred Lee, M.D.
Department of Radiology
St. Joseph Mercy Hospital
Ann Arbor, Michigan

Janis G. Letourneau, M.D.
Associate Professor of Radiology
University of Minnesota
Minneapolis, Minnesota

Wei-Jia Li, M.D.
Department of Urology
Bowman Gray School of Medicine
Wake Forest University
Winston-Salem, North Carolina

A. Lindner, M.D.
Head, Department of Urology
State of Israel-Ministry of Health
The Edith Wolfson Hospital
Holon, Israel

Peter Littrup, M.D.
Director of Research
Department of Radiology
St. Joseph Mercy Hospital
Assistant Professor of Radiology and Urology
Wayne State University
Ann Arbor, Michigan

Deborah Longley, M.D.
Assistant Professor of Radiology
University of Minnesota
Minneapolis, Minnesota

Manuel Maynar, M.D.
Head of Vascular and Interventional Radiology Unit
N. S. del Pino Hospital
Canary Islands, Spain

David L. McCullough, M.D.
Department of Urology
Bowman Gray School of Medicine
Wake Forest University
Winston-Salem, North Carolina

Curtis Mettlin, Ph.D.
Department of Cancer Control and Epidemiology
Roswell Park Memorial Institute
Buffalo, New York

Euan Milroy, F.R.C.S.
Consultant Urologist
The Middlesex Hospital
London, England, United Kingdom

W.S. Ng, M.Eng.
Centre for Robotics
Imperial College London
London, England, United Kingdom

A. Patel, M.D.
Department of Urology
Charing Cross Hospital
London, England, United Kingdom

Ramon Perez-Marrero, M.D., F.R.C.S. (C)
Associate Professor of Urology
Department of Urology
Queen's University
Kingston General Hospital
Kingston, Ontario, Canada

Jon L. Pryor, M.D.
Assistant Professor
Departments of Urologic Surgery and Cell
Biology/Neuroanatomy
University of Minnesota
Minneapolis, Minnesota

J.W.A. Ramsay, M.D.
Department of Urology
Charing Cross Hospital
London, England, United Kingdom

Pratap Reddy, M.D.
Professor of Urologic Surgery
Chief, Urology Section-Minneapolis VA Medical Center
University of Minnesota Hospitals
Minneapolis, Minnesota

Kathy Richardson, R.N.
Department of Urology
University of Iowa Hospitals and Clinics
Iowa City, Iowa

P. Royer, M.D.
Department of Urology
Charing Cross Hospital
London, England, United Kingdom

J. Salvador, M.D.
Urology Service
Instituto de Urologia, Nefrologia y Andrologia
Hospital de la Santa Cruz y San Pablo
Escuela de Post-Graduados-Universidad
    Autonoma de Barcelona
Barcelona, Spain

Jay I. Sandlow, M.D.
Resident
Department of Urology
University of Iowa Hospitals and Clinics
Iowa City, Iowa

Claude Schulman, M.D., Ph.D.
Professor of Urology
Cliniques Université de Bruxelles
Hospital Erasme 808, R. Lennik
Bruxelles, Belgium

Abraham Ami Sidi, M.D.
Associate Professor
Department of Urologic Surgery
University of Minnesota
Minneapolis, Minnesota

Judy F. Siegel, M.D.
Resident
Department of Urology
Long Island Jewish Medical Center
New Hyde Park, New York

Arthur D. Smith, M.D.
Chairman, Department of Urology
Long Island Jewish Medical Center
New Hyde Park, New York

Anthony G. Timoney, M.S., F.R.C.S.
Senior Registrar
Department of Urology
The Royal Surrey County Hospital
Surrey, England, United Kingdom

M. Vandenbossche, M.D.
Urologist
Cliniques Université de Bruxelles
Hospital Erasme 808, R. Lennik
Bruxelles, Belgium

J. Vicente, M.D.
Clinic Head
Urology Service
Instituto de Urologia, Nefrologia y Andrologia
Hospital de la Santa Cruz y San Pablo
Escuela de Post-Graduados-Universidad
    Autonoma de Barcelona
Barcelona, Spain

J.E.A. Wickham, F.R.C.S.
Institute of Urology
London, England, United Kingdom

Jerrold Widran, M.D.
Clinical Associate Professor
Department of Surgery-Urology Section
University of Health Sciences
Chicago Medical School
Chicago, Illinois

Howard N. Winfield, M.D.
Assistant Professor of Urology
Department of Urology
University of Iowa Hospitals and Clinics
Iowa City, Iowa

Ralph D. Woodruff, M.D.
Department of Pathology
Bowman Gray School of Medicine
Wake Forest University
Winston-Salem, North Carolina

Benign Prostatic Hypertrophy: Assessment and Screening

Anatomy of the Prostate

Janis Gissel Letourneau, Deborah Longley

A considerable amount of investigation into the normal and pathologic anatomy of the prostate has been undertaken in recent years. Interest in the anatomy of the prostate has been stimulated in part by the dramatic technologic advances in prostatic imaging that have occurred. Undoubtedly, because of the intense interest in prostatic imaging seen in both benign and malignant processes, a sophisticated understanding of the prostate in normal and pathologic conditions is necessary.

A lobar nature of the prostatic gland was emphasized in the older literature.[1] This concept of prostate anatomy has been replaced by one based on histologically distinct anatomic zones.[2] The relative proportion that each of these zones contributes to the overall configuration of the gland changes with age and the variable development of benign prostatic hyperplasia. Knowledge of this zonal anatomy and the propensity of involvement of specific pathologic processes in certain zones is necessary for accurate evaluation of prostatic imaging studies.

Much of the literature correlating prostate histology with the appearance of the gland as defined by ultrasound, computed tomography (CT), and magnetic resonance imaging (MRI) has focused on the identification and staging of prostatic carcinoma and, to a lesser extent, on the characterization of benign prostatic hyperplasia and inflammatory processes.[3-18] Less has been written on the normal sonographic, CT, or MRI appearance of the gland. However, since an understanding of the normal histology of the prostate is critical to interpretation of radiologic studies, this topic is discussed first in this chapter and correlated with imaging studies. The relationship of the zonal prostate anatomy to the development of pathologic processes then is discussed.

NORMAL ANATOMY

The prostate is a small, cone-shaped gland situated just inferior to the bladder neck. It surrounds the posterior urethra. The base, the broadest aspect, of the gland is situated more cranially, the apex more caudally. The paired seminal vesicles are elliptical saccular structures located just cranially and slightly posteriorly to the prostate, with the ejaculatory ducts forming at the confluence of the seminal vesicle ducts and vas deferens. The ejaculatory ducts course through the prostate to empty into the prostatic urethra at the verumontanum.

The current zonal anatomic concept of the prostate gland has been popularized by McNeal.[19-21] He defines four major types of tissue within the gland, periurethral, transitional, fibromuscular, and acinar glandular regions (Fig. 1–1 and 1–2).

The periurethral zone is small, composed of the glands that line the urethra from the neck of the bladder to the verumontanum. The histologic character of the transitional (or preprostatic) zone is similar to that of the peripheral acinar zone. It is located between the anterior fibromuscular zone and the central and peripheral acinar regions. Like the periurethral glandular region, it is related to the preprostatic sphincter and does not extend caudal to the verumontanum. The anterior fibromuscular zone is composed of smooth and striated muscle elements and is located in the most anterior position of the entire craniocaudad extend of the prostate. It is widest at the midprostate level and is least prominent at the apex. It forms the anterior aspect of the prostatic capsule, blending with the smooth muscle fibers of the bladder neck and thinning at the apex.[19-21] Circularly arranged smooth muscle fibers that are continuous with the stromal elements of the gland comprise the rest of the prostatic capsule.[22]

There are two peripherally situated acinar regions of the gland, the central and peripheral glandular zones. The central acinar region lies just posterior to the urethra and is broadest at the base of the prostate and narrowest at the apex. The ejaculatory ducts course through the central glandular region as they traverse obliquely, caudally, and slightly anteriorly to the verumontanum. The predominant acinar region in the

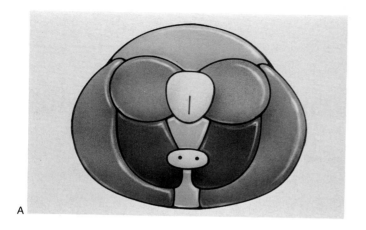
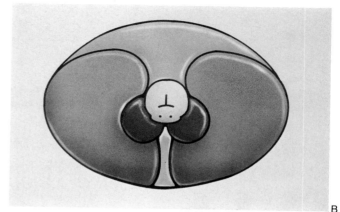
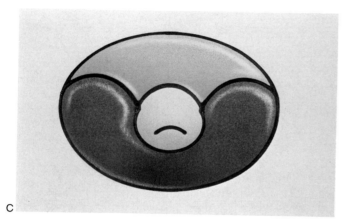
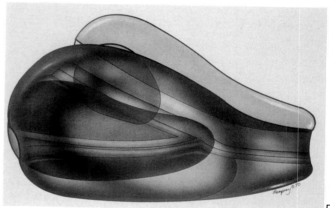

Figure 1–1.   Diagnostic representation of normal anatomy of the prostate. **A.** Transverse section through the base. Note the predominance of central glandular and transitional zones. Paired ejaculatory ducts are seen inferior to the urethra. **B.** Transverse section through the midprostate near the level of the verumontanum shows increasing predominance of peripheral zone. **C.** Transverse section at apex where fibromuscular stroma is present anteriorly and peripheral zone is identified posteriorly. **D.** Lateral view showing zones of the prostate gland, course of urethra, and ejaculatory ducts.

normal prostate is the peripheral zone, constituting approximately 75% of the glandular tissue. The peripheral zone is shaped like an open funnel, surrounding the central acinar region. It is situated largely posterolaterally but also extends anterolaterally at the base of the gland. It constitutes the majority of the prostatic apex.

These zones of the normal prostate can be defined to a variable degree with high-resolution sonography, CT, and MRI.[23–29] By transrectal sonography, the periurethral area is characterized as a hypoechoic region surrounding the prostatic urethra. Likely because of its muscular component, the anterior fibromuscular zone is also somewhat hypoechoic relative to the acinar regions. The central and peripheral glandular regions are of homogeneous, medium echogenicity and may not be separable sonographically. The echoge-

nicity of the transitional zone is intermediate between that of the periurethral and the central and peripheral acinar zones.[23–26]

CT, as it is typically done with 8 or 10 mm slice thicknesses, adds little to our understanding of the complex zonal anatomy of the prostate. Occasionally, however, CT does permit distinction between the more central zones and the peripheral acinar region. Recent technologic developments with MRI, particularly with T2-weighted pelvic imaging and with endorectal coils, have permitted improved capabilities for defining the histologic regions of the prostate and related pathology.[27] With T2-weighted pelvic scanning, the peripheral acinar region has high signal intensity, the anterior fibromuscular region has low signal intensity, and the central glandular region has an intermediate signal

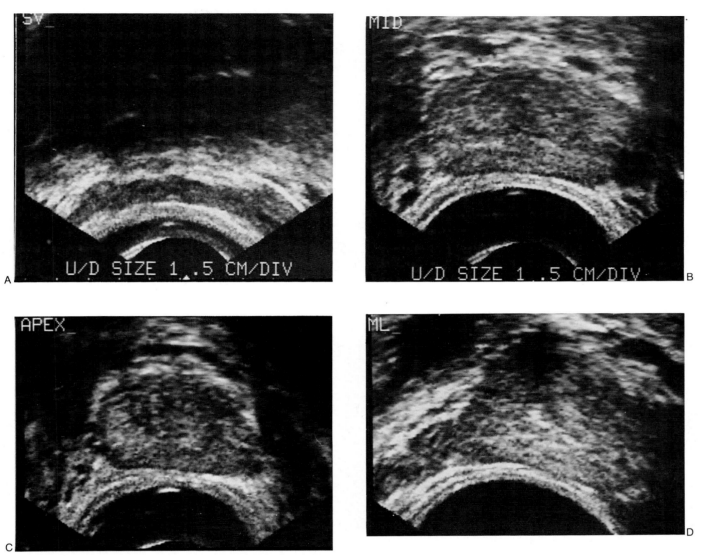

Figure 1–2. Normal anatomy of prostate gland—transrectal ultrasound, 7.0 MHz probe. **A.** Transverse view of seminal vesicles. **B.** Transverse view of midprostate showing more central and peripheral zones. **C.** Transverse view at apex also showing the peripheral zone distinct from the other anatomic zones of the prostate. **D.** Longitudinal view of the right side of the prostate and right seminal vesicle.

intensity. Differentiation of these regions on the basis of signal intensity is not usually possible with T1-weighted sequencing.[27–29]

PATHOLOGIC ANATOMY

An understanding of the zonal anatomy of the prostate is critical to understanding and imaging of prostate pathology because different pathologic processes target different regions of the gland. For example, malignancy and inflammation typically involve the peripheral glandular zone (Fig. 1–3).[30–32] In fact, 70%–80% of prostatic carcinoma arises in the peripheral zone, with the rest of the malignancies arising

from the central glandular and transitional zones. Extension of malignancy within the gland also is determined in part by the zonal structure of the prostate. Similarly, prostatitis predominantly affects the peripheral zone, but severe infection extends throughout the gland and some infections may begin with urethral and periurethral involvement.

Benign prostatic hyperplasia, the concern of this text, primarily affects the transitional zone and, to a lesser degree, the periurethral zone of the gland (Fig. 1–4).[33,34] Because of lateral and posterior displacement of the central glandular region by enlargement of the transitional and peripheral zones, the course of the ejaculatory ducts may be displaced laterally and posteriorly from their usual course. The degree

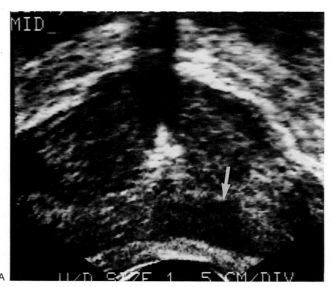 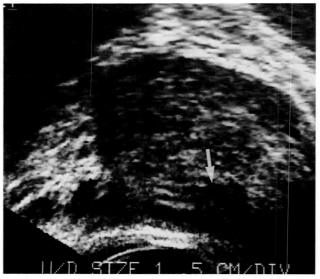

Figure 1–3. Adenocarcinoma of the prostate. A. Transverse view and (B) sagittal view from transrectal ultrasound show a hypoechoic adenocarcinoma in the left peripheral zone. The diagnosis was proved by ultrasound-guided needle biopsy. Note also calcification and adenomatous change centrally.

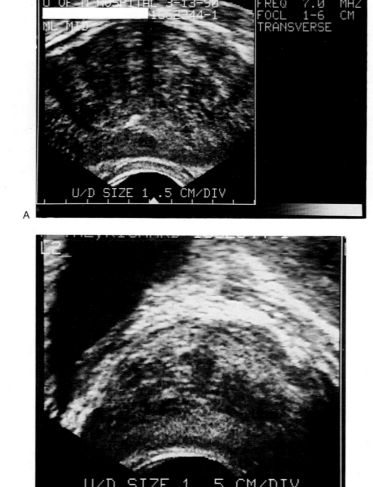 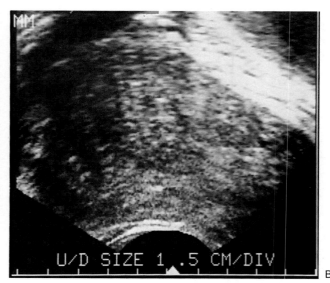

Figure 1–4. Benign prostatic hypertrophy. A. Transverse view from transrectal ultrasound shows an enlarged gland with calcification and adenomatous change in the central gland (from hypertrophied transitional zone). Note homogeneous compressed peripheral zone. B. Longitudinal view at midline again shows enlarged prostate. C. Longitudinal view of the left side of the gland shows inhomogeneous benign adenomatous change.

of hyperplasia and ultimate three-dimensional configuration of the gland are variable. With marked hyperplasia, the central and peripheral acinar zones are compressed and displaced laterally and posteriorly. Alternatively, a hyperplastic prostate can become more heart-shaped or globular in configuration. Hyperplasia also can be responsible for the development of a midline protrusion of prostatic tissue into the bladder base, the so-called median bar. Estimation of gland volume and identification of a median bar configuration can be performed easily with transrectal sonography. These glandular features may be important determinants of therapeutic interventions, as described later in this book. It should be noted that prostatic hyperplasia can occur in the peripheral acinar region, and this occurrence may be a precursor of prostatic carcinoma.[35]

Just as the gross pathologic and histopathologic features of benign prostatic hyperplasia are somewhat variable, so are the imaging characteristics as defined in particular by transrectal sonography and MRI.[8,10,13,14,16,18,23] Prostatic hyperplasia may represent a diffuse or more focal process. In the latter circumstance, focal adenomas, seen as discrete masses, can be identified. A variable degree of associated calcification and cyst formation also can be seen. Compressed and posteriorly displaced corpora amylacea within the central acinar region accentuate the appearance of the surgical capsule with prostatic hyperplasia.

CONCLUSION

The anatomy of the prostate gland is complex. The currently accepted concept of the internal anatomy of the prostate is based on investigations that have revealed different histologic types of tissue organized into well-defined zones. These regions are described commonly as periurethral, transitional, fibromuscular, and central and peripheral glandular. There is also good histopathologic evidence that different disease processes preferentially affect different zones of the gland. Although extensive histopathologic investigation into prostatic pathology is ongoing, it is likely that the rapidly evolving technologies of noninvasive prostate imaging, such as transrectal sonography and MRI, will complement this research in enhancing our understanding of the normal and diseased gland.

REFERENCES

1. Lowsley OS. The gross anatomy of the human prostate gland and contiguous structures. *Surg Gynecol Obstet* 1915;20:183–192
2. McNeal JE. Regional morphology and pathology of the prostate. *Am J Clin Pathol* 1968;49:347–357
3. Platt JF, Bree RL, Schwab RE. The accuracy of CT in the staging of carcinoma of the prostate. *AJR* 1987;149:315–318
4. Thornhill BA, Morehouse HT, Coleman P, Hoffman-Tretin JC. Prostatic abscess: CT and sonographic findings, *AJR* 1987;148:899–900
5. Barloon TJ, Foderaro AE, Kramolowsky EV. Giant prostate carcinoma: computed tomography findings and review of previous reports. *J Comput Tomogr* 1988;12:49–53
6. Bezzi M, Kressel HY, Allen KS, et al. Prostatic carcinoma: staging with MR imaging at 1.5 T. *Radiology* 1988;169:339–346
7. Friedman AC, Seidmon EJ, Radecki PD, Lev-Toaff A, Caroline DF. Relative merits of MRI, transrectal endosonography and CT in diagnosis and staging of carcinoma of prostate. *Urology* 1988;31:530–537
8. Griebel J, Hess CF, Schmiedl U, Koelbel G. MR characteristics of prostatic carcinoma and benign prostatic hyperplasia at 1.5 T. *J Comput Assist Tomogr* 1988;12:988–994
9. Di Trapani D, Pavone C, Serretta V, Cavallo N, Costa G, Pavone-Macaluso M. Chronic prostatitis and prostatodynia: ultrasonographic alterations of the prostate, bladder neck, seminal vesicles and periprostatic venous plexus. *Eur Urol* 1988;15:230–234
10. Allen KS, Kressel HY, Arger PH, Pollack HM. Age-related changes of the prostate: evaluation by MR imaging. *AJR* 1989;152:77–81
11. Andriole GL, Coplen DE, Mikkelsen DJ, Catalona WJ. Sonographic and pathological staging of patients with clinically localized prostate cancer. *J Urol* 1989;142:1259–1261
12. Carter HB, Hamper UM, Sheth S, Sanders RC, Epstein JI, Walsh PC. Evaluation of transrectal ultrasound in the early detection of prostate cancer. *J Urol* 1989;142:1008–1010
13. Jones DR, Roberts EE, Griffiths GJ, Parkinson MC, Evans KT, Peeling WB. Assessment of volume measurement of the prostate using per-rectal ultrasonography. *Br J Urol* 1989;64:493–495
14. Kahn T, Bürrig K, Schmitz-Drager B, Lewin JS, Fürst G, Modder U. Prostatic carcinoma and benign prostatic hyperplasia: MR imaging with histopathologic correlation. *Radiology* 1989;173:847–851
15. Lee F. Transrectal ultrasound: diagnosis and staging of prostatic carcinoma. *Urology* 1989;33:5–10
16. Schiebler ML, Tomaszewski JE, Bezzi M, Pollack HM, Kressel HY, Cohen EK, et al. Prostatic carcinoma and benign prostatic hyperplasia: correlation of high-resolution MR and histopathologic findings. *Radiology* 1989;172:131–137
17. Shinohara K, Wheeler TM, Scardino PT. The appearance of prostate cancer on transrectal ultrasonography: correlation of imaging and pathological examinations. *J Urol* 1989;142:76–82
18. Tzai TS, Chang CL, Yang CR, Hwang IS, Chang CH, Wu HC. Transrectal sonography of the prostate and seminal vesicles on patients with hemospermia. *J Formosan Med Assoc* 1989;88:232–235
19. McNeal JE. The prostate and prostatic urethra: a morphologic synthesis. *J Urol* 1972;107:1008–1016
20. McNeal JE. Normal and pathologic anatomy of prostate. *Urology* 1981;17:11–16
21. McNeal JE. Normal histology of the prostate. *Am J Surg Pathol* 1988;12:619–633
22. Ayala AG, Ro JY, Babaian R, Troncoso P, Grignon DJ. The prostatic capsule: does it exist? *Am J Surg Pathol* 1989;13:21–27
23. Jones DR, Griffiths GJ, Parkinson MC, Evans KT, Roberts EE, Davies RLI, et al. Structure and per-rectal ultrasonography of prostatic disease using cadaver specimens. *Br J Urol* 1989;64:611–617
24. Kaye KW, Richter L. Ultrasonographic anatomy of normal prostate gland: reconstruction by computer graphics. *Urology* 1990;35:12–17
25. Shinohara K, Scardino PT, Carter SStC, Wheeler TM. Patho-

logic basis of the sonographic appearance of the normal and malignant prostate. *Urol Clin North Am* 1989;16:675–691

26. Villers A, Terris MK, McNeal JE, Stamey TA. Ultrasound anatomy of the prostate: the normal gland and anatomical variations. *J Urol* 1990;143:732–738

27. Schnall MD, Lenkinski RE, Pollack HM, Imai Y, Kressel HY. Prostate: MR imaging with an endorectal surface coil. *Radiology* 1989;172:570–574

28. Gevenois PA, Salmon I, Stallenberg B, van Sinoy ML, van Regemorter G, Struyven J. Magnetic resonance imaging of the normal prostate at 1.5 T. *Br J Radiol* 1990;63:101–107

29. Schnall MD, Bezzi M, Pollack HM, Kressel HY. Magnetic resonance imaging of the prostate. *Magn Reson Q* 1990;6:1–16

30. McNeal JE. Origin and development of carcinoma in the prostate. *Cancer* 1969;23:24–34

31. McNeal JE, Redwine EA, Freiha FS, Stamey TA. Zonal distribution of prostatic adenocarcinoma: correlation with histologic pattern and direction of spread. *Am J Surg Pathol* 1988;12:897–906

32. Doble A, Carter SStC. Ultrasonographic findings in prostatitis. *Urol Clin North Am* 1989;16:763–772

33. McNeal JE. Origin and evolution of benign prostatic enlargement. *Invest Urol* 1978;15:340–345

34. McNeal JE. Anatomy of the prostate and morphogenesis of BPH. *Prog Clin Biol Res* 1984;145:27–53

35. McNeal JE, Bostwick DG. Intraductal dysplasia: a premalignant lesion of the prostate. *Hum Pathol* 1986;17:64–71

2

Clinical Assessment of Benign Prostatic Hypertrophy/Bladder Outlet Obstruction

Ramon Perez-Marrero

Benign prostatic hypertrophy (BPH) is the most common neoplastic growth in man. It requires some form of treatment in about 20% of all males by the age of 80 years, most often for the relief of troublesome obstructive or irritative symptoms.[1] Traditionally its diagnosis is made on clinical grounds, with a careful assessment of the symptom complex, and confirmed on physical examination and often cystoscopy and radiographic imaging. Urologist have been diagnosing this condition for many years and obtaining good success with traditional treatments.[2] Recently some concern has been raised regarding the accuracy and reproducibility of a diagnosis made in this fashion[3,4] and the safety of some traditional treatment methods.[5] At the same time, new diagnostic and treatment modalities have emerged, making a review of our clinical assessment tools timely.

In this chapter, we review the clinical assessment of bladder outlet obstruction. Subsequent chapters deal with urodynamic assessment and screening for prostatic malignancy.

ANALYSIS OF SYMPTOMS

We rely heavily on assessment of patients' symptoms to make the diagnosis of BPH. A careful history will elicit a variety of symptoms of outflow obstruction, often designated as the *prostatism complex*. This symptom complex includes both irritative and obstructive symptoms, but the term *prostatism* most often is used to describe the obstructive ones. These are not specific of BPH but may be seen in other types of outflow obstruction, such as urethral stricture, bladder neck contracture, and carcinoma. Similarly irritative symp-

toms may be due to other processes, such as bladder stones, bladder cancer, infection, and foreign bodies. These other entities must be ruled out.

The classic obstructive symptoms of BPH include hesitancy, intermittency, diminished caliber, and force of the stream, difficulty terminating urination, postvoid dribbling, and a feeling of incomplete emptying. Since these symptoms progress slowly over a long period of time, patients may compensate for them without being fully aware of their presence. Frequency, nocturia, urgency, and urge incontinence may not be directly attributable to the degree of obstruction and are termed *irritative symptoms*. These symptoms may be due to a decrease in effective bladder volume or to local irritation factors caused by the expanding adenoma. Nocturia is in part due to a reversal in the cricadian rhythm of urine production seen in elderly men, some of whom may excrete as much as two thirds of their daily urine volume at night.[6]

Hematuria, urinary tract infections, and urinary retention are other presentations of BPH. Gross hematuria in men over the age of 60 years is most commonly due to BPH. This is usually terminal, but it also can occur throughout the stream. It probably arises from dilated veins in the prostatic urethra caused by compression from the enlarging adenoma. Nevertheless, although these veins may be evident in cystoscopy, this assumption should not be made until other causes of hematuria are ruled out.[7] Urinary tract infections often are caused by urinary stasis and elevated residuals seen in men with BPH and produces dysuria in addition to other irritative voiding symptoms. They can worsen other symptoms of BPH, and it is necessary to treat these infections before an adequate assessment of the severity of the prostatism is made. Approximately 20% of patients with BPH will experience urinary retention. Once a patient has gone into retention, it is very likely that he will have another episode within a year. Paradoxically, very few patients go into retention while awaiting their prostatectomy.

All these symptoms of BPH are quite variable and often have spontaneous remission for varying periods of time. Several symptom scores have been proposed to standardize and semiquantitate their recording. These scores usually group symptoms into obstructive and irritative and give a value to their severity. We have found the one proposed by Boyarski et al. to be very useful in our clinical practice.[8] It is not yet clear whether such an accurate recording of symptoms improves their clinical relevance in diagnosis or therapeutic decision making. Several authors have found little correlation between these scores and urodynamic evidence of obstruction or presence of detrusor instability,[9,10] but most agree that a preponderance of irritative symptoms mandates further assessment.[11]

We believe that careful assessment of patients' symptomatology will continue to be important in the diagnosis and management of BPH. A standardized method of recording these symptoms will be invaluable in improving patient follow-up and in analyzing their response to different therapeutic modalities. Symptom scores not only may help us tailor our diagnostic approach to the patient but, in conjunction with other diagnostic tools, may help us in the rational application of old and new treatment modalities to this disease process.

DIGITAL RECTAL EXAMINATION

Palpation of the prostate is an important part of the clinical assessment. It gives us an idea of its consistency and may uncover an occult malignancy. Assessment of prostatic size is more difficult and not as reproducible.[12] We can palpate only a portion of the prostatic surface and can be fooled by anterior or intravesical growth, by obesity, and by local inflammation. There seems to be very little correlation between rectal estimation of prostatic weight and the severity of symptoms or degree of outflow tract obstruction.[13] In fact, prostatic size alone may have little to do with symptomatology or degree of obstruction. Other factors, such as the elasticity of the capsule and the number and activity of periprostatic neuroreceptors, may be more important,[14] but, a properly performed digital rectal examination is still quite valuable to rule out other pathologic conditions and as an adjunct to cystoscopy in estimating prostatic size.

CYSTOSCOPY

Cystoscopy has been and continues to be the cornerstone of urologic practice. In BPH, cystoscopy can rule out strictures and other outflow tract pathology and can give us some information about the detrusor. When taken in conjunction with a digital rectal examination, it can give us a more accurate assessment of prostatic size by taking into account the shape of the prostatic urethra and the degree of obstruction (intrusion) of the adenoma.[15]

In our center, we perform cystoscopy for BPH after the patient has emptied his bladder for a flow rate assessment, obtaining in this way a visual impression of the prostatic obstruction, of the degree of trabeculation, and a measurement of residual urine. When performed with a simultaneous digital rectal examination, a fairly accurate estimate of prostatic volume can be made that correlates fairly well with transrectal ultrasonography estimates.[13] This information allows us to tailor additional investigations and is helping us develop a rational way in which to allocate patients to different treatment modalities. Today, with excellent flexible cystoscopes, preoperative cystoscopy is very feasible and well tolerated and should be part of every evaluation for symptoms of prostatism.

RESIDUAL URINE

Many urologists use an elevated residual urine as an indication of the severity of the prostatic obstruction and the degree of detrusor decompensation,[15] although some authors have questioned the value of this measurement.[4] They point out that there is little reproducibility in consecutive measurements and no correlation between an elevated residual and other measurements of obstruction. We take a different view of residual urine measurements. We believe that they are primarily a reflection of detrusor decompensation and, as such, can help us tailor our investigations. We only rely on measurements in the presence of a full bladder and express our results as a percentage of total bladder volume (TBV).

$$\text{Residual + voided volume = TBV}$$

In this way, we usually obtain reproducible results. All elevated residuals are confirmed with repeated measurements. Residuals over 50% of TBV can indicate significant detrusor decompensation and, in our practice, are an indication for further urodynamic testing.

UPPER TRACT IMAGING

Traditionally, the workup of BPH has included some form of upper tract imaging. An intravenous pyelogram (IVP) yields very little information about prostatic enlargement but does give us incidental information about the upper tract. It occasionally can reveal an unsuspected median lobe but really adds very little to the cystoscopic assessment.[16] Ultrasonography recently has gained popularity for upper tract screening in BPH. We prefer to do an ultrasound of the upper tract with postvoid views of the pelvis for residual urine and have found it useful in our clinical assessment.

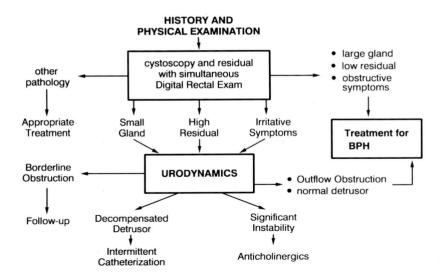

Figure 2–1. Diagnostic algorithm for bladder outflow obstruction.

TRANSRECTAL ULTRASONOGRAPHY

Transrectal ultrasonography has provided us with a very accurate way to determine prostatic volume.[17] Whether this accuracy is necessary for clinical decision making is still uncertain. We have found that prostatic size assessed by digital rectal palpation and cystoscopy is sufficiently accurate for most clinical situations, and we use transrectal ultrasonography primarily in our research protocols and to screen for malignancy when indicated.

CLINICAL EVALUATION

We assess all of our patients symptomatically and perform a cystoscopy with simultaneous measurement of residual urine and digital–rectal palpation. Patients with clear-cut obstructive symptoms, enlarged prostate by cystoscopy and rectal examination, and moderate residuals can be offered one of the many modalities of treatment for outflow obstruction without further evaluation. If there is some doubt in our minds about the etiology of the symptoms, particularly if a very small gland is found or there is moderate to high residual, chronic retention, or mainly irritative symptoms, we perform a more thorough urodynamic assessment (Fig. 2–1).

CONCLUSION

The clinical assessment of BPH has been and remains a very important urologic tool. It has been the basis for therapeutic decisions for many years and has produced excellent surgical results in 85%–90% of cases.[18] New diagnostic tools, such as complex urodynamics and transrectal ultrasound, are being used in an attempt to enhance our ability to select appropriate candidates for surgery. It is not yet clear whether they will improve our results. New treatment modalities have emerged and are making our therapeutic decision making more difficult. Only by subjecting our patients to as careful and vigorous an assessment as clinically feasible and by recording our findings in a standardized fashion will we be able to evaluate these new diagnostic and treatment modalities and eventually formulate a rational plan for their use. We believe that even in light of these new technologies, a careful history and physical examination and a urologically trained eye and finger will form the cornerstone of any future therapeutic algorithm for BPH.

REFERENCES

1. Berry SJ, Coffey DIS, Walsh PSC, Ewing LL. Development of benign prostatic hyperplasia with age. *J Urol* 1984; 132:474–479
2. Birkhoff JD. Natural history of benign prostatic hypertrophy. In: Hinman F Jr (ed). *Benign Prostatic Hypertrophy*. New York: Springer-Verlag, 1983:5–9
3. Abrams PH, Griffith DJ. The assessment of prostatic obstruction from urodynamic measurements and from residual urine. *Br Urol* 1979;SI:129–134
4. Bruskewitz RC, Iversen P, Madsen PO. Value of postvoid residual urine determination in evaluation of prostatism. *Urology* 1982;20:602–604
5. Roos NP, Wennberg YE, Malenka DJ, et al. Mortality and reoperation after open and transurethral resection of the prostate for benign prostatic hyperplasia. *N Engl J Med* 1989;320:1120–1124
6. Kirkland JL, Lye M, Levy DW, Banerjee AK. Patterns of urine flow and electrolyte excretion in healthy elderly people. *Br Med J* 1983;287:1665–1667
7. Shah PJR. Clinical presentation and differential diagnosis. In: Fitzpatrick J, Kanp R (eds.) *The Prostate*. New York: Churchill-Livingston, 1989:91–102
8. Boyarsky S, Jones G, Paulson DF, Prout GR Jr. A new look at

bladder neck obstruction by the Food and Drug Administration regulators: guidelines for investigation of benign prostatic hypertrophy. *Trans Am Assoc Genitourin Surg* 1977;68:29

9. Castro JE, Griffiths HJL, Shackman R. Significance of signs and symptoms in benign prostatic hypertrophy. *Br Med J* 1969;2:598–601

10. Abrams PH, Fenley RCL. The significance of symptoms associated with bladder outflow obstruction. *Urol Int* 1978;33:171–174

11. Blaivas JG. Urodynamics: The second generation. *J Urol* 1983;129:783

12. Meyhoff HH, Hald T. Accuracy in preoperative estimation of prostatic size. *Scand J Urol Nephrol* 1981;15:45–51

13. Andersen JT, Nordling J, Walter S. Prostatism I. The correlation between symptoms, cystometric and urodynamic findings. *Scand J Urol Neophrol* 1979;13:229–236

14. Furuya S, Kumamoto Y, Yokoyama E, Tsakamoto T, Izumi T, Abiko. Alpha-adrenergic activity and urethral pressure in prostatic zone in benign prostatic hypertrophy. *J Urol* 1982;128:836–839

15. Andersen JT, Norlding J. Prostatism II. The correlation between cystourethroscopy, cystometric and urodynamic findings. *Scand J Urol Nephrol* 1980;14:23–27

16. Abrams PH. Use of intravenous urogram in diagnosis. In: Hinman F Jr (ed). *Benign Prostatic Hypertrophy*. New York: Springer-Verlag, 1983:605–609

17. Mori Y. Measurement of the normal prostate size by means of transrectal ultrasonotomography. *Jpn J Urol* 1982;73:767–781

18. Bruskewitz RC, Larsen EH. The clinical evaluation of benign prostatic hypertrophy and prostatism in benign prostatic hyperplasia. *Proceedings of a Workshop of NIH*. Bethesda, MD: NIH Publications, 1985;2:231–235

3

Practical Urodynamic Approach to Bladder Outlet Obstruction

Edgardo F. Becher, Abraham Ami Sidi

The diagnosis of bladder outlet obstruction is not always obvious from the medical history and the findings of a physical examination and radiologic and endoscopic tests because bladder emptying problems and irritative symptoms are not necessarily related to bladder outlet obstruction.[1] However, a series of well-chosen and properly performed urodynamic procedures combined with such evaluations can identify the underlying pathophysiology in most cases of lower urinary tract dysfunction.

A urodynamic evaluation of a male with obstructive symptoms can establish or confirm a diagnosis of outlet obstruction. Multichannel urodynamic studies or video urodynamic studies can determine the site of obstruction. The several useful urodynamic tests are presented in this chapter, and their relative importance in the diagnosis of bladder outlet obstruction is discussed.

UROFLOWMETRY

Measurement of the urinary flow rate, called uroflowmetry, is the single most useful test in diagnosing and screening for bladder outlet obstruction. Uroflowmetry is a simple and noninvasive urodynamic test. It determines urine flow rate, defined as the volume of urine (in milliliters) expelled from the bladder per unit of time (seconds). In this test, a funnel is used to direct the flow of urine to a transducer, which is placed under a commode. The most common transducers are the gravimetric, which calculates the flow by weighing the urine mass, the momentum exchange, which calculates the effect of the inertia of the urinary stream over a rotating disc, and the dipstick, which measures changes in the urine capacitance.

The ideal conditions for this test are a comfortably full bladder, use of the usual voiding position, and maximum privacy for the patient. To obtain an accurate measurement of flow, more than one voiding usually is necessary. Often, flow cannot be measured accurately because of the patient's anxiety, voiding in an unfamiliar environment, and psychologic influences that may lead to inhibition of bladder contraction, abdominal straining, and lack of pelvic floor relaxation. If this appears to be the case, the patient should be questioned as to whether the tested flow was representative of a typical voiding.

Uroflow results are most accurate for voided volumes of between 200 and 400 mL because the urinary flow rate is dependent on the volume voided.[2] Uroflowmetry determines voided volume, peak flow rate, average flow rate, flow time, and time to peak flow. The peak flow rate is the best parameter reflecting the degree of outflow obstruction. The peak urinary flow rates below which bladder outlet obstruction is likely, for several age groups, are listed in Table 3–1.

The flow rate, which is proportional to the intravesical volume, will be affected by differences in intravesical volume, assuming that detrusor contraction velocity remains the same. To incorporate the effect of volume on flow, one should use the nomogram developed by Siroky et al.,[3,4] which correlates the peak or average flow rate with intraves-

Table 3–1.   Minimum values for peak urinary flow

	PEAK FLOW (mL/sec)	
Age (years)	Male	Female
<45	21	25
45–60	15	18
>60	13	15

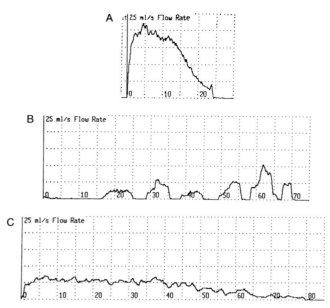

Figure 3–1.   Three urine flow patterns. A. Bell-shaped curve characteristic of normal flow. B. Interrupted curve characteristic of abdominal straining. C. Flat tracing characteristic of prostatic obstruction. (From ref. 17.)

ical volume. A patient with bladder outlet obstruction will have a peak flow of more than 2 standard deviations below the mean adjusted for intravesical volume (voided volume + residual volume).

The shape of the uroflow curve varies according to voiding pattern (Fig. 3–1). The curve for normal, nonobstructed flow is bell shaped, and the curve representative of outlet obstruction is flat with a low peak flow rate and a prolonged voiding time. Straining during voiding produces an irregular, spiked pattern, and low outflow resistance may produce a curve with a very high peak flow rate achieved in a short voiding time.

The urinary flow is the end result of several factors, including the quality of the detrusor contraction, the degree of outlet relaxation, and the urethral patency. Therefore, a low peak flow rate, although suggestive of bladder outlet obstruction, cannot be considered pathognomonic because neurogenic or myogenic damage to the detrusor can mimic an obstructive uroflow curve. On the other hand, a normal uroflow curve does not always exclude obstruction. A small number of males with obstructive and irritative symptoms may have a high-flow obstruction with peak flow above 15 mL/sec and high voiding pressure.[5] For these males, a study of the pressure and flow relationship will establish the diagnosis.

Uroflowmetry is a good and reliable screening test, especially when it is combined with a measurement of postvoiding residual urine volume. However, for a more accurate diagnosis in equivocal cases, uroflowmetry must be combined with simultaneous measurement of voiding pressure.

CYSTOMETROGRAPHY

Cystometrography (CMG) determines the pressure/volume relationships in the bladder during filling. This test is performed by filling the bladder with water or carbon dioxide via a urethral catheter.[6] The intravesical pressure, which is the combined pressure generated by the detrusor contraction and the surrounding abdominal pressure, is transmitted by a transducer to a chart recorder. When a fluid is used to fill the bladder, a dual-lumen catheter or two small catheters may be used, one to fill the bladder and the other to measure the pressures. It is important to measure the intraabdominal pressure, which is accomplished via a rectal catheter,[7] so that the true detrusor pressure can be determined by electronic subtraction of the abdominal from the intravesical pressure.

Cystometrography provides information on bladder capacity, compliance, stability, and sensation. Cystometrography of a low-compliance bladder demonstrates a progressive increase in pressure in response to filling (Fig. 3–2). This can be caused by neurogenic or structural damage, such as fibrosis or that produced by radiation therapy. An unstable bladder (Fig. 3–3) exhibits uninhibited detrusor contractions that may reflect outlet obstruction, neuropathy, infection, or intravesical pathology, such as carcinoma in situ.

Although cystometrography provides information primarily on the filling and storage phases of micturition, it also provides extremely valuable information for a patient with bladder emptying symptoms, such as frequency, nocturia, and slow stream, which may result not only from obstruction but also from a low-compliance or low-capacity bladder. Demonstration of a voluntary and sustained detrusor contraction at the end of the filling phase (Fig. 3–4) in a patient with a low peak flow rate supports the diagnosis of outlet obstruction and predicts proper bladder emptying once this problem is resolved.

Cystometrography should be performed on a patient with symptoms of bladder outlet obstruction to identify cystometrographic patterns characteristic of such symptoms and to assess the presence of an adequate voluntary detrusor contraction. In a patient with urinary retention, demonstration of an adequate detrusor contraction by cystometrography is suggestive of bladder outlet obstruction.

URETHRAL PRESSURE PROFILE

The static urethral pressure profile (UPP) is the measured pressure change that occurs along the urethra as a catheter is slowly withdrawn from the bladder at a constant rate. The resulting curve (Fig. 3–5) identifies the maximum urethral pressure, the maximum urethral closure pressure (the difference between the maximum urethral pressure and the intravesical pressure), total profile length, and functional length (the length of the urethra along which the urethral pressure exceeds the intravesical pressure).

When large groups of patients are considered, there may

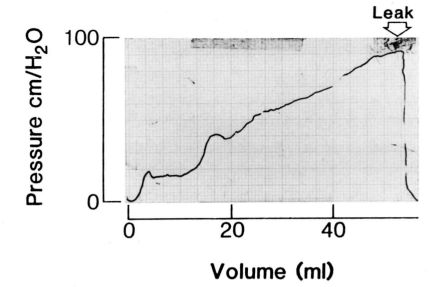

Figure 3–2. Cystometrogram showing a linear increase in intravesical pressure in response to filling, which is characteristic of a low-compliance bladder. (From ref. 17.)

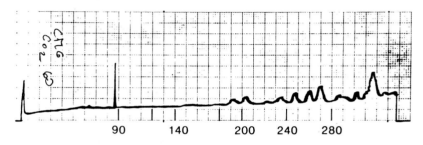

Figure 3–3. Cystometrogram showing uninhibited detrusor contractions characteristic of an unstable bladder. (From ref. 17.)

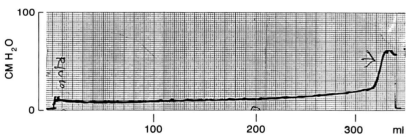

Figure 3–4. Cystometrogram showing a voluntary detrusor contraction at the end of filling. (From ref. 17.)

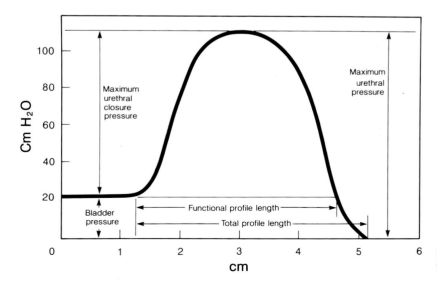

Figure 3–5. Urethral pressure profile parameters. (From ref. 17.)

be a statistically significant difference in the static UPP for patients with obstruction as compared to those without obstruction. In an individual, however, this profile provides no clues to diagnosis. The test is inaccurate for the diagnosis of bladder outlet obstruction because it does not measure the changes in intraurethral pressure that occur during voiding.[8] Therefore, in our opinion, the static UPP is of limited usefulness, although it may be valuable to compare preoperative and postoperative profiles when procedures to increase or decrease outlet resistance, such as bladder neck suspension, placement of an artificial urinary sphincter, or sphincterotomy, have been performed.

The micturitional UPP represents simultaneous measurement of bladder and urethral pressures during voiding.[9] Measurements are recorded while the urethral portion of the catheter is slowly withdrawn from the posterior urethra during voiding. During normal micturition, intravesical and proximal urethral pressures are equal. In the presence of obstruction, a pressure gradient develops across the obstructed site and can be detected by a dual transducer-tipped catheter. The micturitional pressure profile is important in determining the exact site of obstruction, whether in the bladder neck, prostate, or urethra. However, this time-consuming test requires expensive instruments and expertise to perform. Therefore, it is reserved for extremely complex cases.

SPHINCTER ELECTROMYOGRAPHY

Sphincter electromyography (EMG) measures the bioelectric potentials generated in the striated urinary sphincter. During the filling phase in a normal lower urinary tract, increased electromyographic activity reflects increased tone of the sphincteric and pelvic floor muscles (interference pattern). During the voiding phase, absence of electromyographic activity reflects relaxation of the striated sphincter that occurs in synergy with detrusor contraction. Failure of the sphincter to relax in coordination with detrusor contraction during voiding is defined as detrusor–sphincter dyssynergia (Fig. 3–6). This condition occurs in patients with suprasacral spinal cord lesions[10] and constitutes a functional outlet obstruction without structural (anatomic) abnormalities.

Sphincter electromyography is used to determine denervation and synergistic action of the detrusor and sphincter. Direct (needle) electromyography[11] can determine both parameters and is especially useful for the measurement of single motor unit potentials when a neurologic etiology for urinary incontinence is suspected. Indirect (surface) electromyography can be performed using electrocardiography patches, an anal plug, or catheter transducers and can be sufficient for a crude assessment of detrusor–sphincter synergy.

The indication for performing sphincter electromyography on a patient with bladder-emptying problems is limited to

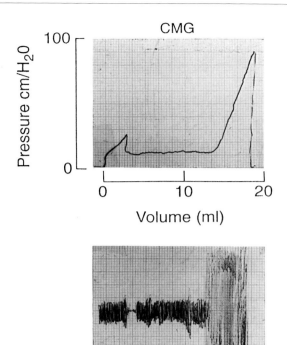

Figure 3–6. Simultaneous cystometrography and electomyography showing an early detrusor contraction with an increase in electromyographic activity (detrusor–sphincter dyssynergia). (From ref. 17.)

documentation of detrusor–sphincter dyssynergia, and, therefore, this test should not be performed in the absence of neuropathy.

VOIDING PRESSURE–FLOW STUDY

A voiding pressure–flow study determines whether a low urinary flow results from impaired detrusor contractility or outlet obstruction. A low urinary flow rate is not diagnostic of bladder outlet obstruction even if it is associated with a high residual urine volume.[12] Infravesical obstruction is characterized by a low urinary flow rate in the presence of a high, sustained detrusor pressure. On the other hand, low urinary flow with a low intravesical pressure is present in patients with impaired detrusor contractility.

In this test, intravesical, abdominal, and detrusor pressures are recorded simultaneously as uroflowmetry is performed (Fig. 3–7). A small-caliber urethral catheter or a suprapubic needle is used to record voiding pressures. In the presence of neuropathy, simultaneous sphincter electromyography assesses the coordination of detrusor contraction with external sphincter relaxation.

In a normal patient, the detrusor contraction should be sustained during voiding and should occur at a pressure of

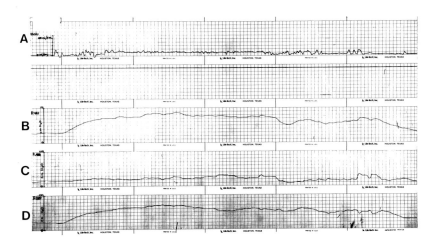

Figure 3–7. Voiding pressure–flow study showing abnormally high voiding pressure and a low peak uroflow curve in a patient with prostatic obstruction. **A.** Uroflowmetry. **B.** Intravesical pressure. **C.** Intraabdominal pressure. **D.** Detrusor pressure. (From ref. 17.)

approximately 40 cm of water. Parameters determined by the voiding pressure–flow test are the urethral opening pressure, which is the detrusor pressure at which voiding starts, maximum voiding pressure, and detrusor pressure at peak flow. The voiding pressure–flow study is a valuable test when the diagnosis of bladder outlet obstruction is equivocal, such as in high flow obstruction.[5] However, this test does not determine the site of obstruction.

Impaired detrusor contractility or detrusor areflexia may result from underlying psychogenic, myogenic, or neurogenic etiologies or a combination. The urodynamic diagnosis of bladder outlet obstruction in the presence of detrusor areflexia is extremely difficult because the urodynamic tests are affected by the inability to void. In these situations, an attempt should be made to establish the underlying cause of impaired detrusor contractility.[13] For the large, decompensated, acontractile bladder, a second evaluation after decompression is warranted when detrusor tone and contractility are regained.

VIDEO URODYNAMICS

Video urodynamics combines the various urodynamic procedures with simultaneous fluoroscopic evaluation of the lower urinary tract.[14] Using contrast material as the filling medium, all phases of micturition can be investigated by displaying the results of cystometrography, electromyography, and pressure–flow studies with the fluoroscopic image.

Although video urodynamics provides the most comprehensive information on the lower urinary tract, it is time consuming and expensive and requires expertise to perform. Its role in the evaluation of outlet obstruction is to determine the exact anatomic location of the obstruction,[15] that is, at the bladder neck, prostate, or sphincter. Without this test, it is impossible to know whether a radiographic finding of a functional obstruction, such as a closed bladder neck, occurs during voiding. Video urodynamics allows correlation of dynamic real time fluoroscopic imaging with a functional urodynamic evaluation. Video urodynamics is especially valuable for the diagnosis of complicated urinary incontinence,[16] for the evaluation of young patients with an equivocal diagnosis of obstruction, and for those with persistent symptoms after surgery and lower urinary tract symptoms resulting from neurovesical dysfunction.

CONCLUSION

A urodynamic evaluation must be tailored to the patient based on the information obtained during the preliminary evaluation. Every patient with symptoms of bladder outlet obstruction should be evaluated initially with uroflowmetry and measurement of the residual urine volume, provided the patient is able to void. In the presence of abnormal results for uroflowmetry, a low residual urine volume, and findings supportive of prostatic obstruction, no further urodynamic evaluation is needed. If the residual urine volume is high, assessment of detrusor activity is mandatory and can be accomplished via a simple cystometrography or a more complex pressure–flow study. In young patients or in those in whom the diagnosis is equivocal, outlet obstruction can be verified by a pressure–flow study. Also, in young patients, video urodynamics or a micturitional urethral pressure profile determines the exact location of obstruction. In the presence of neuropathy, sphincter electromyography confirms or rules out detrusor–sphincter dyssynergia as a cause of infravesical obstruction.

Urinary retention is a problematic situation for which urodynamic evaluation is affected by the inability to void. In these cases, the presence of a detrusor contraction at the end of simple filling cystometrography is suggestive of bladder outlet obstruction.[17]

Urodynamic evaluation can determine the presence and site of bladder outlet obstruction. The complexity of the urodynamic test needed varies with the patient, the instruments available, and the examiner's expertise. From a practical standpoint, most patients with symptoms of bladder outlet obstruction can be evaluated successfully using uro-flowmetry, measurement of residual urine volume, and cystometrography.

REFERENCES

1. Katz GP, Blaivas JG. A diagnostic dilemma: when urodynamic findings differ from the clinical impression. *J Urol* 1983;129:1170–1174
2. Abrams P, Feneley R, Torrens M (eds). Urodynamic investigations. *Urodynamics.* 1983;3:31–40
3. Siroky MB, Olsson CA, Krane RJ. The flow rate nomogram: I. Development. *J Urol* 1979;122:665–668
4. Siroky MB, Olsson CA, Krane RJ. The flow nomogram: II. Clinical correlation. *J Urol* 1980;123:208–210
5. Gerstenberg TC, Andersen JT, Klarskov P, Ramirez D, Hald T. High flow infravesical obstruction in men: symptomatology, urodynamics and the results of surgery. *J Urol* 1982;127:943–946
6. Jorgensen L, Lose G, Anderson JT. Cystometry: H_2O or CO_2 as filling medium? A literature survey of the influence of the filling medium on the qualitative and the quantitative cystometric parameters. *Neurourol Urodynam* 1988;7:343–350
7. McCarthy TA. Validity of rectal pressure measurements as indication of intra-abdominal pressure changes during urodynamic evaluation. *Urology* 1982;20:657–660
8. Wein AJ. The pitfalls of urodynamics. In: Mundy AR, Stephenson TP, Wein AJ (eds). *Urodynamics Principles, Practice and Application.* New York: Churchill-Livingstone, 1984;15:150–153
9. Yalla SV, Sharma GVRK, Barsamian EM. Micturitional static pressure profile: a method of recording urethral pressure profile during voiding and implications. *J Urol* 1980;124:649–656
10. Diokno AC, Koff SA, Bender LF. Periurethral striated muscle activity in neurogenic bladder dysfunction. *J Urol* 1974; 112:743–749
11. Siroky MB. Electromyography: needle. In: Barrett DM, Wein AJ (eds). *Controversies in Neuro-urology.* New York: Churchill-Livingstone, 1984:93–102
12. Abrams PH, Griffiths DJ. The assessment of prostatic obstruction from urodynamic measurements and from residual urine. *Br J Urol* 1979;51:129–134
13. Sidi AA, Dykstra DD, Peng W. Bethanechol supersensitivity test, rhabdosphincter electromyography and bulbocavernosus reflex latency in the diagnosis of neuropathic detrusor areflexia. *J Urol* 1988;140:335–337
14. Tanagho EA, Miller ER, Meyer FH, Corbett RK. Observations on the dynamics of the bladder neck. *Br J Urol* 1966;38:72–84
15. Webster GD, Older RA. Video urodynamics. *Urology* 1980;16:106–114
16. Becher EF, Sidi AA. Evaluating the incompetent outlet. In: Webster Webster GD, Stone AR (eds). *Problems in Urology: Urinary Incontinence.* Philadelphia: JB Lippincott, 1990; 41:1–8
17. Becher EF, Sidi AA. Urodynamic evaluation of bladder outlet obstruction. *Semin Intervent Radiol* 1989;6:22–27

4

State of the Art: Transurethral Resection of the Prostate

Jay I. Sandlow, Howard N. Winfield

Transurethral resection of the prostate (TURP) is the second most common surgical procedure performed on men over the age of 50. It accounts for 38% of all major urologic interventions and is responsible for nearly one quarter of a urologist's annual total workload.[1]

Although the operative mortality of prostatic resection has decreased considerably from 2.5% to 0.2% in the last 25 years, the morbidity of the procedure has remained relatively constant. Recently, the indications and long-term effects of TURP have come into question. With the advent of less invasive alternative methods of treatment, this procedure may become less frequent in years to come.[2]

Nevertheless, with the multitude of technical advances, such as improved optics, more efficient electrocautery units, and more compact equipment, combined with safer methods of anesthesia and postoperative care, TURP remains the gold standard against which all other treatment modalities are measured.

THE HISTORY OF TRANSURETHRAL RESECTION

In 1806, Sir William Blizard cut out segments of prostatic tissue transurethrally, using a knife through a perineal urethrostomy. He noted improvement in the patient's ability to void but was quite dismayed with the ensuing complications of bleeding and infection.[3] This was followed in the 1870s by French surgeons, who used sharpened lithotrites to incise the prostatic obstruction. However, hemorrhaging was again a problem due to lack of instrumentation to obtain a tamponade effect.[4]

Several advances, all made independently, led to the creation of the resectoscope. In 1879, Thomas Edison invented the incandescent lamp. This subsequently was incor-

porated into a cystoscope by Bousseau du Rocher in 1885 and, 2 years later, by Nitze and Leiter, each working separately. However, it was not until 1900 that Wappler and Otis introduced the cystoscope to American surgeons.[4]

In 1908, DeForest and Beer presented an electrical generator that could be connected to a cystoscope, with resultant cutting ability. Wappler and Wyeth eventually altered this approach, in 1924, leading to the development of a scope with an oscillating current, which they called *endotherm cutting current*. Although this represented an improvement over previous instruments, the device continued to have difficulties cutting under water. Wappler continued his efforts and in 1931 presented the *complex oscillator*, which was, in fact, capable of cutting tissue submerged in water. Unfortunately, it was unable to coagulate, and bleeding remained a serious problem. However, with the addition of a spark gap unit, originally developed by Bovie, a workable transurethral instrument was created that was capable of both cutting and coagulating tissue under water.[4]

Independent of these developments, Hugh H. Young first developed a fenestrated prostatic punch instrument in 1908. Subsequent revisions by Rose in 1925 and Bumpus in 1926 led to direct vision transurethral surgery using three major components: an incandescent lamp with direct vision, a high-frequency cutting and coagulation current, and a fenestrated tube. Modifications by Maximillan Stern, including replacement of the cutting knife with a tungsten wire loop, led to the development of the precursor of today's resectoscope. In 1931, Theodore Davis reported on his first 230 cases of prostatic resection using this instrument. He cited consistently adequate results without any postoperative deaths. In 1932, McCarthy introduced further modifications, including the foroblique lens system, magnification of the visual field, and a semicircular cutting loop.[4]

Until 1947, sterile water was used as the irrigant during resections. However, Creevy and Webb noted significant morbidity due to intravascular hemolysis and, therefore, advocated the use of an isotonic 4% glucose solution.[5] Series from the Mayo Clinic confirmed these observations and have led to present-day resection solutions.[6] A 1.5% glycine solution is now the osmotic agent of choice.

From the 1950s until the 1970s, there were only minor changes and improvements reported in the development of the resectoscope. Since then, fiberoptic vision and video-camera technology combined with continuous flow resectoscopes have made TURP not only an effective and efficient method of relieving prostatic obstruction but also a procedure of great surgical satisfaction.

INDICATIONS FOR TRANSURETHRAL RESECTION

The indications for TURP are variable, but there are certain absolute criteria. Males who have urinary retention, hydronephrosis with associated azotemia due to long-standing obstruction, recurrent urinary tract infections as a result of urinary stasis in the bladder, significant hematuria from an enlarged prostate gland, or severe symptoms of outflow obstruction are definite candidates for prostatic resection. More subtle or less emergent indications for TURP are listed in Table 4–1.

Preoperative evaluation should include a detailed history outlining typical symptoms of prostatism (Table 4–2). Rapid onset of prostatism may be indicative of carcinoma of the prostate and should be excluded. Physical examination may demonstrate a distended bladder, and digital rectal examination should assess the size, consistency, and firmness of the prostate. It should be noted that the size of the prostate does not correlate with the symptoms of prostatism nor with the postoperative outcome following TURP.[7–9] However, size of the prostate is important in deciding whether TURP is feasible. A prostate greater than 60–70 g is best managed by open suprapubic or retropubic prostatectomy.

After examination of the urine to rule out the presence of pyuria, bacteriuria, microhematuria, or glucosuria, it has been our policy to perform cystourethroscopy. This allows adequate inspection of the urethra to determine the presence or absence of strictures and to assess the length of the prostatic urethra as well as the degree of lobar (bilobar or trilobar) obstruction. Finally, the bladder is examined to determine the degree of trabeculation, cellule, or diverticular formation and to rule out the presence of stones or tumors. A postvoid residual urine is determined at the time of cystoscopy. There is considerable controversy in the literature regarding the need for cystoscopy in evaluating patients before TURP. It is known that there are men with severe bladder outlet obstruction who are asymptomatic, whereas some patients with marked obstructive symptomatology show little or no visual endoscopic prostatic obstruction.[10] We feel more comfortable visualizing the entire lower urinary tract before TURP so that surprises are not discovered at the time of anesthesia.

If the patient has no urologic history of infection, stones, or tumors and the urinalysis is unremarkable, upper tract imaging studies are not obtained. The cost effectiveness and risk–benefit ratios would suggest that IVP is not justified in the otherwise healthy male.[11] Renal ultrasound is a safe procedure, but the cost probably is not justified.

Serum electrolytes, creatinine, blood urea nitrogen, CBC, and coagulogram are obtained prior to administration of anesthesia. The prostatic enzymes—prostatic specific antigen (PSA) and acid phosphatase (PAP)—are poor screening tests for carcinoma of the prostate. Up to 21% of patients with BPH will have elevated PSA levels.[12] Thus, unless the urologist is suspicious of carcinoma, these enzymes should not be routinely obtained.

Optional tests include uroflowmetry, urodynamics (cystometrogram, pressure–flow, urethral pressure profile), and transrectal ultrasound of the prostate. Unless the diagnosis is unclear or if the patient is part of a research study, these investigations are not routinely required.

It is important to determine to what extent the symptoms of prostatic obstruction interfere with the patient's day-to-day activities. In some cases, a watchful waiting period may seem reasonable. If TURP appears to be the most logical

---

Table 4–1. Indications for Transurethral Resection of the Prostate in Management of BPH

ABSOLUTE	STRONG	MINIMAL
Renal failure secondary to bladder outlet obstruction Bilateral hydroureteronephrosis Recurrent urinary tract infections due to stasis of urine in bladder Bladder calculi Significant hematuria due to prostate after eliminating other sources Urinary retention or overflow incontinence after ruling out other causes	Large postvoid residuals (>200 mL) Symptoms that significantly interfere with day and nighttime activities Significant bladder diverticuli, cellule, or trabeculation suggesting severe outlet obstruction	Variable or mild symptoms of prostatism Subnormal uroflow studies Large prostate on digital rectal, ultrasound, or cystoscopic examination

Table 4–2. Symptoms of Prostatism

OBSTRUCTIVE	IRRITATIVE
Weak stream	Frequency
Abdominal straining	Nocturia
Hesitancy	Urgency
Intermittent stream	
Incomplete bladder emptying	
Terminal dribbling	

choice, the patient is informed of all the risks and complications of this procedure as well as the other alternative forms of treatment, such as balloon dilation or pharmacotherapy.

The potential complications associated with TURP are listed in Table 4–3. A study by Roos et al. examined the morbidity and mortality associated with TURP and open prostatectomy. Surprisingly, the long-term mortality in males undergoing TURP was greater than that associated with open prostatectomy, and there did not appear to be any correlation with the size of the prostate. Nearly half of the deaths were related to cardiovascular events.[13] Subsequent reexamination of the patient characteristics and adjusting for differences in medical conditions still could not explain this alarming discovery associated with TURP.[14] There does not appear to be any apparent biologic explanation for these differences. It has been suggested that the irrigant used during TURP may be a myocardial irritant, resulting in cardiovascular injury. The American Urological Association is in the process of initiating a major prospective study examining the outcomes of different forms of treatment for symptomatic BPH. Hopefully, this study will further illuminate this very disturbing finding.

METHODS OF TURP

It would be incorrect to state that there is only one way to perform a TURP. Some surgeons begin the resection anteriorly and work down, whereas others start on the floor of the prostatic urethra and resect upward. However, there are a few fundamental points that all resectionists must understand. First, it is imperative to be cognizant of the surgical anatomy of the prostate with respect to the vascular supply and the surgical capsule. Second, the relationship of the verumontanum and the external sphincter must be appreciated. Finally, the proximity of the ureteric orifices to the bladder neck or median lobe of the prostate (subcervical) must be determined prior to beginning the resection.

The first detailed description of the vasculature of the prostate was by Flocks in 1937.[15] Examining cadavers, he determined that the prostatic artery was a branch of the inferior vesical artery. It divided into two major branches of arteries—the capsular and the central (urethral) vessels. The capsular branch passes superficially along the posterolateral surface of the prostate to supply two thirds of its substance. It then penetrates the gland to supply the periurethral portion of the prostate only at the level of the verumontanum. The central (urethral) vessels penetrate the substance of the prostate at the vesicoprostatic junction, at the 4 o'clock and 7 o'clock positions on each side. They then turn distally to supply the entire periurethral portion of the prostate. Thus, early control of the central branches of the prostatic artery may significantly reduce blood loss and make resection easier. At the termination of the TURP, careful inspection for hemostasis at the bladder neck and level of the verumontanum may prevent postoperative hemorrhage.

Benign prostatic hyperplasia implies hyperplasia of the stromal (smooth muscle and fibrous) and epithelial components of the prostate, which develop in the periurethral region. This growing tissue compresses the true prostatic tissue peripherally, resulting in the surgical capsule. This thin capsule is composed of compressed prostatic acini between muscular and fibrous tissue. During a TURP, it is important to recognize this capsule as a smooth fibrous white layer. Prostatic adenomatous tissue has a crusty, snowlike appearance. The surgical goal is to resect all the adenomatous tissue while preserving the surgical capsule. An important clue that the surgeon has reached the surgical capsule is

Table 4–3. Complications Associated with Transurethral Resection of the Prostate

INTRAOPERATIVE	POSTOPERATIVE—IMMEDIATE	POSTOPERATIVE—DELAYED
Hemorrhage—arterial/venous	Persistent hemorrhaging	Hemorrhaging at 2–3 weeks postoperative
Significant periprostatic extravasation of irrigant	Dilutional hyponatremia (TUR syndrome)	Bladder neck contracture
Venous intravasation of irrigant	Sepsis and urinary tract infection	Urethral stricture
Perforation of prostatic capsule	Urinary incontinence	Ureteric orifice injury—stenosis or vesicoureteral reflux
Perforation at vesicourethral junction	Urinary retention due to incomplete resection, blood clots, or residual prostatic chips in bladder	Incontinence—stress, urgency
Bladder perforation		Epididymitis
Injury to ureteric orifices	Deep vein thrombosis and pulmonary emboli	Ejaculatory duct obstruction—pain
Injury to external urethral sphincter		Impotence
Injury to anterior urethra	Disseminated intravascular coagulation/secondary fibrinolysis	Inadequate resection requiring repeat TURP
Inadequate evacuation of prostatic tissue (large)	Irritative bladder symptoms	Increased risk of cardiovascular event
Surgical burns to patient or surgeon		

the visualization of arterial bleeders pulsating at 90 degrees to the capsule. Prior to reaching this level, bleeders come off diffusely and at various angles. Resecting through the surgical capsule reveals fatty tissue and may result in significant venous sinus bleeding, with absorption of irrigant into the intravascular space and excessive extravasation of fluid into the periprostatic space. Intravasation of the glycine solution may lead to hypervolemia, hyponatremia, and the TUR syndrome.

The verumontanum is an important landmark situated on the floor of the prostatic urethra. The embryologic utricle as well as the ejaculatory ducts open on the lateral slope of the verumontanum, whereas the prostatic ducts open at its base. The apex of the prostate envelops the verumontanum. Resecting much beyond the verumontanum may injure the external urethral sphincter, resulting in stress urinary incontinence. This is especially true anteriorly as the external sphincter leans forward toward the verumontanum. Preservation of this important landmark prevents injury to the external sphincter should repeat TURP be required.

Finally, identification of the ureteric orifices is crucial in preventing injury to these structures during TURP. Should injury occur, vesicoureteral reflux or ureteral obstruction may result. Unfortunately, in the presence of a significant median lobe that extends intravesically (subcervical), the ureteric orifices may be hidden or displaced. In this situation, great care must be taken in slowly taking down the median lobe starting laterally and resecting down toward the floor of the bladder neck. Should injury occur to the ureteric orifices, placement of an internal ureteric catheter for several weeks may prevent excessive scarring.

The final goal of a TURP is the resection of all adenomatous tissue circumferentially from the bladder neck back to the verumontanum and down to an intact surgical capsule. Preservation of the verumontanum, external sphincter, bladder wall, and ureteric orifices should be realized. The resection should require less than 60 min, and blood transfusions should be the exception.

As mentioned earlier, there are numerous methods of performing a TURP, and each urologist should develop his or her own style. Each surgeon should recognize that a different approach may be required for larger adenomas than for smaller ones.

It has been shown that smaller prostates (less than 25 g) are more susceptible to the development of bladder neck contracture.[16] Therefore, our approach is to preserve the lip of the bladder neck circumferentially and to avoid excessive coagulation in this area. Alternatively, avoidance of the prostatic tissue at the bladder neck region between the 11 o'clock and 1 o'clock positions may prevent contractures. Resection is otherwise routine back to the verumontanum.

Prostate sizes greater than 40 g require an experienced endoscopist to prevent complications and to obtain an adequate resection. Our approach is initially to define the bladder neck circumferentially to identify the surgical capsule early in the procedure and hopefully interrupt the central, periurethral major prostatic branches. Then, employing long, sweeping cuts, the adenoma is resected back to the verumontanum, starting at the 6 o'clock position and sweeping up to the 11 o'clock position. A similar technique is performed on the contralateral lobe. Near the end of the procedure, the tissue at the roof (12 o'clock) is resected from the bladder neck back to the verumontanum. Bleeding vessels should be controlled throughout the resection so as not to cause undue distortion of vision and blood loss. At the termination of the procedure, prostatic chips are irrigated out of the bladder, and a careful inspection for hemostasis is performed. A 22–24 F 3-way 30-mL balloon Foley catheter is inserted. Our approach is the use of continuous bladder irrigation overnight to keep blood clots from developing in the bladder. In an uncomplicated TURP, the Foley catheter is removed on the first postoperative day, and antibiotics are administered perioperatively until the patient is discharged. Studies concerning the use of antibiotics at the time of TURP are confusing and poorly controlled.[17] Thus, our antibiotic regimen is empirical but targeted at reducing urinary tract infection at the time of the resection as well as during the time of catheterization.

Techniques of resection have been described by Nesbit, Barnes, Alcock, and Flocks.[18] A description of each of these techniques is beyond the scope of this manuscript. However, it behooves all novice endoscopists to familiarize themselves with these methods to understand which approach may work best in different circumstances.

TECHNICAL ADVANCES

A major development in endoscopy was presented in 1975 by Iglesias et al., who described the development of the continuous flow resectoscope. This instrument relied on the simultaneous suction of effluent from the bladder allowing for a continuous inflow of irrigant. The proposed advantages of this system consisted of uninterrupted resection, better vision due to the continuous inflow of clear irrigant, and lower intravesical pressures (10 mm Hg). As a result, it was expected to lead to less absorption of irrigant fluid and shorter operating time.[19]

In 1983, Widran modified the Iglesias continuous flow resectoscope by developing a controlled continuous flow device. This device maintains flow as well as the intravesical pressure by pumping fluid both into and out of the bladder. An automatic shutoff valve prevents excessive bladder pressures due to obstruction of the outflow port.[20] Advantages of the Widran device included the ability to adjust both the inflow and outflow rates, rather than depending on the force of gravity for inflow and vacuum suction for outflow. The automatic shutoff of inflow when a specified pressure is reached was designed to further reduce fluid absorption.

Despite claims of superiority, however, there have been no studies to demonstrate that continuous flow resection provides a major advantage over standard resection. Flechner and Williams compared continuous flow and conventional resectoscopes for differences in blood loss, fluid absorption, resection time, and blood chemistry. There was no significant difference in any of these parameters, and operator preference was identified as the most important factor.[21] A study by a Swedish group led by Hahn found significantly lower fluid absorption as measured by ethanol-marked 1.5% glycine irrigant. There did not, however, appear to be any significant difference in resection time or blood loss.[29] It appears that continuous flow irrigation resectoscopes work best in the hands of those who feel comfortable using the instrument.

In 1984, O'Boyle et al. introduced the concept of videoprostatectomy, a technique that currently is spreading throughout the urologic community.[22] With improved fiberoptics, video cameras, and continuous flow equipment, video TURP has become a technically feasible and safe procedure. Video TURP is performed by attaching a full-beam, lightweight camera chip to the eyepiece of the resectoscope (preferably continuous flow). The operative image is transmitted to a large TV monitor via the video controller system. With the surgeon in the standing or sitting position, the TV monitor is visualized, and the resection proceeds in the usual fashion. There is an initial tendency to look directly through the resectoscope as the operator perceives a different two-dimensional appearance of the prostate. However, with a little persistence, the technique comes rapidly, and the resection is comparable to a standard TURP.

The advantages of video TURP are (1) less craning and twisting of the neck, (2) less risk of facial and ocular splashing with blood and uriniferous fluids, and (3) tremendous potential for teaching resident and operating room personnel in the technique of transurethral resection. The staff surgeon can feel much more comfortable as a junior resident proceeds with those initial bites at a TURP. The residents learn quickly how the staff perform the technique of TURP.

Widran compared the results of 200 video TURPs to 400 conventional TURPs using the controlled continuous flow resectoscope. There were no significant differences in the amount of tissue resected, blood loss, resection time and rate, or operative complications. However, the advantages previously mentioned should lead to more widespread use of video TURP.[23]

THE ROLE OF TURP TODAY

Modern technology has produced a vast array of instrumentation designed to improve the urologist's ability to treat bladder outlet obstruction. However, although it appears that the picture on the video screen is becoming clearer, the indications for TURP are getting hazier. At this time, many patients are concerned with more than just the ability to void with an adequate stream. The public is demanding less invasive procedures, with shorter hospitalization and recovery time. Today, the urologist has a number of options from which to choose. Pharmacotherapy in the form of selective alpha-blocking agents or 5-alpha-reductase inhibitors currently is undergoing double-blind, placebo-controlled, randomized studies. Initial studies seem to indicate about a 30% improvement rate.[24,27] Transurethral balloon dilation has attracted a tremendous amount of attention, but its role in the management of BPH also is unclear. There have been no randomized, placebo-controlled studies with balloon dilation.[26,27] Transurethral incision of the prostate (TUIP), as pioneered by Orandi, is effective for patients with small adenomas or individuals with significant bladder neck hyperreflexia.[28] The major advantages of these minimally invasive or noninvasive forms of treatment are preservation of ejaculation, reduced or eliminated hospital stay, and minimal convalescence.

With this array of alternative forms of management for BPH, it is difficult for both the urologist and the patient to choose the best treatment plan. The American Urological Association has undertaken the challenge of comparing some of these alternatives to the gold standard—transurethral resection of the prostate. A proposed 5-year study hopefully will improve our understanding of the natural history of BPH as well as determine the most appropriate and cost-effective treatment for each patient. In addition, the morbidity and mortality questions associated with TURP will be addressed. Urologists of the 1990s have the convenience of superb endoscopic equipment to make transurethral resection an operation of great satisfaction and enjoyment. However, they also face the realization that TURP is not the only treatment option, and it is their responsibility to familiarize themselves with the newer, less invasive options in the management of BPH.

REFERENCES

1. Holtgrewe HL, Mebust WK, Dowd JB, et al. Transurethral prostatectomy practice aspects of the dominant operation in American urology. *J Urol* 1989;141:248–253
2. Mebust WK, Holtgrewe HL, Cockett ATK, et al. Transurethral prostatectomy: immediate and postoperative complications. A cooperative study of 13 participating institutions evaluating 3,885 patients. *J Urol* 1989;141:243–247
3. Nesbit RM. A history of transurethral prostatectomy. *Rev Mex Urol* 1975;35:349–362
4. Mebust WK. Transurethral prostatectomy. *Urol Clin North Am* 1990;17:575–576
5. Creevy CD, Webb EA. A fatal hemolytic reaction following transurethral resection of the prostate gland: a discussion of its prevention and treatment. *Surgery* 1947;21:56–66
6. Emmett JL, Gilbaugh JH Jr, McLean P. Fluid absorption during transurethral resection: comparison of mortality and morbidity after irrigation with water and non-hemolytic solutions. *J Urol* 1969;101:884–889
7. Castro JE, Griffith HJL, Shackman R. Significance of signs

and symptoms in benign prostatic hypertrophy. *Br Med J* 1969;2:598–601

8. Andersen JT, Nordling J, Walter S. Prostatism. I. The correlation between symptoms, cystometric and urodynamic findings. *Scand J Urol Nephrol* 1979;13:229–236

9. Jensen KME, Bruskewitz RC, Iversen P, et al. Significance of prostatic weight in prostatism. *Urol Int* 1983;38:173–178

10. Graversen PH, Gasser TC, Wasson JH, et al. Controversies about indications for transurethral resection of the prostate. *J Urol* 1989;141:475–481

11. Bauer DL, Garrison RW, McRoberts JW. The health and cost implications of routine excretory urography before transurethral prostatectomy. *J Urol* 1980;123:386–389

12. Optenberg SA, Thompson IM. Economics of screening for carcinoma of the prostate. *Urol Clin North Am* 1990;17:719–737

13. Roos NP, Wennberg JE, Malenka DJ, et al. Mortality and reoperation after open and transurethral resection of the prostate for benign prostatic hyperplasia. *N Engl J Med* 1989;320:1120–1123

14. Malenka DJ, Roos NP, Fisher ES, et al. Further study of the increased mortality following transurethral prostatectomy: a chart-based analysis. *J Urol* 1990;144:224–228

15. Flocks RH. Arterial distribution within the prostate gland: its role in transurethral prostate resection. *J Urol* 1937;37:524–548

16. Greene LF, Robinson HP. Postoperative contracture of the vesical neck. VI. Prophylaxis and treatment. *J Urol* 1966;95:520–525

17. Chodak GW, Plaut ME. Systemic antibiotics for prophylaxis in urologic surgery: a critical review. *J Urol* 1979;121:695–699

18. Mauermayer W. *Transurethral Surgery*. New York: Springer-Verlag, 1983:193–240

19. Iglesias JJ, Sporer A, Gellman AC, et al. New Iglesias resectoscope with continuous irrigation, simultaneous suction and low intravesical pressure. *J Urol* 1975;114:929–933

20. Widran J. Controlled continuous flow method for transurethral resection. *Urology* 1983;21:130–131

21. Flechner S, Williams RD. Continuous flow and conventional resectoscope methods in transurethral prostatectomy: comparative study. *J Urol* 1982;127:257–259

22. O'Boyle PJ, Lumb GN, Appleton GVN. Videoprostatectomy. In: *Endourology, Third Congress Issue*. Karlsruhe Verlag, 1984:323–324

23. Widran J. Video transurethral resection. Report of 200 cases. *Br J Urol* 1990;65:357–361

24. Lepor H. Nonoperative management of benign prostatic hyperplasia. *J Urol* 1989;141:1283–1289

25. McConnell JD. Androgen ablation and blockade in the treatment of benign prostatic hyperplasia. *Urol Clin North Am* 1990;17:661–670

26. Reddy PK, Wasserman N, Castaneda F, et al. Balloon dilation of the prostate for treatment of benign hyperplasia. *Urol Clin North Am* 1988;15:529–535

27. Goldenberg SL, Perez-Marrero RA, Lee LM, et al. Endoscopic balloon dilation of the prostate: early experience. *J Urol* 1990;144:83–88

28. Orandi A. Transurethral incision of prostate (TUIP): 646 cases in 15 years—a chronological appraisal. *Br J Urol* 1985;57:703–707

29. Hahn RG, Algottson LA, Tornebrandt K. Comparison of ethanol absorption during continuous and intermittent flow irrigation in transurethral resection. *Scand J Urol Nephrol* 1990;24:27–30

5

Prostate Cancer Screening: Current Trends and Future Implications

Peter J. Littrup, Fred Lee, Curtis Mettlin

Until recently, research about the natural history and development of both prostate cancer and benign prostatic hyperplasia provided no compelling basis for pursuing early detection or alternative treatment possibilities. The excitement and controversy surrounding current prostate cancer research follow on the heels of recent advances in ultrasound, improved staging and biopsy techniques, magnetic resonance imaging (MRI), and serologic tests. With these new technologies, early detection of prostate cancer may become more cost-effective on a diagnosed per cancer basis than is the case for either breast or cervical cancer screening. Data continues to accrue regarding the optimal combination of prostate specific antigen (PSA), digital rectal examination (DRE), and transrectal ultrasound (TRUS).

Carcinoma of the prostate is now the cancer most common in men and the second leading cause of male cancer deaths in the United States.[1] Prostate cancer is therefore a good candidate for improved control by early detection and, if diagnosed at a localized stage, survival rates for both radical prostatectomy and radiation therapy are excellent.[2,3] Prostatic carcinoma is a slow growing tumor at its onset and metastatic potential is related to size and degree of differentiation.[4-7] In current practice however, most patients have advanced disease at the time of diagnosis by DRE.[8]

The autopsy incidence of prostate cancer in men over age 50 frequently is reported at 30%, though fewer than 1% of the population have overt clinical manifestations.[9] Autopsy incidences, therefore, do not accurately reflect the spectrum of clinical disease since 60% of tumors found at autopsy are less than 0.5 mL. These tumors have little clinical significance, except in younger men.[7] Patients who may benefit from screening will have tumor sizes ranging from 0.5 to 3.0

mL, i.e., potentially curable lesions. Tumors with volumes of 0.5 to 3.0 mL comprised only 5% of the autopsy series and one-fifth of the cancer group.[7]

Seventy percent of prostate cancers arise in the peripheral zone, 20% in the transitional zone, and 10% within the central zone.[9] Up to 40% of cancers may arise anterior to the midline of the prostate[10] and are out of reach of the examining finger. Tumor size is the factor most related to patient survival,[6,7] however, tumor volume determination by the DRE is inaccurate.[11] Lacking any large, randomized trials at this time, screening for prostate cancer can only refer to the early detection of prostate cancer in an otherwise asymptomatic patient, rather than subsequent reduction in population death rates. Questions which address important concerns about screening include: "Are there diagnostic tests that can reliably identify the majority of clinically important cancers and not 'latent,' insignificant disease?" and "Given the lack of results from randomized trials, are we able to justify any large scale early detection efforts in light of public and economic pressures?"

HISTORY OF THE DIGITAL RECTAL EXAMINATION

Routine screening for prostate cancer was advocated as early as 1905 by Young[12] and reemphasized by Kimbrough in 1956.[13] Gilbertsen reported a large series of 5856 men screened with 28,407 routine DREs and found 75 cancers, for an overall detection rate of 1.3%.[14] He interpreted the equivalent survival rates of these 75 men compared to the normal population as being synonymous with a cure of the disease. Data regarding the clinical stage at the time of diagnosis, and details of subsequent therapy were not sufficiently reported to allow critical analysis. Partly on the basis of this early experience, the DRE assumed its role as the gold standard in prostate cancer detection.

Thompson et al. investigated the results of routine screening[15] and its impact on stage distribution of prostate cancer.[16] In a screening population of 2005 men, a detection rate of 0.8% was achieved and 88% of the cancers were considered clinically localized.[15] However, 66% of patients who underwent surgery were upstaged to either stage C (capsular penetration) or D1 (nodal metastases) disease. The follow-up article[16] demonstrated a significantly increased percentage of patients with clinically localized disease, however, pathologic upstaging to C or D1 disease continued to occur in 60% of patients. Chodak's screening series yielded 11 cancers in 811 men (1.4%), with five men considered stage B (palpable, focal nodule). Negative lymphadenectomy was available in only 2 of these 5 patients, while the remaining patients were already at advanced stages.[17] The expected increase in more localized cancer stages was not demonstrated and the stage distribution was similar to national percentages found by the American College of Surgeons in non-screened populations.[18]

It has been shown that some optimally positioned cancers of 0.2 mL in volume may be palpable,[19] however, the preceding screening series represent more accurately the limited ability of DRE to detect pathologically localized cancers. Another limitation is the variability between the assessments of individual clinicians, making the DRE difficult to reproduce and standardize for screening. Two major problems in interpreting any screening study include lead time and length bias.[20]

Lead time bias produces an artificial estimate of increased survival time because a screening cancer may simply be diagnosed at an earlier date without decreasing eventual mortality from the disease. Lead time bias may be theoretically removed if a randomized, large screening group demonstrates fewer deaths from the disease than a matched control group. *Length bias* is a selection artifact that disproportionately detects malignancies with inherently slower growth. The longer the preclinical duration of the disease, the stronger the length bias. Prostate cancer has been estimated to take up to 10 years to reach a volume of 1 mL,[9] thereby increasing length bias. In an older population with a higher prevalence of other pathologic conditions, it may be difficult for any diagnostic test to demonstrate a clear reduction in prostate cancer mortality. Even if lead time bias was eliminated in a long-term study, the innate length bias in screening for prostate cancer could provide continued controversy in the ultimate cost-efficacy debate.

TRUS AND PROSTATE CANCER

The advent of high frequency transducers provided the necessary improvement in spatial resolution to allow for a detailed view of internal prostate anatomy. The majority of papers published prior to 1986 utilized ultrasound transducers operating at 3.5 MHz and 4.0 MHz. These images of the prostate produced criteria for cancer that relied on evaluation of the external contours of the gland for asymmetry, prostate diameter, and distortion of the capsule.[21,22] With newer 5 MHz and 7 MHz transducers, the basic zonal concept of the prostate was rediscovered and the criteria for early prostate cancer were dramatically altered.[23] Tumor size could be estimated from the greatest measurable dimensions by TRUS[24-26] and produced more objective evaluation of tumor volume, subsequent growth, and/or response to therapy. Despite the encouraging use of MRI for assessing lymph node status and staging advanced disease,[27,28] detailed images of internal prostatic architecture and tumor size are frequently obscured or degraded by small hemorrhages and/or blood products from recent biopsies. The limited availability and high cost of MRI also mitigate against its use for screening or primary evaluation of suspicious lesions.

Most cancers appear hypoechoic relative to the adjacent peripheral zone.[23-26,29-33] Early prostate cancer can be classified into three growth patterns: nodular, nodular with infiltrating components, and predominantly infiltrative[34] (Figure 5–1). As neoplasms enlarge, they tend to invade the adjacent parenchyma in a pattern of least resistance, engulfing adjacent tissue and becoming relatively isoechoic.[26] The hypoechoic appearance of prostate cancer is thus dependent upon the density of cancer per unit area. The contours of both the prostate and surgical capsules are important morphologic landmarks in the evaluation of neoplastic disease. Therefore, an isolated hypoechoic lesion must be taken in context with its effect upon local architectural distortion in order to obtain optimal diagnostic performance and higher predictive values.[24,33,35]

TRUS and Early Detection

The report by Lee and colleagues[35] was an early comparative study suggesting the superior sensitivity of TRUS over the DRE in the detection of early prostate cancer. That effort screened 784 men, detected 22 cancers and demonstrated double the detection rate for TRUS over the DRE (2.6% vs. 1.3%). The statistical values obtained for the prevalence of carcinoma are shown in Table 5–1. Seventy-seven percent (17/22) of TRUS screening cancers were considered potentially curable (less than 1.5 cm in average diameter), and only 17% (1/6) were upstaged by subsequent radical prostatectomy. The two cancers missed by TRUS were large infiltrating lesions which destroyed the normal internal architecture, a sign the investigators now consider as highly suspicious. Non-palpable cancers were 1.2 cm in average diameter, i.e., clinically significant, yet potentially curable. Using the results obtained from this study, the screening costs of detecting an early prostate cancer by TRUS and the DRE were calculated to be essentially equivalent.[36]

Increasing positive predictive values with increasing

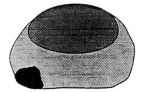

Nodular

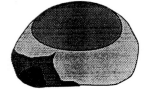

**Nodular +
Infiltrative**

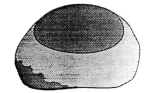

Infiltrative

Figure 5–1. Graphic representation of the variable morphologic appearance of prostate cancer.[34]

TRUS lesion size has been noted in both screening and clinical biopsy series.[33,35] This supports the assumption that directed biopsy produces more tumor per biopsy core, thereby rendering better tumor volume data, and runs counter to the suggestion that more cancers are found by ultrasound simply because more biopsies are recommended.[37] In addition, equivalent positive predictive values for TRUS and the DRE suggest that the TRUS biopsy criteria do not produce excessive biopsies relative to the DRE. While it is true that systematic biopsies may increase the diagnostic yield for cancer,[37] random biopsy involves the greatest risk of diagnosing insignificant, incidental tumors. Limiting the use of systematic biopsy may reduce criticism concerning insignificant tumor detection and the associated treatment dilemmas. These issues are especially troublesome when systematic biopsy cores reveal less than 2 mm of cancer. When the level of suspicion for cancer is high based on prostate-specific antigen (PSA) and hypoechoic and/or architectural abnormalities are not seen by TRUS, biopsy of only the regions of anatomic weakness, (i.e., parenchyma surrounding the superior and inferior vascular bundles, as well as the apex and bladder neck at the level of the anterior fibromuscular stroma) may be indicated. The intention of doing this is to biopsy only regions where the majority of cancers originate and escape from the prostate and avoid detection of smaller lesions located more centrally in the transition zone.[25]

Not all comparisons of DRE and TRUS have shown TRUS to be significantly more sensitive than the DRE. However, some of these reports compared the accuracy of TRUS and the DRE using low MHz transducers with preselected patient populations,[22,38] or used populations with significant portions of elderly patients who most likely would not even have benefitted from screening.[37] Patient populations were prese-lected for palpable abnormalities[38] or were urologic referrals for suspected prostate pathology.[23] Technical expertise and knowledge of anterior gland evaluation by TRUS also becomes suspect when DRE detects more cancers than TRUS,[37] particularly when TRUS appeared to have been performed with adequate equipment.

The American Cancer Society–National Prostate Cancer Detection Project (ACS–NPCDP) is a multicenter multidisciplinary study evaluating TRUS, DRE and PSA in a large cohort of men not previously suspected of having prostate cancer. This project only evaluates individuals aged 55 to 70 years, and it has demonstrated that the estimated sensitivity of TRUS is significantly greater than the digital rectal exam[39] (Table 5–1). The first year report from this demonstration program showed that 85% (44/52) of cancers were detected by TRUS while 63% (33/52) had positive DRE. Five additional cancers were diagnosed subsequently by elevated PSA, although most had suspicious TRUS in retrospect when follow-up biopsy was performed. The lower positive predictive value for TRUS compared to the prior screening study by Lee et al. may represent an initial learning curve for TRUS in these first year results. TRUS suffers from the same limitations to mass implementation as the DRE, that is, unavoidable operator dependent performance. Major issues in standardizing technique, equipment, criteria, and level of suspicion remain to be resolved. PSA may thus serve as a more objective initial screening parameter and improve the diagnostic performance of DRE and TRUS.

PROSTATE-SPECIFIC ANTIGEN

PSA is a highly immunogenic glycoprotein produced solely by the prostate and was initially used only as an indicator of

Table 5–1. Statistical Parameters for TRUS & DRE Screening

	TRUS		DRE	
CANCER DETECTION RATES	Lee et al. 2.6%	ACS-NPCDP 1.8%	Lee et al. 1.3%	ACS-NPCDP 1.4%
Sensitivity	91%	71%	45%	58%
Specificity	94%	89%	97%	96%
Positive predictive value	31%	15%	34%	28%
Negative predictive value	99%		98%	

tumor volume and clinical disease progression following therapy for prostate cancer.[40-45] The use of PSA for early detection was considered limited by the false positive elevations produced by benign prostatic hyperplasia (BPH).[41-45] PSA was then found to increase the positive predictive value for TRUS-guided biopsy of hypoechoic lesions of the prostate.[33,46] PSA levels are elevated approximately 0.3 ng/mL per gram of BPH tissue compared with 3.0 ng/mL per gram of cancer.[44] A prostate with BPH and a gland volume of 60 mL may thus have a PSA value indistinguishable from a normal sized, 30 mL gland harboring a 3 mL cancer. Studies done with radical prostatectomy specimens also show that prostate weight is the most important, non-cancer variable in PSA elevation.[45]

Debate exists over the upper limits of normal for both monoclonal (m-PSA) and polyclonal (p-PSA) PSA results. The manufacturer's recommended upper limits of normal for m-PSA is 4.0 ng/mL (Tandem-R, Hybritech Inc., San Diego, CA) and for p-PSA, 2.5 ng/mL (Pros-Check, Yang Laboratories, Bellevue, WA). Selecting the appropriate cut-off between normal and abnormal PSA values significantly influences published estimates of sensitivity and specificity, as well as the number of patients referred for TRUS. A large study of cancers by Partin et al. demonstrated patients with BPH to have m-PSA values indistinguishable from those with localized prostate cancer.[42] The BPH patients did not have TRUS evaluation, however, and it is possible that undetected, non-palpable cancers occurred in that group despite a negative transurethral resection. Approximately 45% of the pathologically confined cancers and 25% of patients with non-confined prostate cancer demonstrated m-PSA values $\leq$ 4.0 ng/mL. If their suggested decision level for m-PSA of 2.8 ng/mL were used instead of 4.0 ng/mL, only 29% of organ confined and 12% of non-confined disease would have had normal values.

In contrast, early reports using p-PSA and the manufacturer's recommended value of 2.5 ng/mL demonstrated elevated values in approximately 90% of cancer patients.[33,44,45] Both PSA assays measure the same analyte (r = 0.98) and the discrepancy between assay values appears to stem from differences in calibration standards producing values 1.6 to 1.85 times higher for the polyclonal assay.[46,47] These laboratory derived values are similar to the 1.5 to 1.75 conversion factors used to compare separate populations within the ACS-NPCDP.[49,50] In other words, the p-PSA decision level of 2.5 ng/mL should be compared to an m-PSA value of approximately 1.4, while the m-PSA decision level of 4.0 ng/mL should correspond to a p-PSA value of approximately 7.0 ng/mL. In any event, it is clear that the manufacturer's current recommendations of normal values need to be reassigned and a consensus reached on universal calibration standards. The American Cancer Society plans to hold a workshop on standards for PSA interpretation in the coming year.

At the inception of the ACS-NPCDP, the investigators hoped that obtaining accurate gland volume measurements would produce insight into BPH development and potential effects on PSA results. The correlation of TRUS gland volume and PSA results was initially limited to patients with normal TRUS and DRE.[49,50] Both studies produced PSA decision levels based on gland volume ranges (Table 5-2, Figure 5-2) and were the first to incorporate TRUS in the selection of normal patients. Men with PSA values above the 95th percentile decision levels (Table 5-2) were estimated to have a nine-fold increased risk of prostate cancer.[49] Approximately 60% (1042/1695) of patients had gland volumes $\leq$35mL (Figure 5-2) with relatively minimal BPH distortion. Figure 5-3 demonstrates that an m-PSA decision level of 4.0 ng/mL may represent a disproportionately elevated PSA value for over half of all screening patients using the 90th percentile. Two objective variables, PSA and TRUS gland volume, have thus identified a potential high risk cancer group and better defined abnormal PSA values for the majority of screening patients.

In order to individualize a patient's PSA relative to gland volume, it may be desirable to modify the approach of gland volume grouping to the concept of predicted PSA.[51] Basically, predicted PSA operates on the premise of PSA production per gram of BPH tissue which was calculated to be 0.2 ng/mL. Predicted PSA functioned near the 95th percentile and objectively allowed approximately 70% of cancer detection to occur in only 10% of the population. The use of predicted PSA has greatly increased our confidence level for biopsy recommendation of subtle TRUS lesions in patients where serum PSA exceeds the predicted value. This ap-

Table 5–2. Mean PSA Levels with Standard Deviation (SD) and 95th Percentile Decision Levels for the Four Gland Volume Ranges Derived from Two ACS-NPDCP Centers[49]

MONOCLONAL PSA (m-PSA), ng/mL				
Prostate Volume (mL)	n	Mean	SD	95th % x + (1.65 × SD)
0–30	158	1.3	1.1	3.1
31–40	75	1.9	1.2	3.9
41–50	35	3.0	2.1	6.5
>50	30	5.0	3.9	11.4
Total	298	2.0	2.1	5.5

POLYCLONAL PSA (p-PSA), ng/mL				
Prostate Volume (mL)	n	Mean	SD	95th % x + (1.65 × SD)
0–30	117	2.1	2.6	6.4
31–40	69	3.1	2.8	7.7
41–50	40	5.6	7.8	18.5
>50	29	8.5	6.3	18.9
Total	255	3.6	4.8	11.5

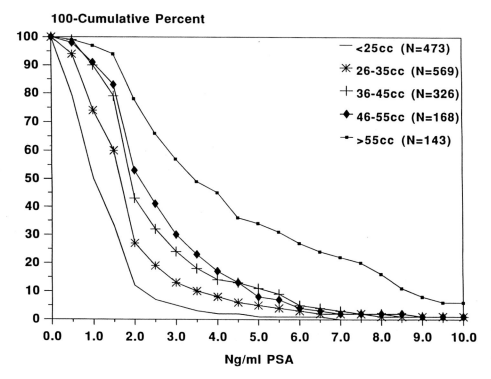

Figure 5–2. PSA levels from total ACS-NPCDP data in presumed normal men (N = 1595) according to TRUS gland volume ranges (monoclonal and transformed polyclonal values combined).[50]

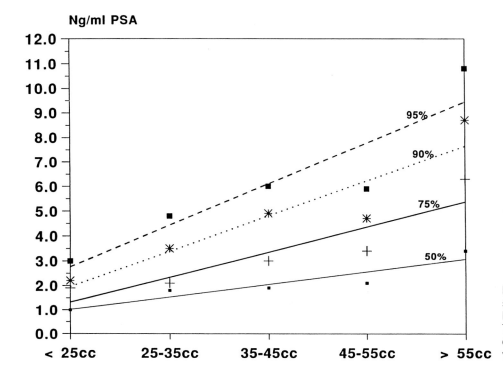

Figure 5–3. PSA levels in presumed normal men and best-fit trend lines by percentile rank according to TRUS gland volume ranges (monoclonal and transformed polyclonal values combined).[50]

proach also decreases the number of low yield biopsies in patients with markedly elevated PSA but proportional gland enlargement. Cancer detection rate remained high while significantly increasing the positive predictive value of TRUS using the formulas

Predicted monoclonal PSA = 0.12 ng/mL/gm × TRUS volume (mL).

Estimated TRUS lesion size can be derived from

Mean TRUS diameter = $^3\sqrt{}$Tumor volume
= $^3\sqrt{}$(Excess mPSA/2.0 ng/mL/gm cancer),

where excess PSA = serum PSA − predicted PSA.

PSA AND EARLY DETECTION

One screening study to date using PSA as the initial screen found 37 cancers in 1653 men for a detection rate of 2.2%.[52] Patients with two consecutive m-PSA results greater than 4.0 ng/mL then received DRE and TRUS. Patients were biopsied based on TRUS or DRE findings alone. No patient with a PSA > 10.0 ng/mL had an abnormal TRUS. No biopsies were performed in the group of patients with PSA results between 4.0 and 10.0 ng/mL if the DRE and TRUS were normal. The DRE missed 12 cancers and TRUS missed 16 cancers such that PSA appeared to have the best specificity, positive predictive value and accuracy using the 4.0 ng/mL decision level. The methods and results of this study also demonstrate the operator dependent nature of TRUS. Since PSA results were not stratified according to TRUS gland volume, it is difficult to interpret their findings for patients with values between 4 and 10 ng/mL. Forty-one percent of their cancer patients with PSA levels of 4.0 to 10.0 ng/mL already had extracapsular extension of tumor. This correlates well with prostatectomy series where 43% of patients also had non-confined disease.[42] Catalona et al. states, "We detected both advanced and localized cancer in the study group and thus far have not demonstrated increased detection of early prostate cancer with PSA screening."[52] PSA at a decision level of 4.0 ng/mL may thus be the most accurate test for the clinical detection of prostate cancer, however, new data is emerging which suggests that lower decision levels may be considered for future screening attempts.

In a series of 1002 men randomly selected from electoral rolls of Quebec City and its vicinity, DRE, TRUS and PSA were performed on all men and a total of 57 cancers were detected.[53] Using statistical parameters for the cancer prevalence in that study, the optimal decision threshold for PSA was determined to be 3.0 ng/mL. The sensitivity, specificity, positive predictive value (PPV) and negative predictive value (NPV) for PSA at this 3.0 ng/mL were 80.7%, 89.6%, 24.1% and 98.6%, respectively. If PSA were to be used as the initial screen, 19% of the whole cohort had PSA values above 3.0 ng/mL and 46 cancers would have been detected subsequently by DRE and/or TRUS. If the 4.0 ng/mL level were used, 12% of the cohort would have been considered

abnormal and only 41 cancers would have been detected. The relative increase in cancer detection using PSA at 3.0 ng/mL instead of 4.0 ng/mL thus appeared greater than the increase in patients designated as having "elevated" PSA values. However, 6 of 11 cancers with values below 3.0 ng/mL also had abnormal DRE.

When PSA is used as the initial screening filter,[52] repeat PSA determinations could be used to eventually detect cancers missed on the first pass.[53,54] This assumes a direct correspondence of PSA level to tumor volume and growth rate, yet pathologic correlation with clinically benign specimens suggest that PSA levels do not increase significantly until tumors reach a size of 1 mL.[55] Even for follow-up, the lower the PSA decision level, the greater the cancer sensitivity and percent of patients with organ confined disease. Indeed, 77% (30/39) of cancers detected in Partin's series between 2.8 and 4.0 ng/mL were organ confined, compared to only 54% (71/132) being confined with PSA values 4.0 to 10.0 ng/mL. Continued elevations or significant interval increases in PSA over time may actually be more important than absolute PSA values.

The decision to screen for prostate cancer using any or all available tests to decrease eventual mortality are important public health and economic issues. Examining the cancers found thus far in the ACS-NPCDP, the potential impact of combined screening with PSA, TRUS, and DRE can be seen[56] (Figure 5–4, Table 5–3). There is an even distribution of cancers over the PSA ranges of 0 to 4.0, 4.0 to 10.0 and >10.0 ng/mL. A third of cancers (29/88) may be missed using a decision level of 4.0 ng/mL, similar to other reports.[42,47,53] TRUS detected 90% (26/29) of cancers with PSA ≤ 4.0 while the DRE detected 52% (15/29). TRUS appeared to perform better at lower values of PSA and DRE detection remained constant for all PSA ranges.

Table 5–3 provides further insight into cancer detection according to PSA level. Half of all biopsies in the ACS-NPCDP were performed on lesions with PSA values less than 2.0 ng/mL for a total PPV of only 3.9%. For PSA values 2.1 to 4.0 ng/mL, the PPV for both TRUS and DRE improved significantly and 66% (10/15) of cancers below 4.0 ng/mL occurred here. This suggests that statistics in other reports which group all PSA results below 4.0 ng/mL[46,52] may need further evaluation. To illustrate, the ACS-NPCDP data could be viewed such that 18 TRUS examinations are required to find 1 cancer when the DRE is negative and m-PSA ≤ 4.0 ng/mL (Figure 5–4). However, this could also be broken down to represent 34 TRUS for PSA ≤ 2.0 and only 9 TRUS required to find 1 cancer for PSA 2.1 to 4.0 ng/mL, given a normal DRE.

Clinical detection of early prostate cancer requires the addition of PSA to any screening approach and relegates TRUS to further assessment of any abnormalities suspected by DRE or TRUS. Currently, it is prudent to continue advocating thorough DRE performed by an experienced examiner with the addition of PSA at 4.0 ng/mL. In this

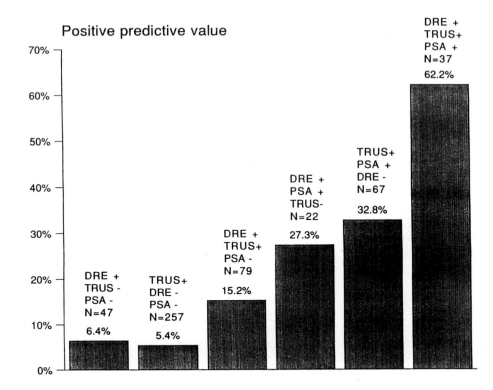

Figure 5–4. Positive predictive values according to combination of TRUS, DRE, and PSA. Positive PSA defined as >4.0 ng/mL.

manner, DRE should still detect half of all lesions with PSA ≤ 4.0 ng/mL and produce an estimated sensitivity for the PSA + DRE combination of 83% (66% + 17%). Using previous screening cost formulations[36] and the cancer incidence and detections rates from the ACS-NPCDP,[39] the cost per cancer detected for TRUS alone, DRE alone and the PSA + DRE approach mentioned above are $9,611, $4,029 and $5,081 respectively.

Despite this rough cost estimate, more cancers will be detected using PSA + DRE than with TRUS alone, and for nearly half the price! DRE could be done much cheaper[36] when used alone for mass screening, however, detection would be significantly reduced and many (40–50%) cancers would already have spread beyond the prostate. Even in its secondary role, TRUS could be done cheaper by using gland volume ranges to establish high risk groups among those with elevated PSA. Effective TRUS screening could then be done by well trained technicians who perform the routine evaluation for suspicious lesions, obtain a gland volume and compare it with the volume adjusted 95th percentile for PSA. A physician may then need to personally scan only those patients with a suspicious lesion for possible biopsy, or those with a volume adjusted PSA level above the 90 to 95th percentile in order to confirm or deny the presence of a subtle tumor missed by the technician. This could greatly lower the professional time and cost component for TRUS screening and hopefully not decrease TRUS sensitivity alone.

SUMMARY

Screening for prostate cancer represents a clinical dilemma with no clear evidence to suggest decreased mortality from

Table 5–3. Positive Predictive Value of TRUS & DRE According to PSA for All Biopsies Performed to Date in the ACS-NPCDP[56]

EXAMINATION RESULTS	PSA (ng/mL)							
	0–2.0		2.1–4.0		4.0–10.0		>10.0	
	n	%	n	%	n	%	n	%
TRUS+, DRE−	5/172	2.9	9/85	10.6	12/49	24.5	10/18	55.6
DRE+, TRUS−	1/36	2.8	2/11	18.1	4/15	26.7	2/7	28.6
DRE+, TRUS+	4/50	8.0	8/29	27.6	8/19	42.1	15/18	83.3
DRE−, TRUS−	0	0	0	0	1/3	33.3	7/8	87.5
Total DRE+	5/86	5.8	10/38	26.3	12/34	35.3	17/25	68.0
Total TRUS+	9/222	4.1	17/114	14.9	20/68	29.4	25/36	69.4
All Combination	10/258	3.9	19/121	15.7	25/86	29.1	34/51	66.6

any diagnostic test. We now possess new knowledge regarding optimal combinations of DRE, TRUS, and PSA. While DRE and TRUS may be too subjective and PSA nonspecific, their combined predictive values not only identify those at high risk, but also those patients where continued frequent screening may not be cost effective. A monoclonal PSA decision level of no greater than 4.0 ng/mL should be used since 40% of cancers detected from 4.0 to 10.0 ng/mL already have extracapsular extension. Assuming that DRE is performed by experienced examiners, the combination of PSA and DRE should produce cost-effective early detection and minimize missed cancers of less than 4.0 ng/mL. TRUS should be reserved for those patients with either PSA elevations and/or DRE abnormalities. The use of TRUS gland volume data to further modify PSA decision levels, such as the predicted PSA concept, may also improve TRUS biopsy criteria and predictive values. Prostate cancer detection can now be objectively limited to a small percentage of the population and select for earlier, more localized, disease. The ultimate decrease in mortality from screening remains to be demonstrated in randomized trials or observed only after decades of increased public awareness about prompt early detection combined with effective, definitive therapy.

REFERENCES

1. Boring CC, Squires TS, Tong T, Luberta J. Cancer statistics, 1992. *CA* 1992;42:19–38
2. Paulson DF, Lin GH, Hinshaw W, Stephani S. The Uro-Oncology Research Group. Radical surgery versus radiotherapy for adenocarcinoma of the prostate. *Urol* 1982;128:502–504
3. Pilepich MV, Bagshaw M, Asbell SO, et al. Radical prostatectomy or radiotherapy in carcinoma prostate–the dilemma continues. *Urol* 1987;30:18–21
4. McNeal JE. Origin and development of carcinoma in the prostate. *Cancer* 1969;23:24–34
5. Scott R Jr., Mutchnik DL, Laskowski TZ, Schmalhorst WR. Carcinoma of the prostate in elderly men: incidence, growth, characteristics, and clinical significance. *J Urol* 1969;101:602–607
6. Culp OS, Meyer JJ. Radical prostatectomy in the treatment of prostate cancer. *Cancer* 1973;32:1113–1118
7. McNeal JE, Kindrachuk RA, Freiha FS, et al. Patterns of progression in prostate cancer. *Lancet* 1986;1:60–63
8. Gittes RF, Chu TM. Detection and diagnosis of prostate cancer. *Semin Oncol* 1976;2:123–130
9. McNeal JE. The prostate gland: morphology and pathobiology. *Monogr Urol* 1988;9:36–54
10. McNeal JE, Price HM, Redwine EA, et al. Stage A versus stage B adenocarcinoma of the prostate: morphological comparison and biological significance. *J Urol* 1988;139:61–65
11. Speigelman SS, McNeal JE, Freiha FS, et al. Rectal examination in volume determination of carcinoma of the prostate: clinical and anatomical correlations. *J Urol* 1986;136:1228–1230
12. Young HH. The early diagnosis and radical cure of carcinoma of the prostate: being a study of 40 cases and presentation of a radical operation which was carried out in four cases. *Bull Johns Hopkins Hosp* 1905;16:315–318
13. Kimbrough JC. Carcinoma of the prostate: five year follow-up of patients treated by radical surgery. *J Urol* 1956;76:287–290
14. Gilbertsen VA. Cancer of the prostate gland. Results of early diagnosis and therapy undertaken for cure of the disease. *JAMA* 1971;215:81–84
15. Thompson IM, Ernst JJ, Gangai MP, Spence R. Adenocarcinoma of the prostate: results of routine urological screening. *J Urol* 1984;132:690–692
16. Thompson IM, Rounder JB, Teague JL, et al. Impact of routine screening for adenocarcinoma of the prostate on stage distribution. *J Urol* 1987;137:424–426
17. Chodak GW, Schoenberg HW. Early detection of prostate cancer by routine screening. *JAMA* 1984;252:3261–3264
18. Murphy GP, Natarajan N, Pontes JE, et al. The national survey of prostate cancer in the United States by the American College of Surgeons. *J Urol* 1982;127:928–932
19. Stamey TA, McNeal JE, Freiha FS, Redwine E. Morphometric and clinical studies on 68 consecutive radical prostatectomies. *J Urol* 1988;139:1235–1241
20. Cole P, Morrison AS. Basic issues in population screening for cancer. *J Natl Cancer Inst* 1980;64:1263–1272
21. Watanabe H, Saitoh M, Mishina T, et al. Mass screening program for prostatic diseases with transrectal ultrasonotomography. *J Urol* 1977;117:746–747
22. Chodak GW, Wald V, Parmer E, et al. Comparison of digital examination and transrectal ultrasonography for the diagnosis of prostatic cancer. *J Urol* 1986;135:951–954
23. Lee F, Gray JM, McLeary RD, et al. Transrectal ultrasound in the diagnosis of prostate cancer: location, echogenicity, histopathology, and staging. *Prostate* 1985;7:117–129
24. Lee F, Littrup PJ, McLeary RD, et al. Needle aspiration and core biopsy of prostate cancer: comparative evaluation with biplanar transrectal ultrasound guidance. *Radiology* 1987;164:515–520
25. Shinohara K, Scardino PT, Carter SC, Wheeler TM. Pathologic basis of the sonographic appearance of the normal and malignant prostate. *Urol Clin N Am* 1989;16:675–692
26. Lee F, Siders DB, Torp-Pedersen ST, Kirscht JL, McHugh TA, Mitchell AE. Prostate cancer: transrectal ultrasound and pathology comparison—a preliminary study of outer gland (peripheral and central zones) and inner gland (transition zone) cancer. *Suppl Cancer* 1991;67:1132–1142
27. Hricak H, Dooms GC, Jeffrey RB Jr, et al. Prostatic carcinoma: staging by clinical assessment, CT, and MR imaging. *Radiology* 1987;162:331–336
28. Bezzi M, Kressel HY, Allen KS, et al. Prostatic carcinoma: staging with MR imaging at 1.5 T. *Radiology* 1988;169:339–346
29. Lee F, Gray JM, McLeary RD, et al. Prostatic evaluation by transrectal sonography: criteria for diagnosis of early adenocarcinoma. *Radiology* 1986;158:91–95
30. Rifkin MD, Friedlang GW, Shortliff L. Prostatic evaluation by transrectal endosonography: detection of carcinoma. *Radiology* 1986;158:85–90
31. Dahnhert WF, Hamper UM, Eggleston JC, et al. Prostatic evaluation by transrectal sonography with histopathologic correlation: the echopenic appearance of early carcinoma. *Radiology* 1986;158:97–102
32. Torp-Pedersen S, Lee F, Littrup PJ, et al. Transrectal biopsy of the prostate guided with transrectal US: longitudinal and multiplane scanning. *Radiology* 1989;170:23–27
33. Lee F, Torp-Pedersen S, Littrup PJ, et al. Hypoechoic lesions of the prostate: clinical relevance of tumor size, digital rectal examination, and prostate-specific antigen. *Radiology* 1989, 170:29–32
34. Kastendieck H, Alternahr E. Cyto- and histomorphogenesis of

the prostate carcinoma. A comparative light and electron-microscopy study. *Vichows Arch Pathol Anat* 1976;370: 207–24

35. Lee F, Littrup PJ, Torp-Pedersen S, et al. Prostate cancer: comparison of transrectal ultrasound and the digital rectal examination for screening. *Radiology* 1988;168:389–394
36. Torp-Pedersen S, Littrup PJ, Lee F, et al. Early prostate cancer: diagnostic costs of screening transrectal US and digital rectal examination. *Radiology* 1988;169:351–354
37. Palken M, Cobb OE, Simons CE, et al. Prostate cancer: comparison of digital rectal examination and transrectal ultrasound for screening. *J Urol* 1991;145:86–92
38. Clements R, Griffiths GJ, Peeling WB, et al. How accurate is the index finger? A comparison of digital and ultrasound examination of the prostatic nodule. *Clin Radiology* 1988;39:87–89
39. Mettlin CJ, Lee F, Drago J, Murphy GP, et al. The American Cancer Society National Prostate Cancer Detection Project - Findings on the detection of early prostate cancer in 2425 men.
40. Killian CS, Yang N, Emrich LJ, et al. Prognostic importance of prostate-specific antigen for monitoring patients with stages B2 to D1 prostate cancer. *Cancer Res* 1985;45:886–891
41. Stamey TA, Yang N, Hay AR, McNeal JE, Freiha FS, Redwine E. Prostate-specific antigen as a serum marker for adenocarcinoma of the prostate. *N Engl J Med* 1987;317:909–916
42. Partin AW, Carter HB, Chan DW, et al. Prostate specific antigen in the staging of localized prostatic cancer: influence of tumor differentiation, tumor volume and benign hyperplasia. *J Urol* 1990;143:747–752
43. Lange PH, Ercole CJ, Lightner DJ, Fraley EE, Vessella R. The value of serum prostate-specific antigen determinations before and after radical prostatectomy. *J Urol* 1989;141:873–879
44. Stamey TA, Kabalin JN. Prostate-specific antigen in the diagnosis and treatment of adenocarcinoma of the prostate. I. Untreated patients. *J Urol* 1989;141:1070–1075
45. Stamey TA, Kabalin JN, McNeal JE, et al. Prostate-specific antigen in the diagnosis and treatment of adenocarcinoma of the prostate. II. Radical prostatectomy treated patients. *J Urol* 1989;141:1076–1083
46. Cooner WH, Mosley BR Rutherford CL, et al. Clinical application of transrectal ultrasonography and prostate-specific antigen in the search for prostate cancer. *J Urol* 1988;139:758–761
47. Chan DW, Bruzek DJ, Oesterling JE, et al. Prostate-specific antigen as a marker for prostatic cancer: a monoclonal and a polyclonal immunoassay compared. *Clin Chem* 1987;33: 1916–1920
48. Hortin CL, Bahnson RR, Daft M, et al. Differences in values obtained with 2 assays of prostate-specific antigen. *J Urol* 1988;139:762–765
49. Littrup PJ, Kane RA, Williams CR, et al. Determination of prostate volume with transrectal US for cancer screening–Part 1: comparison with prostate-specific antigen assays. *Radiology* 1991;178:537–542.
50. Kane RA, Littrup PJ, Babaian R, et al. Prostate-specific antigen levels in 1695 men without evidence of prostate cancer. *Cancer* 1992;69:1201–1207
51. Lee F, Littrup PJ, Loft-Christensen L, et al. "Predicted" prostate specific antigen results using transrectal ultrasound gland volume: Differentiation of benign prostatic hyperplasia and prostate cancer. *Cancer* 1992;(in press)
52. Catalona WJ, Smith DS, Ratliff TL, et al. Measurement of prostate-specific antigen in serum as a screening test for prostate cancer. *N Engl J Med* 1991;324:1156–61
53. Labrie F, Dupont A, Suburu R, et al. Serum prostate specific antigen as pre-screening test for prostate cancer. *J Urol* 1992; 147:(in press)
54. Stamey TA. Editorial comment. *J Urol* 1992; 147:(in press)
55. Brawn PN, Speights VO, Kuhl D, et al. Prostate-specific antigen levels from completely sectioned, clinically benign, whole prostates. *Cancer* 1991;68:1592–99
56. Babaian RJ, Mettlin C, Kane R, Murphy GP, et al. The relationship of prostate-specific antigen to digital rectal examination and transrectal ultrasonography. *Cancer* 1992;69: 1195–1200

Prostatic Urethroplasty with Balloon Catheter

6

History of Prostatic Dilation (Prostatic Divulsion)

Santiago Isorna, Flavio Castañeda, Ben C. Berg

Since antiquity, dysuria has plagued mankind, and physicians and others practicing the healing arts have directed much of their efforts toward alleviating obstructive urinary symptoms. Instruments resembling catheters[1] have been identified in Egyptian hieroglyphics from about 3000 BC, and similar bronze instruments were discovered during the excavations of Herculaneum and Pompeii.[2]

The first description of benign prostatic hypertrophy (BPH) is attributed to the mystic Susruta, the Hindu Hippocrates, who practiced during the Brahman Period of Indian medicine (sixth–third centuries BC).[3] Even before anatomic studies were pursued, Hippocrates (460–375 BC) established a clear clinical differentiation between dysuric processes caused by a bladder neck tumor and those caused by the "stone ailment."[4]

The word prostate (from the Greek *prostates,* meaning one who stands before) is attributed to Herophilus, an anatomist of the ancient Greek School of Alexandria (300 BC).[5]

Pliny the Elder (first century AD)[6] recommended the first medical treatment for prostatism, which consisted of drinking potions of pulverized snail shells. A succession of equally fantastic remedies followed. Aretaeus recommended worms in honey, and Paul of Aegina prescribed warm blood from an old male goat, scorpion oil, and selvatic carrots and pumpkin seeds, which contain, in fact, large amounts of vitamin E. A large number of equally ridiculous remedies consisting of infusions, poultices, and potions of insects, plants, and miracle waters were used until a few centuries ago because of the lack of a better solution and the fear of undergoing surgery. Some of these remedies still are used in rural areas.

Until the Renaissance, few surgical procedures and concepts of urinary obstruction were developed, with the exception of the classic descriptions by Celsus (30 BC–50 AD) and Galen (130–200 AD), a few notable medieval physicians like Paul of Aegina (eighth century AD), and such Arab physicians as Rhazes of Baghdad (about 860–925 AD) and Abulcasis (eleventh century AD).[2,3] However, these practitioners were masters at catheterization and designing instruments using different materials, including flexible ones.

Francisco Diaz (1590),[7] one of the most important figures of Spain's Golden Age, is considered the father of urology.[8-10] Contemporary and fellow countryman of the literary genius Cervantes, author of *El Quijote,* Diaz was the surgeon of Emperor Felipe II.[11] He wrote the first urology book, *Tratado Nuevamente Impresso de Todas las Enfermedades de los Rinones, Vexiga, y Carnosidades de la Verga y Urina* (Fig. 6–1) [or *Newly Printed Treatise about All the Diseases of Kidneys, Urinary Bladder and Fleshiness of the Penis and Urine.*][12] In this book, pathologic prostatic growth is described and differentiated from other urethral pathologic processes for the first time. Diaz designed and used many different instruments (Fig. 6–2), among which was the "cutting instrument" he used to perform an inner urethrotomy, a surgical procedure he also developed.[13] A similar instrument was used by Ambroise Paré, his contemporary and the founder of modern surgery. Paré was one of the first to perform transurethral surgery.[14]

Until the first half of the nineteenth century, when Guyon, the founder of modern urology,[15] and his colleagues were active, BPH was not differentiated from other prostatic pathologic processes.[16] During this time, many procedures were developed to treat BPH that went beyond simple catheterization to focus specifically on the resolution of the prostatic obstruction rather than on treating urethral stenosis. Later in the same century, Freyer (1870) performed, accidentally, the first surgical treatment for BPH. All these procedures are the forerunners of the instrumental treatment

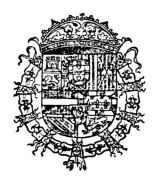

Figure 6–1. Cover of the first known edition of the urologic pathology book written by Francisco Diaz in 1588. It is the first known urology treatise.

techniques used today. Among them are the instruments of Civiale, Mercier, and Guthrie, who used a two-armed instrument, one arm of which held the bladder neck and the other allowed cool resection or ablation of the posterior anterior commissure (Figs. 6–3, 6–4).[2,17] A similar instrument, but one that incorporated for the first time the electric cut, is Bottini's "new thermogalvanic cauterizer and cutter" (Fig. 6–5).[18] Bottini's procedure represents the first transurethral resection (TUR). It was a blind procedure, since Nitze's instrument[19] incorporating direct vision, the cystoscope, was not perfected until 1877. Two years later, Marion[20] introduced his "cutting benique" [benique tranchant] (Fig. 6–6), demonstrating that the anterior commissurotomy by cool cut has a permanent place in the treatment of cervicoprostatic obstructive processes.

In regard to the development of balloon dilation procedures, we must look to the past for techniques with similar mechanisms. In a previous report,[21] we identified two different balloon dilation mechanisms: (1) anterior prostatic commissure disruption, allowing detachment of obstructive prostatic lateral lobes, and (2) distention of hypertrophic prostatic tissue and its capsule (true prostate) by loosening and separating the untied prostatic lobes during urination. We think therefore, that the appropriate name for this procedure using Castañeda's balloon is divulsion rather than dilation.

The techniques already described are based on the first mechanism, the section or disruption of the anterior prostatic commissure. We now turn to procedures that specifically target prostatic space dilation or BPH compression. One of the most picturesque of these was described by Mercier as a possible treatment. It consists of producing posterior pros-

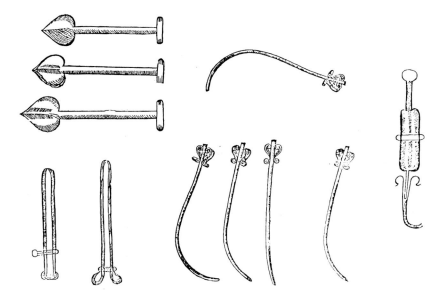

Figure 6–2. Instruments used or invented by Francisco Diaz and included in his urology treatise.

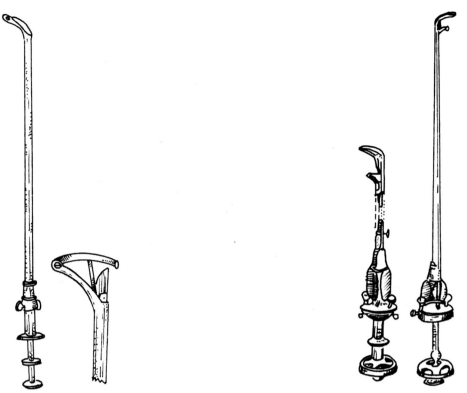

Figure 6–3. Instrument designed by Civiale.

Figure 6–4. Excisor designed by Mercier.

tatic compression or flattening by introducing a rigid urethral catheter up to the urinary bladder and an ivory instrument into the rectum.[22]

Sir Henry Thomson, the great English urologist of the Victorian Age, published *Practical Treatise of Urinary Tract Diseases.*[2] In this extraordinary book, there is an instrument resembling Castañeda's balloon catheter. This is a rigid instrument with a curved distal tip that incorporates something resembling a dilatable globe, possibly made of animal gut (Fig. 6–7). Thomson called it an "air or water dilator,"

and it is thought to have been used for bladder neck and prostatic urethra distention. Nearly all the urologic gadgets of the time are illustrated in this book. Thomson expanded the concept of prostatic compression. He wrote

"Es evidente que precisa ejercer una accion compresiva mucho mas fuerte que la de una sonda, aun del mas grueso calibre, si se quiere obtener algun resultado en la reduccion del volumen del organo, o en la dilatacion del cuello de la vejiga obstruido en parte."

Figure 6–5. Bottini's diathermic prostatic cutter. By approximating the two arms, it accomplishes tissue resection by electric energy, using a platinum and iridium incandescent grip.

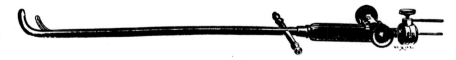

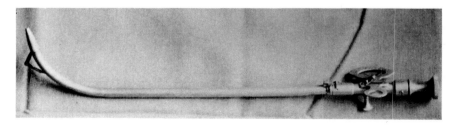

Figure 6–6. Marion's cutting benique (benique tranchant). (Courtesy of Dr. Ponce Socorro.)

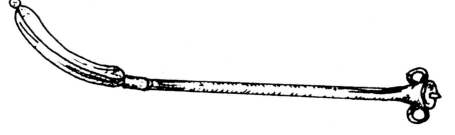

Figure 6–7. Air or water dilator. (Reproduced in ref. 2 without attribution.)

["It is evident that a greater compressive force is needed that could possibly be applied by the largest possible sound, if any result is expected in the reduction of the organ size, or in the dilation of the partially obstructed bladder neck."]

The American surgeon Physick devised a procedure that "employed a small sack made of bull gut that was introduced into the bladder and then was filled with a fluid introduced from the external open end, and then pulled out inflated through the bladder and urethra." This procedure,[23] successfully performed, is strongly reminiscent of the traction needed during distention using Castañeda's balloon.

Leroy d'Etoiles,[24] looking for the same effect, first tried compression of the posterior bladder neck and prostate with a metal catheter tilted vigorously backward up to the urinary bladder. Later, he designed another metal catheter to get the same effect axially (Fig. 6–8). Other noteworthy instruments were Mercier's ingenious prostatic depressor[25] (Fig. 6–9) and Deisting's divulsor[26] (Fig. 6–10), which has been promoted more recently by Aboulker and Steg.[27] Others were Thomson's divulsor (Fig. 6–11) and Leroy d'Etoiles'

excisor (Fig. 6–12). Although these procedures were mechanical and without radiologic guidance, their action was extraordinarily close to the mechanism of Castañeda's procedure for BPH.

In 1938, Frank[28] reported a large patient series in which he performed digital disruption of the anterior prostatic commissure using surgical cystostomy. This gives us an idea of how we opt for very limited action even when surgery is required because of the mortality associated with complete surgical resection for BPH. On the other hand, it confirms the efficacy of simple disruption in alleviating obstructive symptoms.

This brief review should remind us of our predecessors, and by putting their knowledge and methods into historic perspective, we can fully appreciate their giant efforts. At the same time, the application of these early ideas to modern methods and technology may provide patients who are concerned with the morbidity and mortality of surgical techniques for BPH with new alternatives that are more comfortable, cheaper, and safer.

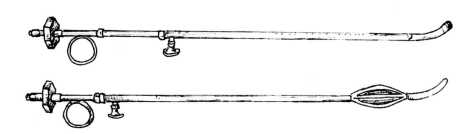

Figure 6–8. Leroy D'Etoiles' dilator.

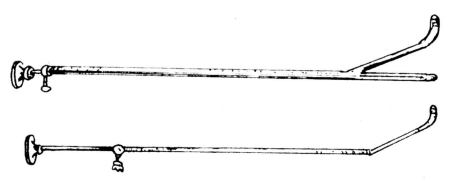

Figure 6–9. Mercier's prostatic depressor.

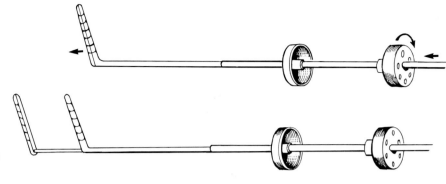

Figure 6–10. Deisting's prostatic divulsor.

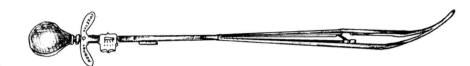

Figure 6–11. Thomson's divulsor.

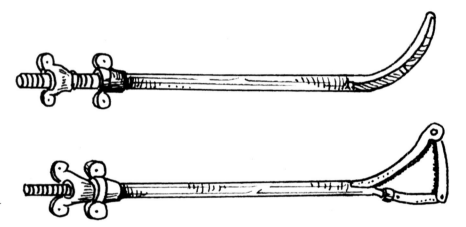

Figure 6–12. Leroy D'Etoiles' excisor.

REFERENCES

1. Hulbert JC. Benign prostatic hyperplasia. *Semin Intervent Radiol* 1989;6:8–9
2. Thomson H. *Tratado Practico de las Vias Urinarias.* Madrid: Bailliere, 1876
3. Pellici G. *Iter Urologico.* Madrid: Zambeletti Espana S.A., 1982
4. Nogueira-March JL. Cancer de Prostata: Diagnostico, Clasificacion y Variedades. Discurso de entrada en la Real Academia de Medicina y Cirugia de Galicia. Spain, 1983
5. Schultze-Seemann F. The historical contribution of European urology to scientific progress in the field of prostatic neoplasia. In: Jacobi GH, Hohenfellner R (eds). *Prostate Cancer.* Baltimore: Williams & Wilkins, 1982
6. Plinio. Historia Naturalis. Libro 28. Cap. 19. In: Pellici G (ed). *Iter Urologico.* Madrid: Zambeletti Espana S.A., 1982
7. Molla y Rodrigo R. *Tratado de Todas las Enfermedades de los Pinones, Vexiga y Carnosidades de la Verga, y Urina del Dr. Francisco Diaz. Estudio Preliminar Acerca del Autor y Sus Cobras.* Biblioteca Clasica de la Medicina. Madrid: Imprenta Julio Cosano, 1922
8. Morton L. *Garrison and Morton's Medical Bibliography: An Annotated Check-List of Texts Illustrating the History of Medicine,* 2nd ed. New York: Argosy Book Stores, 1961:364
9. Sanchez R, Bush RB. Francisco Diaz (1510?–1590). *Invest Urol* 1968;6:227–230
10. Bush RB, Bush IN. *Francisco Diaz and the World of Sixteenth Century Urology.* Section of History of Medicine. The Chicago Medical School, 1970
11. Maganto E. *El Doctor Francisco Diaz y su Epoca.* Barcelona: Eduard Fabregat, 1990
12. Diaz F. *Tratado Nuevamente Impresso de Todas las Enfermedades de los Rinones, Vexiga, y Carnosidades de la Verga y Urina.* Madrid: Impreso por Francisco Sanchez, 1588
13. Gross DJ. Practical treatise on the diseases, injuries and malformations of the urinary bladder, the prostate gland and the urethra. Philadelphia, 1851. In: Pulgvert A (ed). Comentario nuevo a un libro viejo. *Actas Urol Esp* 1977;1:231–238
14. Purpon I. Iniciadores de la prostatectomia transuretral. In: *Prostatectomia Transuretral Endoscopica.* Madrid: Queromon Editores, 1979
15. Minder J. Indole y finalidad de la Urologia. In: *Tratado de Urologia.* Barcelona: Modesto Uson, 1948

16. Maisonnet J. Tumores benignos de la prostata. In: *Nuevo Tratado de Patologia Quirurgico*. Barcelona: 1937;4:948–1001

17. Gutierrez R. In: Lewis B (ed). *History of Urology*. Baltimore: Williams & Wilkins, 1933;2:137–186

18. Bottini E. *Di un Nuovo Cauterizzatore ed Incisore Termogalvanico Contro le Tsouri da Ipertropfia Prostatica*. Bologna, 1874, cited by Hurry FE. *Urinary Surgery,* 2nd ed. Bristol: John Wright and Co., 1895

19. Nitze M. *Lehrbuch der Kystoskopie ihre Technik und Klinische Bedeutung*. Wiesbaden: Verlag von Bergmann JF, 1907

20. Marion G. *Tralte d'Urologie,* 3rd ed. Paris: Masson et Cie, 1935;2:1270–1271

21. Isorna S, Maynar M, Belon JL, Pulido-Duque JM, Martell R, Nogueira JAF, Castañeda F. Prostatic urethroplasty: endoscopic findings. *Semin Intervent Radiol* 1989;6:46–56

22. Mercier LA. *Recherches sur les Valvules du Col de la Vessie.* Paris: 1850

23. Parrish J. Surgical observations. In: Thomson H (ed). *Tratado Practico de las Enfermedades de las Vias Urinarias*. Madrid: Bailliere, 1876:258

24. Leroy d'Etoilles J. Expose des procedes pour guerir la puierre. In: Thomson H (ed). *Tratado Practico de las Enfermedades de las Vias Urinarias*. Madrid: Bailliere, 1876:664

25. Mercier LA. *Recherches sur le Traitement des Voies Urinaries.* Paris: 1856:474–475

26. Deisting N. Transurethral dilatation of the prostate: a new method in the treatment of prostatic hypertrophy. *Urol Int* 1956;2:158–171

27. Aboulker P, Steg A. La divulsion de la prostate: d'apres 218 observations personnelles. *J Urol Nephrol* 1964;70:337–364

28. Frank O. Die Sprengung des Prostataringes. *Med Wochenschr* 1938;21:777–782

7

Experimental Studies and Basis of Retrograde Transurethral Urethroplasty with Balloon Catheter

*Flavio Castañeda, David Hunter,
Wilfrido R. Castañeda-Zúñiga, Kurt Amplatz*

Encouraged by the results of dilation techniques used in the past for the relief of bladder outlet obstruction from benign prostatic hyperplasia (BPH) and to take advantage of the development and refinement of the balloon catheter, we undertook an experimental study of prostatic urethral dilation in dogs.[1] We assessed the feasibility of the procedure and tried to determine the optimal extent and duration of balloon inflation required for optimal results.

A subsequent follow-up animal and human study was done to find the mechanism of prostatic urethroplasty.[2] This showed that separation of the anterior prostatic commissure was the most important mechanism of prostatic obstruction relief.

MATERIALS AND METHODS

In the first phase of a three-phase study, we attempted to find the optimal balloon size and duration of inflation that would provide long-lasting results. In the second phase, the technique was used to evaluate the acute, subacute, and long-term effects on the urethra and prostate.

Because of its convenient size, ready availability, and similarity in urethral structure (Fig. 7–1) to humans, the dog was chosen as the experimental model. Twenty-eight mongrel dogs ranging in weight from 18 to 22 kg were used for the study, 18 dogs in the first phase and 10 in the second. Although it is difficult to determine a dog's age by physical

examination alone, an attempt was made to obtain older dogs because the frequency of benign prostatic hypertrophy increases with age in dogs (Fig. 7–2A, B) as well as in humans. The dogs were under general and local anesthesia, and fluoroscopy was used for guidance. The technique is basically the same as described for humans in Chapter 10.

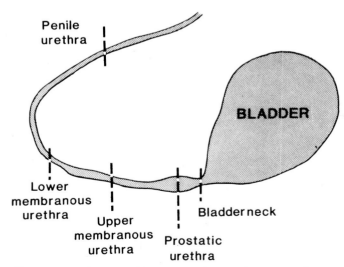

Figure 7–1. Diagram of the canine lower urinary tract shows the acute angle between the penile and membranous urethra that makes catheterization with large catheters extremely difficult. (From ref. 1.)

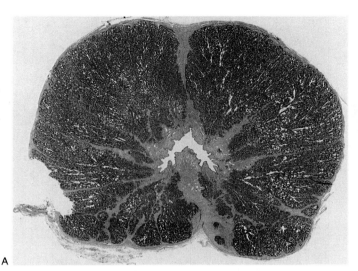
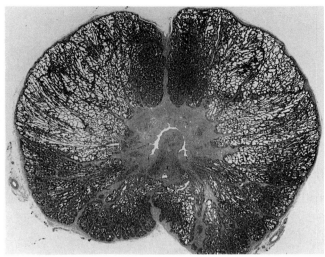

A   B

Figure 7–2. **A.** Transverse section of a canine prostate with minimal hyperplastic changes compared to an older dog (**B**), which shows characteristic diffuse epithelial and glandular proliferation throughout the prostate. This is in comparison to human BPH, which specifically arises within the periurethral tissues and is characterized primarily by stromal hyperplasia.

For the first phase of the study, to evaluate the ideal balloon diameter and inflation time needed to obtain long-lasting dilation of the prostatic urethra, we chose to dilate the first 3 dogs with an 8-mm balloon for 9 min (three inflations at 3 min each). Because no significant dilation occurred, we used the same sized balloon and 10 min inflation in the next 3 dogs and a 10-mm balloon for 10 min in 4 more dogs. Because there was still no significant increase in urethral diameter, we used a 15-mm balloon for 10 min in the next 4 dogs and two 10-mm balloons for 10 min in 2 more dogs. Two dogs did not undergo dilation and were used as controls to obtain baseline histology.

In the second phase, 10 dogs underwent dilation with a 20-mm balloon for 10 min. Of these, 2 dogs were sacrificed immediately, 2 at 2 weeks, 2 at 3 months, and 2 at 6 months. One died at 8 months secondary to rupture of its bladder during cystography, and 1 died of gastric volvulus 14 months after dilation.

After excision, the histologic sections were examined microscopically for urethelial alteration, fibromuscular and glandular hyperplasia or atrophy, and inflammatory changes.

The goal of the third phase of the study was to find the principal mechanism of bladder outlet obstruction relief in benign prostatic hypertrophy by prostatic urethroplasty with a balloon catheter.

We performed this procedure on 6 normal older dogs using a 30-mm prostatic urethroplasty balloon. Baseline and follow-up urethrograms were obtained. Three animals were killed immediately, and 3 were killed 3 months after urethroplasty. The bladder, prostate, and urethra were studied by gross pathologic examination for integrity of the prostatic capsule, commissures, and urethra.

The human study of this third phase involved 10 patients with benign prostatic hypertrophy who were candidates for transurethral resection (TUR). All patients willing to undergo prostatic urethroplasty instead of TUR of the prostate were included without regard to their medical condition. Each patient had a physical examination, cystoscopy, uroflowmeter assessment, retrograde and voiding cystourethrography, and transrectal sonography before the procedure. A 30-mm urethroplasty balloon was used. Immediately after the procedure, retrograde cystourethrography, voiding cystourethrography, and cystoscopy were repeated.

RESULTS

Significant dilation was not produced with balloons 15 mm in diameter or smaller, and the dilation achieved tended to decrease to baseline levels with time. With the use of two 10-mm balloons or a single 20-mm balloon, the results were long lasting.

In the 12 dogs in which dilation up to 20 mm was performed (Fig. 7–3A, B, C), the urethral diameter ranged from 3.1 mm to 4.1 mm before dilation and from 16.1 mm to 18.5 mm immediately afterward. These changes in urethral diameter were statistically significant, as calculated by Student's t-test ($p < 0.005$). There was no significant decrease in diameter at 14 months (Table 7–1).

None of the dogs suffered urinary retention or incontinence at any time. Mild transient hematuria was common but invariably cleared within 24 h.

Prostatic tissue from animals killed immediately after dilation showed partially denuded urothelium with mild subepithelial congestion and minimal focal hemorrhage

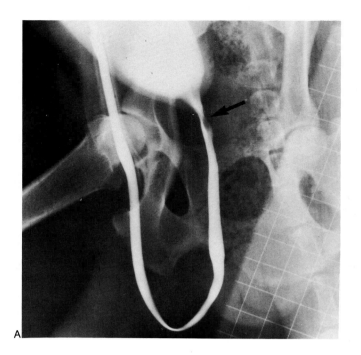

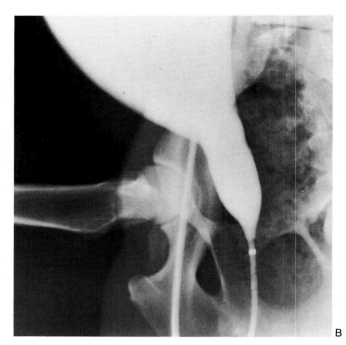

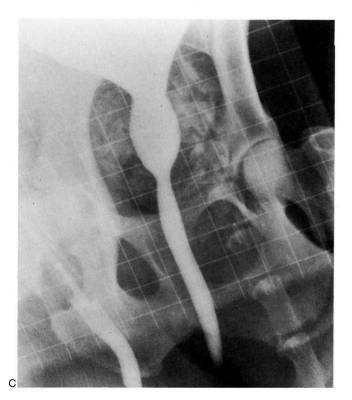

Figure 7–3.   **A.** Baseline retrograde urethrogram in a canine before balloon dilation. Please note the very long anterior urethra with its sharp acute angulation in its midportion, which makes catheterization difficult, especially with large catheters. Black arrows show the position of the verumontanum. **B.** Radiographic image showing a 20-mm balloon catheter fully inflated in the prostatic urethra. **C.** Six-month follow-up retrograde urethrogram showing persistent significant increase of the prostatic urethral caliber. The superimposed grid has 1-cm squares.

Table 7–1.   Results of Retrograde Transurethral Dilation in 26 Dogs[a]

| DOG | BALLOON SIZE (mm) | DURATION OF INFLATION (min) | URETHRAL DIAMETER (mm) | | | | | |
| | | | | | At Follow-up | | | |
			Predilation	Immediately Postdilation	1 month	6 months	1 year	Change (%)
1	8	3 (X3)	3.0	3.0				0
2	8	3 (X3)	3.2	3.3				3
3	8	3 (X3)	3.1	3.0				0
4	8	10	2.9	3.0				3
5	8	10	3.0	3.0				0
6	8	10	3.3	3.2				0
7	10	10	3.6	5.0	3.7			39
8	10	10	3.1	4.2	3.0			35
9	10	10	3.2	5.2	3.3			63
10	10	10	3.1	4.9	3.2			58
11	15	10	3.2	6.7	4.6	4.1		109
12	15	10	3.1	7.2	5.2	3.8		132
13	15	10	3.0	6.7	4.7	3.3		123
14	15	10	3.6	6.9	5.3	3.7		92
15	10 (X2)	10	3.6	16.2	16.2	16.1		350
16	10 (X2)	10	3.7	16.1	16.0	16.1		335
17	20	10	4.1	18.2	[b]			344
18	20	10	3.6	17.9	[b]			397
19	20	10	3.3	16.7	[c]			406
20	20	10	3.8	17.1	[c]			350
21	20	10	3.3	17.9	17.8	[d]		442
22	20	10	3.8	18.1	17.7	[d]		376
23	20	10	3.1	17.6	16.8	16.9	[e]	468
24	20	10	3.3	18.2	17.9	17.8	[e]	452
25	20	10	3.1	18.1	18.2	18.1	[f]	484
26	20	10	3.6	18.5	18.3	18.4	18.2	414

[a]From ref. 1
[b]Killed immediately after dilation.
[c]Killed at 2 weeks after dilation.
[d]Killed at 3 months.
[e]Killed at 6 months.
[f]Died at 8 months as a result of bladder rupture.

(Fig. 7–4). Tissue from dogs killed at 2 weeks showed that the urothelium was largely restored (Fig. 7–5). Sections of gland parenchyma removed 2 weeks to 1 year after dilation showed the usual histologic spectrum of BPH, including proliferative, atrophic, and inflammatory changes.[3] Gross pathologic examination of the prostate after balloon urethroplasty showed disruption of the anterior prostatic commissure with separation of the prostatic lobes in 4 of the 6 dogs. In 1 dog, disruption of both anterior and posterior prostatic commissures was seen. In 1 dog, no disruption was found. In 1 of the dogs with anterior disruption only and in the dog with both anterior and posterior disruption, the disruption extended all the way through the external prostatic capsule. In the dogs sacrificed at 3 months, the divulsion of the prostatic lobes persisted, and the transitional epithelium covered the entire prostatic tissue surface, including the divulsed commissures (Fig. 7–6) and the inner surface of the capsule.

In all 10 patients, urethrograms suggested that separation of the commissures had occurred. The caliber of the prostatic urethra increased in both oblique views but remained slitlike in the anteroposterior projection (Fig. 7–7). Cystoscopy showed divulsion of the prostatic lobes, primarily consisting of disruption of the anterior prostatic commissures (Fig. 7–8). There was no evidence of the tears extending beyond the prostatic capsule on either radiographic contrast-enhanced or cystoscopic studies. In 1 patient in whom cystoscopy was repeated 1 month after the procedure, persistent separation of the prostatic lobes was found.

DISCUSSION

These encouraging results from the initial two phases suggested that clinical human trials were warranted[4,5] and that no deleterious effects on the urethra or prostate should be expected. Also, the technique was relatively easy once certain guidelines were met, such as avoiding the external urinary sphincter and the use of large dilation diameters to obtain long-lasting results.

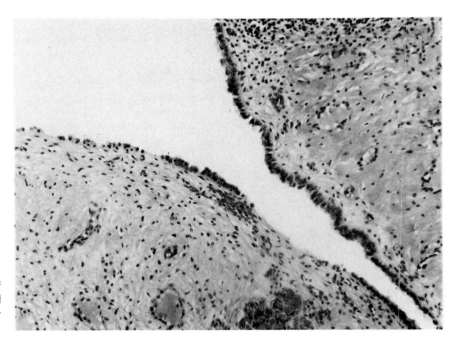

Figure 7–4. Histologic section of prostatic urethra from a dog killed immediately after dilation shows denuded epithelium. (From ref. 1.)

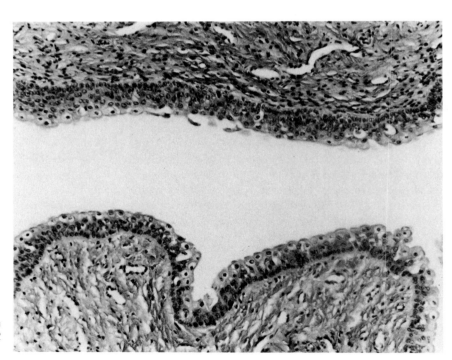

Figure 7–5. Prostatic urethelium has completely regenerated by 2 weeks.

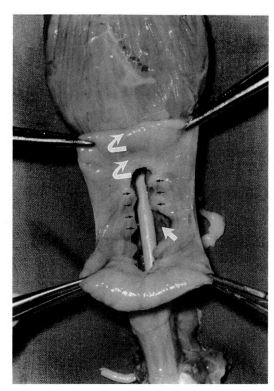

Figure 7–6.   Postmortem specimen from a dog 3 months after balloon urethroplasty. Prostate and urethra have been sectioned transversely through the posterior aspect of the prostate. Section halves have been pulled apart and are viewed posteriorly. Note intact posterior prostatic commissures (curved arrows) and persistent divulsed anterior commissure (black arrows), which is covered by urothelium, including inner surface of prostatic capsule (large white arrow). A catheter is in place in the urethra. (From ref. 2.)

The original discovery that forceful separation or divulsion of the lobes of the prostate occurs as a result of urethral dilation was made by early investigators who used either metal dilators or transvesical digital disruption.[6–8] Because we used a balloon catheter, which exerts a radial force on the prostatic tissue as opposed to the ventrodorsal force exerted by early metal dilators,[7,8] we thought the mechanism of

action of prostatic urethroplasty might be different, especially as we were using much less dilation (25–30 mm as opposed to 40–80 mm). We thought that the prostatic tissue would be better compressed by balloon urethroplasty because of the radial forces exerted by the balloon catheter and because of the progressive shrinkage of the prostate suggestive of atrophy seen in an earlier study with MRI.[9] We thought these two factors were the main mechanisms by which the obstruction was relieved (Fig. 7–7). We also postulated that after the procedure, there would be some degree of atrophy of the prostatic gland caused either by posttraumatic capillary thrombosis with subsequent ischemic atrophy or by another unknown mechanism. No histologic proof has been obtained because of the invasiveness of the necessary biopsies.

The fact that divulsion occurred in humans after balloon urethroplasty was suggested to us during the immediate follow-up retrograde cystourethrogram in which rotational cineimaging of the prostatic urethra was performed from one oblique projection to the other, going through the anteroposterior projection. This showed that the caliber of the prostatic urethra had increased substantially in one oblique projection. In the anteroposterior projection, however, the lumen was only a slit. As the cine unit continued rotating to the other oblique position, the diameter again was noted to increase in size. This asymmetry was not seen in the baseline studies.

Evidence of divulsion was not obtained during earlier animal studies[1] because the largest balloon catheter that could be introduced through the urethra in a retrograde fashion was 20 mm in diameter. The newer, lower profile catheters made it possible to advance 30-mm balloons through the urethra without difficulty.

We think that the tears of the commissures in humans as compared with dogs did not extend beyond the prostatic capsule. In an earlier study, there was no MRI evidence of abnormalities outside the prostate gland. The reason for this is unknown, but it may be that the prostate is larger in humans and that perhaps human tissues are more compliant.

On the basis of the results of this study and the evidence presented by earlier researchers, we think the separation of the prostatic commissures plays a major role in the relief of bladder outlet obstruction.

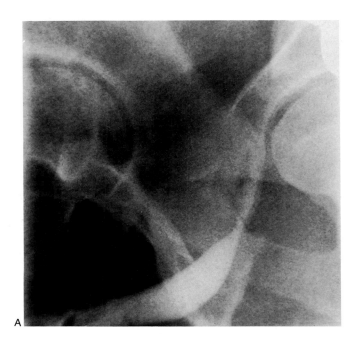
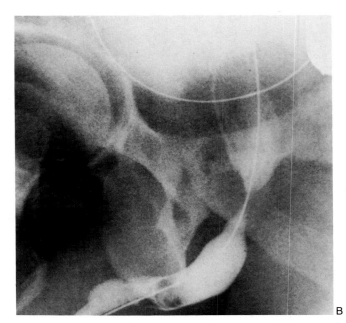
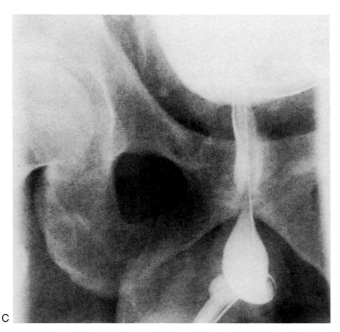
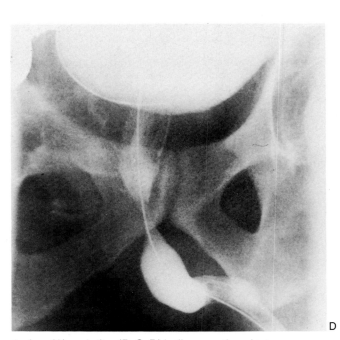

Figure 7–7.   Retrograde urethrograms of prostatic urethra before (**A**) and after (**B, C, D**) balloon urethroplasty. **A.** Predilation retrograde urethrogram shows narrow and flattened prostatic urethra. **B.** Right posterior oblique projection immediately after dilation shows substantial widening of urethral caliber. **C.** Anteroposterior projection shows that diameter is only a narrow slit. **D.** Left posterior oblique projection shows increased diameter of urethra in this plane. (From ref. 2.)

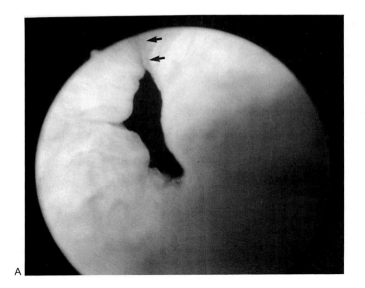

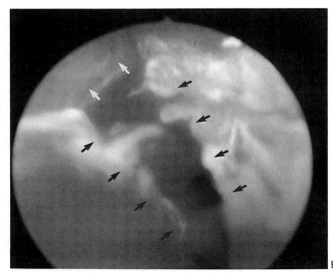

A

B

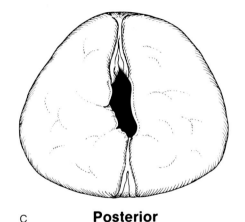

Anterior

Posterior

C

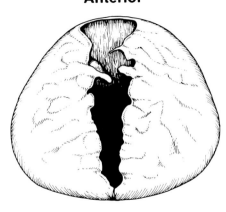

Anterior

Posterior

Figure 7–8. **A.** Cystoscopic image of urethra shows lumen near base of prostate before dilation. Note anterior prostatic commissure (arrows). **B.** Cystoscopic image obtained immediately after dilation shows torn and separated prostatic lobes (black arrows) that resulted from disruption of anterior commissure. Note raw inner surface of prostatic capsule (white arrows), which has remained intact. **C.** Diagrammatic representation of pre- (right) and posturethroplasty (left) cystoscopic images. A preurethroplasty diagram shows intact anterior and posterior prostatic commissures. A posturethroplasty diagram shows divulsion of prostatic commissures, with resultant increase in prostatic urethral caliber. Note ragged margins of tissue at the site of previously intact commissures. (From ref. 2.)

REFERENCES

1. Castañeda F, Lund G, Larson BW, et al. Prostatic urethra: experimental dilation in dogs. *Radiology* 1987;163:645–648
2. Castañeda F, Isorna S, Hulbert J, et al. The importance of separation of prostatic lobes in relief of prostatic obstruction by balloon catheter arethroplasty: studies in dogs and humans. *AJR* 1989;153:1301–1304
3. Jones TC, Hunt RD. *Veterinary Pathology,* 5th ed. Philadelphia: Lea & Febiger, 1983:1571–1575
4. Castañeda F, Reddy P, Wasserman N, et al. Benign prostatic hypertrophy: retrograde transurethral dilation of the prostatic urethra in humans. Work in progress. *Radiology* 1987;163:649–654
5. Castañeda F, Reddy PK, Hulbert JC, et al. Retrograde prostatic urethroplasty with balloon catheter. *Semin Intervent Radiol* 1987;4:115–121
6. Frank O. Die Sprengung des Prostataringes. *Munch Med Wochenschr* 1938;21:777–782
7. Deisting W. Transurethral dilatation of the prostate: a new method in the treatment of prostatic hypertrophy. *Urol Int* 1956;2:158–171
8. Aboulker P, Steg A. La divulsion de la prostate. D'apres 218 observations personnelles. *J Urol Nephrol (Paris)* 1964;70:337–364
9. Johnson SD, Kuni CC, Castañeda F, et al. Magnetic resonance imaging of patients undergoing prostatic balloon dilation. Presented at the annual meeting of the Radiological Society of North America, Chicago, December 1987

8

Overview of Balloon Catheters for Transurethral Dilation of the Prostate

Jon L. Pryor, Edgardo F. Becher, Abraham Ami Sidi

A mainstay of urology has been the treatment of benign prostatic hypertrophy (BPH). An estimated 425,000 prostatectomies were performed for benign disease in the United States in 1989.[1] This translates into major expenses for the American public. In 1985, transurethral resection of the prostate (TURP) was second only to cataract extractions in the number of Medicare dollars spent for surgery.[2]

The prevalence of BPH, a better understanding of its physiology, and incentives for cost control in its treatment have lead to a recent burgeoning of new therapies for BPH, ranging from hyperthermia to alpha-adrenergic blockers.[3,4] Among the nonsurgical techniques for the treatment of BPH is transurethral dilation of the prostate (TUDP). This chapter outlines the steps involved in TUDP and provides an overview of the various balloon catheters available for the procedure.

GENERAL REQUIREMENTS FOR TUDP

Although the exact technique used for TUDP depends on the patient, the type of dilating balloon used and what additional equipment is available, the general steps of insertion, positioning, monitoring the balloon's position, dilation, deflation, and withdrawal are applicable to all cases.

Insertion

Most balloon catheters are relatively stiff and, therefore, are difficult and potentially dangerous to insert without guidance. Consequently, the balloon dilators are inserted either transcystoscopically or over a guidewire.

Positioning

Successful TUDP requires that the balloon be positioned accurately along the entire length of the prostatic urethra, from the bladder neck through the prostatic apex. Accurate positioning is complicated by a tendency for the balloon to migrate proximally from the apex into the bladder during dilation, which potentially can result in partial or unsatisfactory dilation of the prostate. On the other hand, dilating distal to the apex because of incorrect positioning could result in dilation of the external sphincter (rhabdosphincter) and cause incontinence.

Characteristics of the various catheters to aid in the proper positioning of the balloon include radiopaque markers for fluoroscopic positioning, echogenic bands for ultrasonic positioning, buttons and collars for digital transrectal positioning, and markers and auxiliary balloons for endoscopic positioning.

Monitoring the Position

During inflation, the dilating balloon begins to inflate first at the site of least resistance, which is in the bladder. As previously mentioned, this creates a tendency for the balloon to migrate into the bladder, which may lead to incomplete dilation. Therefore, it is vital to monitor the balloon's position during dilation by either direct transcystoscopic visualization, fluoroscopy, ultrasonography, or transrectal palpation of catheter markers. In addition to monitoring the position, special features that help prevent migration have been developed and include a traction collar that is used to pull on the catheter during dilation, a second balloon that is placed in the bulbous urethra to prevent migration, and various balloon sizes to fit the prostate more exactly without protruding into the bladder, thus minimizing the tendency for migration.

Dilation

The balloon is inflated with either sterile water, normal saline, or dilute contrast to a pressure of 3–5 atm depending on the manufacturer's recommendation. This pressure is maintained for approximately 10–15 min. Use of a pressure gauge is always recommended.

Deflation and Withdrawal

The deflated balloon may not have memory and therefore after deflation some balloons do not resume their original diameter and smooth shape. Withdrawal of these balloons could cause mucosal tears and urethral damage. The balloon should be withdrawn gently and slowly. Some catheters have an expandable sleeve over the balloon that helps collapse the balloon.

SPECIFIC BALLOON CATHETERS

There are currently three FDA-approved balloon catheters for TUDP: AMS Optilume, Microvasive-Dowd, and ASI-Uroplasty. Bard manufactures a balloon catheter that is not FDA approved at this time. Table 8–1 lists specifications for the catheters and balloons, and Table 8–2 summarizes special features and insertion techniques. Patient selection, anesthesia, and additional details on insertion techniques are discussed in other chapters in this volume.

American Medical Systems (AMS)

The AMS Optilume (American Medical Systems, Minnetonka, MN) (Fig. 8–1) consists of two balloons, a dilating balloon and a location balloon. The location balloon is positioned distal to the external sphincter and helps prevent migration of the dilating balloon. At the apical end of the dilating balloon is a prominent locator collar that is palpable transrectally and assists in positioning. There are two radiopaque markers on each end of the dilating balloon and a

Table 8–1.   Specifications of Catheters and Balloons for TUDP

	CATHETER LENGTH (cm)	DILATION BALLOON LENGTH (cm)	INFLATED DIAMETER (Fh)	PRESSURE (atm)
AMS Optilume	50	4	90	4
Microvasive	40	5	90	4
ASI Uroplasty	48	Variable (1.5–5)	75	3

Table 8–2.   Special Features and Techniques of Balloon Catheters

	INTRODUCTION TECHNIQUE	POSITIONING AND MONITORING LOCATION	SPECIAL FEATURES
AMS Optilume	Guidewire	Digital Fluoroscopic Endoscopic	Location balloon (40 F) Locator collar
Microvasive	Guidewire	Digital Fluoroscopic Endoscopic Ultrasonic	Positioning nodule (20 F) Traction collar
ASI Uroplasty	Endoscopic	Endoscopic	

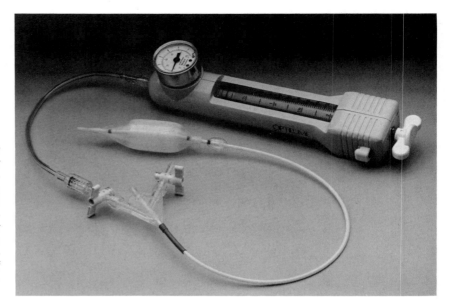

Figure 8–1. The Optilume catheter manufactured by AMS. This catheter has two balloons. Notice that radiopaque markers outline the dilating balloon. A locator collar at the apical end of the dilating balloon is palpable transrectally. Distal to the locator collar is the location balloon, which helps position the catheter and prevent its migration. (Courtesy of American Medical Systems, Minnetonka, MN.)

radiopaque marker at the location balloon. In addition, the Optilume dilating balloon is covered by an expandable silicone sheath that helps collapse the balloon after deflation for atraumatic withdrawal.

Positioning the Optilume balloon catheter may be done by fluoroscopy, palpation, or direct vision techniques. If the catheter is to be placed by fluoroscopic guidance, the patient is placed in the right posterior oblique position. A retrograde urethrogram will establish the location of the external sphincter, which should be marked on the drapes with metallic markers, such as needles. A Councill catheter is then placed into the bladder. A 0.038-inch guidewire is passed through the Councill catheter into the bladder, and the catheter is removed. The Optilume balloon catheter is then inserted over the guidewire. Under fluoroscopic guidance, the radiopaque markers are used to position the location balloon distal to the external sphincter as previously marked on the drapes.

If the catheter is to be positioned by palpation, the patient is placed in the lithotomy position, and the catheter is inserted over a guidewire until both balloons are within the bladder. While the apex of the prostate is palpated transrectally, the catheter is withdrawn until the location balloon can be felt at the apex. The location balloon may need to be partially inflated to be detected by palpation. The catheter is then withdrawn an additional 1.5–2 cm so that the locator collar at the base of the dilating balloon is palpable at the apex of the prostate. The technique for endoscopic positioning is identical to that used for palpation except that the location balloon is positioned transcystoscopically under direct vision.

After the location balloon is positioned correctly, it is filled with approximately 1.3 mL of diluted contrast solution or normal saline, which stabilizes the catheter's position and helps prevent proximal migration of the dilating balloon during dilation. The dilating balloon is inflated to 4 atm and maintained at this pressure for 10 min. The position of the catheter is monitored during dilation by either fluoroscopy, palpation, or direct vision. After dilation, completely deflate both balloons and gently withdraw the Optilume catheter over the guidewire. A Councill catheter is inserted into the bladder, and the guidewire is removed.

Microvasive

The Microvasive-Dowd catheter (Microvasive, Watertown, MA) (Fig. 8–2) has a positioning nodule at the apical margin of the dilating balloon for transrectal digital positioning. There are also markers at the proximal and distal ends of the dilating balloon to monitor its position by fluoroscopy, ultrasonography, or endoscopy. In addition, a handheld traction collar helps maintain the balloon's position during dilation.

A guidewire is placed into the bladder cystoscopically. The cystoscope is removed, and the dilation catheter is inserted over the guidewire until the traction collar is against the patient's urethral meatus. With the operator's finger in the rectum, the catheter is slowly withdrawn until the positioning nodule is palpable at the apex of the prostate. While the finger immobilizes the catheter by pushing on the

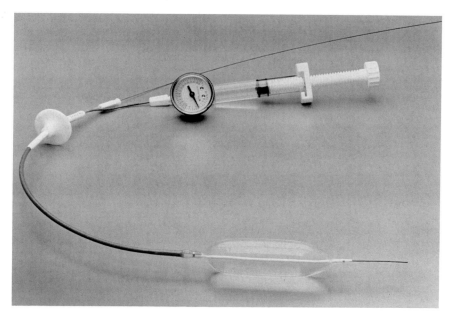

Figure 8–2. The Dowd catheter manufactured by Microvasive. This catheter has a single balloon. Radiopaque markers outline the dilating balloon, and a positioning nodule is located at the apical end. A traction collar is used to keep the balloon from migrating into the bladder. (Courtesy of Microvasive, Watertown, MA.)

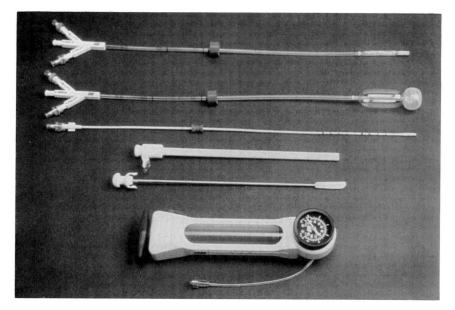

Figure 8–3. The Uroplasty catheter manufactured by ASI. The system from top to bottom: Uroplasty catheter, Uroplasty catheter with Foley and dilation balloons inflated, calibration catheter, 26 F disposable sheath and obturator, and inflation device. (Courtesy of Advanced Surgical Intervention, Inc., San Clemente, CA.)

positioning nodule, an assistant inflates the dilating balloon to 4 atm. The traction collar is pulled gently to help counteract the tendency for the balloon to migrate into the bladder. The position is monitored frequently by palpating the positioning nodule. After 15 min at 4 atm, the balloon is deflated, and the catheter and guidewire are removed together. The catheter is rotated counterclockwise as it is withdrawn so that the balloon wraps tightly around the catheter during removal.

Advanced Surgical Intervention (ASI)

The Uroplasty catheter (Advanced Surgical Intervention, Inc., San Clemente, CA) (Fig. 8–3) is a double balloon system. There is a Foley balloon at the tip of the catheter, proximal to the dilating balloon, that helps position the catheter and maintain its position during dilation. A white marker at the apical end of the dilating balloon assists in transcystoscopic positioning. A calibration catheter is provided for measuring prostatic length and determining the appropriate balloon length. An introduction sheath is provided for atraumatic placement and withdrawal of the catheter.

The Uroplasty catheter is intended to be inserted and its position monitored transcystoscopically. Cystoscopy is performed, and the prostatic length is measured from the bladder neck to the external sphincter using the calibration catheter. This allows an appropriately sized dilation balloon to be selected. The calibration catheter and cystoscope are then removed, and the introduction sheath is inserted into the urethra. The Uroplasty catheter and cystoscope lens are fitted through the end of the sheath, and the Foley balloon at the tip of the catheter is inflated within the bladder. The dilating balloon is positioned under direct vision so that the white marker at the apical end of the balloon is aligned just outside (below) the external sphincter. The dilating balloon is inflated and maintained at a pressure of 3 atm for 10 min. After dilation, the balloon is deflated and removed through the sheath to protect the urethra.

CLINICAL TRIALS

Numerous clinical trials of these catheters have been completed or are ongoing. Dowd and Smith reported on 50 patients who were carefully selected and underwent a stringent pretrial evaluation.[5] More than one third (21 patients) were in complete urinary retention, and nearly two thirds (31 patients) previously had failed a trial of alpha-adrenergic blockers. The patients underwent TUDP using the Microvasive-Dowd catheter. Twenty-nine patients (58%) were dis-

charged from the hospital the day of or the day after the procedure. The remaining 21 patients (42%) were discharged from 2 to 12 days after the procedure. The extended stay in most cases was because of coexistent medical problems. In 36 patients (72%), results were excellent or acceptable. In 7 patients (14%), there was no change in voiding patterns or symptoms, and 7 patients (14%) could not void after the procedure. Dowd and Smith report that no patient for whom the procedure failed benefited from a second dilation.

Klein has reported on 22 patients who were dilated using the Uroplasty catheter and who were followed for at least 1 year.[6] Success was defined as a 50% or greater improvement in their symptom score. In 18 patients (81%), there was initial success, and in 17 patients (76%), symptoms were still improved 1 year after dilation.

Reddy reported on 62 patients with moderate to severe BPH who underwent balloon dilation using the AMS Optilume catheter.[7] Symptoms were improved significantly in 70% of the patients at 6 months and in 58% at 1 year after TUDP. The majority of patients who did not improve had median lobe enlargement. Complications of the procedure were minimal, and no patients required a blood transfusion.

CONCLUSION

TUDP is a relatively straightforward nonsurgical technique that is now part of the urologist's armamentarium for treatment of BPH. There are currently three FDA-approved balloon dilators (AMS, Microvasive, and ASI). There is no evidence that one of these catheters is better than the others. Although each catheter has its own unique features, in all cases the technique involves introduction of the balloon, positioning, monitoring the position, dilation, and balloon deflation and withdrawal. Improvements in balloon dilation will most likely involve determining the optimal balloon size, the duration of inflation, and the subset of patients most likely to benefit from TUDP. Other possible advances include combinations such as TUDP with prostatic stenting or TUDP coupled with hyperthermia.

REFERENCES

1. Wein AJ. Evaluation of treatment response to drugs in benign prostatic hyperplasia. *Urol Clin North Am* 1990;17:631–640
2. Holtgrewe HL, Mebust WK, Dowd JB, Cockett ATK, Peters PC, Proctor C. Transurethral prostatectomy: practice aspects of the dominant operation in American urology. *J Urol* 1989;141: 248–253
3. Lepor H. Nonoperative management of benign prostatic hyperplasia. *J Urol* 1989;141:1283–1289
4. Lindner A, Golomb J, Siegel Y, Lev A. Local hyperthermia of

the prostate gland for the treatment of benign prostatic hypertrophy and urinary retention: a preliminary report. *Br J Urol* 1987;60:567–571

5. Dowd JB, Smith JJ. Balloon dilatation of the prostate. *Urol Clin North Am* 1990;17:671–677

6. Klein LA. Transcystoscopic balloon dilatation of the prostate. In: Olsson CA (ed). *Current Surgical Techniques in Urology.* Wilmington: Medical Publications, Inc., 1990;3:1–8

7. Reddy PK. Role of balloon dilation in the treatment of benign prostatic hyperplasia. *Prostate* (suppl) 1990;3:39–48

9

Prostatic Balloon Dilation: Patient Selection and Evaluation

Howard N. Winfield

On the basis of comprehensive autopsy studies, benign prostatic hyperplasia (BPH) is found rarely in men less than 40 years of age, whereas by the eighth decade of life, the incidence of BPH increases to 85%.[1] The management of BPH constitutes a large proportion of the clinical practice of many urologic surgeons. Transurethral resection of the prostate (TURP) is believed to be the second most common operation paid for by Medicare.[2] The chance of a 50-year-old male requiring a TURP during his lifetime is approximately 10%–25%.[3,4] Despite the magnitude of BPH as a disease entity, it has become apparent over the last few years how little we really understand about its natural history. This dichotomy has become even more evident with the advent of alternative forms of treatment for BPH.

One of the new alternatives is balloon dilation of the prostate. Prostatic dilation has been performed for centuries, using a wide variety of instruments, some of which more closely resemble weapons.[5] However, the use of balloons for dilation of the prostatic urethra was initiated by interventional radiologists in the early 1980s. These physicians were well acquainted with the high-pressure inflation balloons used for dilating narrowed biliary ducts and coronary or peripheral vessels. Burhenne et al. performed prostatic urethral dilation using a high-pressure balloon in a human cadaveric study. Burhenne followed this by self-dilation for his own prostatic obstruction.[6] Initial canine research was performed by Quinn et al., Castañeda et al., and others on the effects of prostatic balloon dilation.[7,8] This technique subsequently was brought into the clinical arena in 1987 and has created a surge of interest over the ensuing years.[9–11]

With greater clinical experience, it has become apparent that balloon dilation of the prostate should not be performed on every patient with symptomatic BPH. This fact is borne out by the results of many centers performing balloon dilation, discussed in other chapters in this book. To date, there are few meaningful data in the peer review literature that address the effectiveness of balloon dilation of the prostate compared to controls or to the accepted gold standard—transurethral resection. This is not to say that balloon dilation does not work in appropriately chosen patients but that its status should be considered investigational at this time.

Since we believe that balloon dilation of the prostate is still an investigational procedure, our preoperative evaluation of the potential candidate is more extensive than that ordinarily required for patients undergoing TURP. In addition, this evaluation must be performed by a urologist, not a radiologist. Urologists are best trained for differentiating patients with BPH from those with urethral stricture disease, neurogenic bladder, malignant processes of the prostate or bladder, or other urologic disorders.

HISTORY

The patient with clinical BPH suffers from some or all of the symptoms of prostatism as described in Table 9–1. Importantly, the symptomatology should be more obstructive than irritative. Irritative symptoms of urgency, dysuria, or

Table 9–1. Symptoms of Prostatism

OBSTRUCTIVE	IRRITATIVE
Weak stream	Frequency
Abdominal straining	Nocturia
Hesitancy, intermittency	Urgency
Incomplete bladder emptying	
Terminal dribbling	

marked frequency of urination may be more suggestive of infection, carcinoma in situ, or neurogenic bladder. Hematuria occasionally is associated with BPH but also may be indicative of urolithiasis or urinary tract malignancies.

The onset of prostatism is an important factor. Men with BPH generally describe a gradual, progressive slowing of urination with increasing difficulty in emptying the bladder. This usually occurs over the course of several years or more. Rapid onset of obstructive urinary symptoms within a 6–12-month period, perhaps associated with irritative voiding symptoms, may be due to carcinoma of the prostate.

Past medical and surgical history identifies patients who may be at high risk for anesthesia. On obtaining this history, it may become apparent that the patient is too sick to have any procedure performed and may be best managed with intermittent or continuous bladder catheterization. It has been our policy not to perform balloon dilation on patients who have had previous transurethral or open prostatectomy. In addition, we prefer that patients chosen for transurethral balloon dilation would otherwise be suitable candidates for TURP and be expected to live for longer than 1 year.

Inquiring into other functional symptoms may reveal symptoms of uremia, renal or bladder infection, or cystolithiasis that may mandate immediate surgery by transurethral resection rather than an investigational procedure, such as balloon dilation. Cardiac or respiratory symptoms may warrant attention prior to surgery. Our impression has been that patients with poorly controlled hypertension manifested the most significant bleeding following balloon dilation and should be well controlled preoperatively. Other bleeding diatheses and intake of aspirin-containing medication should be identified and managed accordingly.

A social history of alcohol abuse may require investigation into clotting ability or bleeding problems. Cigarette smokers are more likely to develop urothelial malignancies. Finally, a history of IV drug abuse, homosexual or promiscuous sexual behavior, hepatitis, or large numbers of previous blood transfusions should make the operator more alert to the risk of acquired immunodeficiency disease (AIDS) or hepatitis transmission.

It is important to obtain a sexual history. In our experience, balloon dilation of the prostate does not interfere with erectile or ejaculatory ability. Patients with these functions before balloon dilation maintain them after the procedure. This has not been the case for TURP, which is known to interfere with ejaculatory ability.

PHYSICAL EXAMINATION

The general appearance of the patient may reveal signs of pallor, edema, or cardiovascular abnormalities that may be representative of significant underlying renal or cardiac disease. Vital signs, including the blood pressure, are important in predicting the patient who may develop problems perioperatively.

A complete examination of all systems is suggested, and abdominal and genital examinations are mandatory. Abdominal examination may reveal visceromegaly suggestive of other disease processes beyond the specialty of urology. The presence of inguinal hernias may suggest further evidence of straining to void. Flank discomfort may indicate urolithiasis, obstructive uropathy, or pyelonephritis. A palpable suprapubic mass most likely indicates a distended bladder that is not emptying correctly due to prostatic obstruction.

The genital examination may reveal scarring or stenosis of the urethral meatus, whereas induration along the ventral aspect of the penis may be secondary to urethral stricture disease. Atrophy of one testis or hardness of the epididymis may be compatible with a previous history of epididymorchitis or lower urinary tract infection.

Rectal examination is mandatory in any evaluation of prostatic disease. The size, shape, and consistency of the prostate should be assessed. The important point to remember is that the size of the prostate does not necessarily correlate with symptoms of prostatism nor with the postoperative outcome from transurethral resection.[12–14] The size of the prostate, however, appears to be an important determinant of success when balloon dilation is the chosen form of treatment. This is discussed in Chapter 16. It is critically important to determine that the prostate is benign on digital palpation. Any doubt whatsoever requires further investigation in the form of transrectal ultrasound and biopsy. It should be remembered that with balloon dilation, tissue is not obtained, as does occur with transurethral or open prostatectomy. Thus, there is less room for error in detecting prostatic carcinoma. Finally, the rectal ampulla should be examined for other masses or lesions.

INVESTIGATIONS

Urinalysis and Culture

Evidence of pyuria and bacteriuria must be evaluated and corrected prior to any intervention. If cultures demonstrate a urinary tract infection, appropriate antibiotics should be initiated. Presence of crystalluria may suggest urolithiasis, and significant hematuria requires further investigation with upper tract imaging and cystourethroscopy. Glucosuria, proteinuria, and bilirubinuria should be recognized.

Uroflowmetry

A typical uroflow study will give the following relevant data: mean and maximum uroflow rates, volume voided, and the shape of the voiding curve depicting the micturition event. It has been our policy to perform uroflowmetry on all potential candidates for balloon dilation of the prostate. In practice, based on the AUA survey of 1989, slightly more than 40% of urologists performed uroflowmetry.[2] Uroflowmetry is a reasonably good and economical screening test for BPH but, alone, should not be considered diagnostic of prostatic obstruction. As has been shown by Sirosky et al., Abrams et al., and others, uroflowmetry is very dependent on the volume of fluid voided and the age and sex of the patient.[15,16] It also is very variable even within the same person. There is no question that patients learn how to perform the uroflow test, thus making repeated studies more accurate and interpretable.

Based on large normogram charts, it is believed that a maximum uroflow rate greater than 15 mL/sec for a voided volume of greater than 125–150 mL suggests that bladder outlet obstruction is not significant. Maximum flow rates less than 10 mL/sec usually correlate with obstruction.[17] Finally, the pattern of flow may be indicative of prostatic obstruction. A prolonged slow stream with evidence of dribbling at the end is typical of BPH. However, this also may be typical of a hypotonic neurogenic bladder. If confusion exists between these two disease entities, a pressure–flow study may clarify the clinical picture. A staccato, interrupted urinary flow pattern associated with a sharp initial peak may indicate a hyperreflexic internal or external urethral sphincter mechanism.

Serial uroflowmetry measurements over the course of a 12–24-month period provide objective data to assess the effectiveness of prostatic balloon dilation.

Residual Urine Measurement

Postvoid residual measurement may be helpful in objectively evaluating the success of treatment.[18] However, it should be realized that residual urine volumes may vary widely in the same patient on repeated measurements and do not necessarily correlate with the degree of obstruction.[19] Our patients have a postvoid residual bladder measurement obtained preoperatively either at the time of cystourethroscopy or on a separate occasion by means of Foley catheterization. At the time of office appointments following dilation, we have found it most convenient and comfortable for the patients to undergo suprapubic ultrasound postvoid residual measurements. Bladder ultrasound is very accurate compared to catheterization but begins to lose its sensitivity in obese patients or when the residual urine gets below 100 mL.[20] The use of the postvoid bladder film as part of the intravenous pyelogram (IVP) examination has been shown to be relatively inaccurate as a tool for measuring postvoid residuals.[21]

Patients who persistently carry a residual urine greater than 300 to 400 mL require further urodynamic evaluation to rule out a hypotonic bladder component. Obviously, patients with detrusor muscle insufficiency will not benefit significantly from any form of treatment and may be served best by a program of intermittent self-catheterization.

Upper Tract Imaging

It has been shown by cost effectiveness and risk–benefit ratios that performing IVP on all patients being evaluated for clinically significant BPH is not justified.[22] Patients who have no past urologic history of infection or stones, absence of pyuria or microhematuria, and otherwise normal physical examination do not warrent upper tract studies. The chance of finding a coexisting abnormality is 15%, and the percentage of these that are clinically significant is considerably less. The risk of a mild, moderate, and severe allergic reaction from the IV contrast medium is 6%, less than 2%, and 0.2%, respectively.[23,24] Renal ultrasound is safer and cheaper but probably not warranted in the healthy patient. Men with any of these risk factors should have upper tract imaging studies in the form of either IVP or renal ultrasound. We have used this approach for our balloon dilation candidates.

Cystourethroscopy

This is a key test for evaluating a patient with prostatism who may undergo balloon dilation and should not be omitted. Cystourethroscopy does not always correlate with symptomatology. There are men with severe bladder outlet obstruction who are asymptomatic and some with marked obstructive symptoms but little or no visual endoscopic prostatic obstruction.[25]

Cystourethroscopy allows the urologist to rule out urethral strictures, assess the length of the prostatic urethra, and measure the postvoid residual urine volume. The degree of bladder trabeculation, cellule, or diverticular formation may be assessed, and bladder stones or tumors may be ruled out. Finally, and most important, patients with significant median lobe enlargement out of proportion to the rest of the prostate do not fare well with balloon dilation. A subcervical median lobe that acts with a ball valve type effect is a contraindication for this procedure and is best managed by transurethral resection.

Prostatic Enzymes

Serum prostatic acid phosphatase and prostate-specific antigen levels have been shown to be poor screening tests for cancer of the prostate but best suited for serial evaluation of patients following radical prostatectomy or radiotherapy. Upward of 21% of patients with BPH will have elevated prostate-specific antigen (>4.0 ng/mL Hybritech assay), thus making it a poor screening test. In general urologic practice, therefore, obtaining these blood tests is not justified unless the patient's history or physical examination is suggestive of prostate cancer.[26]

It has been our belief that since transurethral balloon dilation does not yield any prostatic tissue for histopathology and the procedure is still considered investigational, it would seem prudent to obtain these tests on all candidates. Obviously, any abnormal value will lead to prostatic ultrasound studies and biopsy. We do not know what the effect will be of dilating a prostate that harbors cancer cells, and, therefore, all our patients have serum drawn for prostatic enzymes prior to balloon dilation and at all follow-up visits. We have not used the measurement of prostatic serum enzymes to reflect the degree of prostatic tissue injury that has occurred following the procedure as other authors have advocated.[27]

Transrectal Prostatic Ultrasound

Normally, transrectal ultrasound (TRUS) of the prostate is not performed in patients with prostatism unless there is a suggestion on history or physical examination that may indicate malignancy of the prostate. However, for patients who are scheduled to undergo balloon dilation of the prostate, we routinely perform TRUS of the prostate. The reasons are the following: (1) it allows another measurement parameter of the prostate volume, in addition to rectal and cystoscopic examinations, and (2) it potentially may identify suspicious areas (hypoechoic) of the prostate that may require biopsy to rule out malignancy.[28] It is our goal to rule out cancer of the prostate prior to subjecting any patient to balloon dilation.

Optional Examinations

URODYNAMIC EVALUATION

Urodynamic evaluation, including cystometrogram, urethral pressure profile, pressure–flow studies, and video urodynamics, is not performed routinely in patients selected for balloon dilation of the prostate. We do perform this extensive evaluation in the following situations: (1) very young patients (less than 50 years) with symptoms of prostatism, (2) where there is a question of neurologic or neurogenic bladder disorder, (3) a significant irritative component to the urinary symptoms, (4) excessive bladder capacity (>700 mL) or postvoid residual, and (5) an equivocal or confusing uroflow study. In the AUA 1989 survey, only 40.9% of urologists performed uroflow or more extensive urodynamic studies on patients with prostatism.[2]

It has been our experience that following urodynamic evaluation, we occasionally are more confused than before we started. In healthy elderly males without symptomatic BPH, more than 25%–50% demonstrate uninhibited bladder contractions on cystometrogram.[29] This increases to 50%–60% in men with symptoms of prostatism.[30–32] Thus, the presence of uninhibited bladder contractions should be considered in the light of these known percentages and not necessarily imply that the patient would not benefit from some therapeutic intervention.

PROSTATIC BIOPSY

It has not been our policy to routinely biopsy patients with prostatism who may be candidates for balloon dilation of the prostate. However, any abnormality on routine investigations that may suggest the presence of malignancy of the prostate would most certainly lead to a biopsy using the small diameter biopty needle under TRUS guidance.

Of patients who have undergone biopsy of the prostate before dilation, we have tried to obtain an epithelial–stromal component ratio of the tissue. We are in the process of trying to correlate this ratio to final outcome following dilation. It is my impression that patients with prostates smaller than 30 g with a higher stromal component do better than those with a higher epithelial component. An explanation for this impression is that perhaps the stromal tissue is more likely to tear or split (commissurotomy) with dilation. Epithelial (glandular) tissue tends to be more compliant and resilient, thus resisting a tearing effect with dilation. Again, however, this is pure speculation rather than fact and obviously needs to be proven clinically.

PREOPERATIVE EVALUATION

Assuming after evaluation that the patient is still a candidate for balloon dilation, we arrange for him to be prepared preoperatively. This implies that he undergo general blood tests (CBC, general electrolyte, and enzyme screen), prothrombin, and partial thrombin bleeding times. An electrocardiogram and chest x-ray are obtained if they have not been performed within the previous 6 months. Finally, all patients are seen by the anesthesiologist prior to the operative date. Although we perform balloon dilation under urethral local anesthesia (2% lidocaine jelly) supplemented by IV sedation (fentanyl citrate with or without midazolam), we prefer to have an anesthesiologist stand by to monitor the patient during the case. Since many of the patients who suffer from prostatic obstruction are elderly with cardiac or respiratory problems, we believe this approach is prudent. In a minority of cases, local and IV sedation has been insufficient, and the patient has had to be converted over to a general or spinal anesthetic.

Based on our own experience with transurethral balloon dilation of the prostate, the ideal patient would demonstrate the following characteristics: (1) healthy male older than 50 years, with no significant medical problems, (2) prostatic examination not demonstrating any evidence of malignancy, (3) prostate size less than 35 g, with only lateral lobe obstruction, (4) no median lobe or ball valve subcervical component seen with cystourethroscopy, (5) no significant postvoid residual urine, and (6) a motivated and responsible individual who is willing and capable of keeping follow-up appointments.

It is, of course, rare to find the ideal patient for balloon dilation of the prostate. There are some definite advantages of balloon dilation that should be considered in patient selection. Younger men who wish to preserve their ejaculatory ability should be able to do so with balloon dilation. Older patients with other significant medical or surgical problems may not be candidates for TURP under spinal or general anesthesia. As mentioned before, balloon dilation may be performed under IV sedation and local anesthesia. Thus, these infirm patients may be capable of tolerating this procedure more easily. High-risk patients on catheter drainage have been shown to be rendered catheter free and to benefit on a long-term basis from balloon dilation (Chapter 17). Finally, there are patients who prefer a less invasive form of treatment than TURP and may choose balloon dilation.

CONCLUSION

Transurethral balloon dilation of the prostate is a new and attractive form of treatment for clinically significant BPH. However, to date, only a limited number of studies have been reported in the peer review literature and with only limited periods of follow-up. There have been no placebo-controlled, randomized, prospective studies.[11,27] Thus, the short-term and long-term efficacy of balloon dilation is still unproven. From our own experience, there is no question that it is effective in some patients, but not all.

There are a number of dilating devices commercially available that vary in balloon size, length, and shape. Positioning techniques may depend on fluoroscopic, cystoscopic, or transrectal digital guidance. Balloon dilation of the prostate is technically easy to perform but does have a small learning curve. Thus, all these factors may contribute to the success or failure of the procedure. Undoubtedly, balloon dilation of the prostate will become a reasonable alternative in the management of BPH for the correct patient. This option should be considered only after a thorough properative evaluation and a complete discussion with the patient of the potential risks and benefits.

REFERENCES

1. Berry SJ, Coffey DS, Walsh PC, et al. The development of human benign prostatic hyperplasia with age. *J Urol* 1984;132:474–479
2. Holtgrewe HL, Mebust WK, Dowd JB, et al. Transurethral prostatectomy: practice aspects of the dominant operation in American urology. *J Urol* 1989;141:248–253
3. Lytton B, Emery JM, Harvard BM. The incidence of benign prostatic obstruction. *J Urol* 1968;99:639–645
4. Birkhoff JD. Natural history of benign prostatic hypertrophy. In: Hinman F Jr, Boyarsky, S (eds). *Benign Prostatic Hypertrophy.* New York: Springer-Verlag, 1983:5–9
5. Mercier F. *Recherces sur les Valvules du Col de la Vessie.* Paris: 1850
6. Burhenne HJ, Chisholm RJ, Quenville NF. Prostatic hyperplasia: radiologic intervention. *Radiology* 1984;152:655–657
7. Quinn SF, Dyer R, Smathers R, et al. Balloon dilation of the prostate urethra. *Radiology* 1985;157:57–58
8. Castañeda F, Lund G, Larson BW, et al. Prostatic urethra: experimental dilation in dogs. *Radiology* 1987;163:645–648
9. Castañeda F, Reddy P, Wasserman N, et al. Benign prostatic hypertrophy: retrograde transurethral dilation of the prostatic urethra in humans. *Radiology* 1987;163:649–653
10. Reddy PK, Wasserman N, Castañeda F, et al. Balloon dilation
of the prostate for treatment of benign hyperplasia. *Urol Clin North Am* 1988;15:529–535
11. Klein L, Perez-Marrerro RA, Bowers GW, et al. Transurethral cystoscopic balloon dilation of the prostate. *J Endourol.* 1990;4:115–123
12. Castro JE, Griffith HJL, Shackman R. Significance of signs and symptoms in benign prostatic hypertrophy. *Br Med J* 1969;2:598–601
13. Andersen JT, Nordling J, Walter S. Prostatism. I. The correlation between symptoms, cystometric and urodynamic findings. *Scand J Urol Nephrol* 1979;13:229–236
14. Jensen KME, Bruskewitz RC, Iversen P, et al. Significance of prostatic weight in prostatism. *Urol Int* 1983;38:173–178
15. Siroky MB, Olsson CA, Krane RJ. The flow rate nomogram: I. Development. *J Urol* 1979;122:665–668
16. Abrams P, Feneley R, Torrens M. Urodynamic investigations. In: Abrams P, Feneley R, Torrens M (eds). *Urodynamics.* New York: Springer-Verlag, 1983:28–40
17. Abrams PH. Prostatism and prostatectomy: the value of urine flow rate measurement in the preoperative assessment for operation. *J Urol* 1977;117:70–71
18. Hinman F Jr. Residual urine: measurement and influence on management of obstruction. In: Hinman F Jr, Boyarsky S (eds). *Benign Prostatic Hypertrophy.* New York: Springer-Verlag, 1983:589–596
19. Abrams PH, Farman P, Lawrence JP, et al. Residual urine in prostatism estimated by ultrasound scanning: a simple rule. *Radiography* 1983;49:194
20. Bruskewitz RC, Iversen P, Madsen PO. Value of postvoid residual urine determination in evaluation of prostatism. *Urology* 1982;20:602–604
21. Andersen JT, Jacobsen O, Standgaard L. The diagnostic value of intravenous pyelography in infravesical obstruction in males. *Scand J Urol Nephrol* 1977;11:225–230
22. Bauer DL, Garrison RW, McRoberts JW. The health and cost implications of routine excretory urography before transurethral prostatectomy. *J Urol* 1980;123:386–389
23. Shehadi WH. Contrast media reactions: occurrence, recurrence and distribution patterns. *Radiology* 1982;143:11–17
24. Ansell G, Tweedie MCK, Weset CR, et al. The current status of reactions to intravenous contrast media. *Invest Radiol* 1980;15:S32–S35
25. Graversen PH, Gasser TC, Wasson JH, et al. Controversies about indications for transurethral resection of the prostate. *J Urol* 1989;141:475–481
26. Optenberg SA, Thompson IM. Economics of screening for carcinoma of the prostate. *Urol Clin North Am* 1990;17:719–737
27. Goldenberg SL, Perez-Marrero RA, Lee LM, et al. Endoscopic balloon dilation of the prostate: early experience. *J Urol* 1990;144:83–88
28. Hernandez AD, Smith JA. Transrectal ultrasonography for the early detection and staging of prostate cancer. *Urol Clin North Am* 1990;17:745–757
29. Jensen KME, Bruskewitz RC, Madsen PO. Urodynamic findings in elderly males without prostatic complaints. *Urology* 1984;24:211–213
30. Anderson JT. Detrusor hyperreflexia in benign infravesical obstruction. A cystometric study. *J Urol* 1976;115:532–534
31. Turner-Warwick R, Whiteside CG, Arnold EP, et al. A urodynamic view of prostatic obstruction and the results of prostatectomy. *Br J Urol* 1973;45:631–645
32. Abrams PH, Ferrar DJ, Turner-Warwick RT, et al. The results of prostatectomy: a symptomatic and urodynamic analysis of 152 patients. *J Urol* 1979;121:640–642

10

Balloon Prostatic Urethroplasty Under Fluoroscopic Guidance

Flavio Castañeda, Terry Brady, Joseph Banno, Wilfrido R. Castañeda-Zúñiga

Fluoroscopic guidance for prostatic urethroplasty offers the advantage of real time monitorization throughout the procedure. This is extremely helpful when there is a tendency for the balloon to migrate into the bladder, which might occur inadvertently, with subsequent unsatisfactory results.[1–5] Fluoroscopic guidance also allows for precise determination of landmarks and immediate evaluation of the results obtained, for example, commissurotomy with the subsequent increase in the anteroposterior diameter of the prostatic urethra, so that repeat dilation can be performed if the initial results are not satisfactory.

TECHNIQUE

For this procedure, the patient is placed in a supine position on the table. Optimal imaging and guidance are obtained in either oblique projection. The desired oblique position can be obtained by placing a sponge wedge on either side of the patient, or, if a C-arm fluoroscopy unit is available, the tube can be rotated either way. The latter is preferable since the patient is more comfortable in a flat supine position.

An intravenous line is started before the procedure for the administration of antibiotics and sedatives or for emergency medication if it should become necessary. Broad-spectrum prophylactic antibiotics, such as cephalosporin, ampicillin, or a combination of sulfamethoxasole and trimethoprim, are started before the procedure and continued orally for 5–7 days.

The penis is prepared and draped as it would be for a surgical procedure. Transureteral topical 2% viscous lidocaine (Xylocaine) is applied generously in the urethra. All catheter and guidewire maneuvers are performed under fluoroscopic control.

A baseline retrograde urethrogram is performed to assess the degree of obstruction and to determine the landmarks that would be followed throughout the procedure, for example, position of the external sphincter, length of the prostatic urethra, and position of the bladder floor and neck. This baseline retrograde urethrogram is performed by advancing a 20 F to 22 F Councill catheter to the midanterior urethra or just beyond the meatus, with its balloon filled with 1 mL or 2 mL of dilute contrast material (Fig. 10–1). This ensures snug occlusion of the urethra so that forceful injection of contrast material can be accomplished to achieve maximal distention of the anterior and posterior urethra without retrograde reflux. The catheter can be positioned at the midanterior urethra or just beyond the meatus so that the partially inflated balloon lodges in the fossa navicularis. Once the urethra has been occluded, a retrograde urethrogram is performed with a 60-mL catheter tip syringe (Fig. 10–2). The catheter tip ensures that the connections are snug and leakproof. The position of the external sphincter is determined and marked. This can be done either by putting a small-gauge needle through the skin directed toward and overlapping the position of the external sphincter or by rotating the C-arm so that the position of the external sphincter is overlapped by a known bony landmark, such as the inferior margin of the inferior pubic ramus. At this point, the tube angle and the patient should remain as stable as possible so that the landmarks remain unchanged.

The length of the prostatic urethra is determined so that it may be dilated in its entirety. Some contrast material should be kept in the bladder to identify the bladder base because this is where most of the prostatic bulk lies, and it is extremely crucial to dilate this area adequately. Once this has been accomplished, the Councill catheter balloon is deflated, and

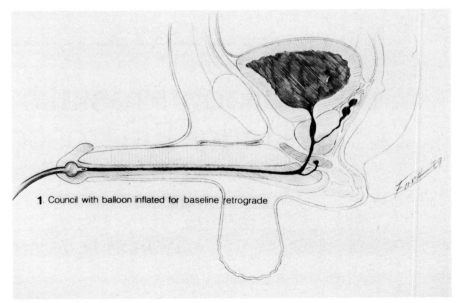

1. Council with balloon inflated for baseline retrograde

Figure 10–1. Method for performing retrograde urethrogram for optimal imaging.

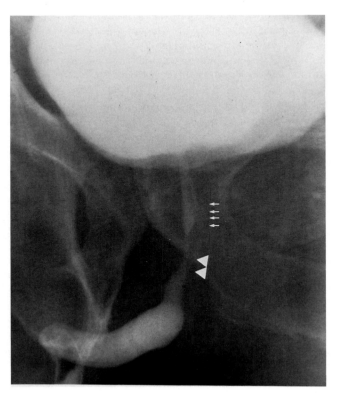

Figure 10–2. Baseline retrograde urethrogram shows the position of the external sphincter (arrowheads), which is at the membranous portion of the urethra. It can be identified by its position, just distal to the characteristic tapering cone shape of the bulbar urethra. The narrow and elongated prostatic urethra (arrows) also is noted.

the catheter is advanced into the bladder (Fig. 10–3). A guidewire is advanced through the lumen of the Councill catheter and curled in the bladder. At this point, the Councill catheter is removed from the bladder and penis. Although not essential, a voiding cystourethrogram can be performed on the table, especially if the patient feels like voiding. This helps to confirm the landmarks (Fig. 10–4).

A generous amount of lubricant is applied to the prostatic urethroplasty balloon catheter before it is advanced over the guidewire. The catheter is advanced so that the proximal balloon marker is placed beyond the external sphincter (Fig. 10–5). At this point, and especially if the patient or the C-arm arc has moved, a repeat retrograde urethrogram can be performed using a small (6 F) pediatric feeding tube, which should be advanced *alongside* the shaft of the catheter to approximately the midanterior urethra. Compression should be applied to the penis so that the proximal urethral channel is occluded adequately and no reflux of contrast material can occur. A repeat injection of contrast material will determine the external sphincter/proximal balloon marker relationship. These repeat retrograde urethrograms can be performed at any time during the dilation procedure, even when the balloon is fully inflated, to ensure that the landmarks have remained unchanged.

The balloon catheter is inflated slowly to its maximal diameter and pressure (Fig. 10–6). Because the patient experiences the most discomfort during the initial inflation, adequate IV sedation should be available. More intense than the pain that the patient experiences is the extreme urge to void. This is the result of the stretching of the muscle and

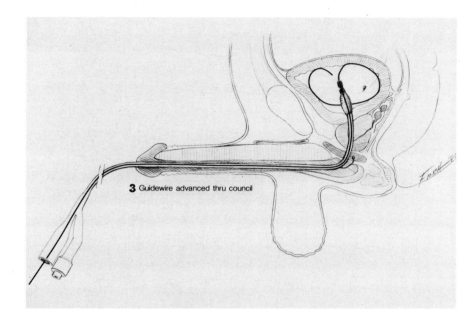

3 Guidewire advanced thru council

Figure 10–3. The Councill catheter has been advanced into the bladder, and through it a guidewire has been introduced and curled in the bladder.

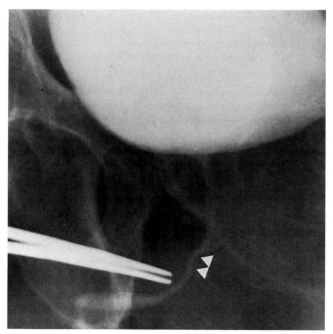

Figure 10–4. Voiding cystourethrogram shows the position of the external sphincter (arrowheads) as well as the narrow prostatic urethra.

nerve fibers of the bladder neck. Because the balloon has a strong tendency to migrate into the bladder, the place of least resistance, strong tension should be applied on the catheter while the balloon is being inflated. If at any point the balloon has migrated into the bladder or distal in the prostatic urethra, it should be deflated and repositioned so that adequate dilation of the entire prostatic urethra, including the apex, may be accomplished. If there is any doubt about the position of the external sphincter, a repeat retrograde urethrogram with the feeding tube should be performed. It may look as if the balloon is being pulled proximal to the external sphincter and anterior urethra. However, the pelvic floor is formed by a group of muscles, tendon attachments, and soft tissues, and the external sphincter is a very strong muscular structure that most likely will not allow the balloon to go through when fully inflated. If there is any doubt, a repeat retrograde urethrogram will show that the relationships are still the same, and it is merely the pelvic floor that is being pulled (Fig. 10–7). After a few minutes of full balloon inflation, the tension required on the catheter shaft will decrease as the compliance of the prostatic and periprostatic tissues increases with the forces applied by the balloon. The balloon should be left in place for approximately 10 min.

There are some instances in which the prostatic urethra is so long that the balloon has to be repositioned more distally to dilate the entire urethra, including the bladder neck. If this is necessary, an extra 5–10 min of dilation should be adequate.

At the completion of the dilation, the balloon is fully deflated and removed, leaving the guidewire in place. During balloon catheter removal, the shaft of the catheter should be turned continuously in the same direction in which the balloon was originally folded, so that the catheter collapses as much as possible, thus avoiding more trauma to the anterior urethra.

The next step is to repeat the retrograde urethrogram to assess the results. The same 20 F to 22 F Councill catheter is advanced *alongside* the guidewire to the midanterior urethra. Again, the Councill catheter balloon is partially inflated with 1 mL to 2 mL of dilute contrast material to ensure snug

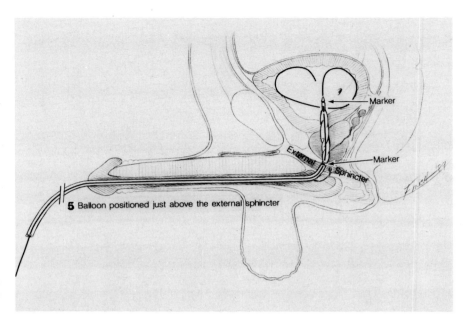

Figure 10–5. Schematic diagram shows the correct position of the balloon catheter.

occlusion of the urethra. (*Note:* If the Councill catheter is advanced *over* the guidewire, the seal between the syringe and the injecting port of the Councill catheter would be faulty, allowing leakage of contrast material and precluding a

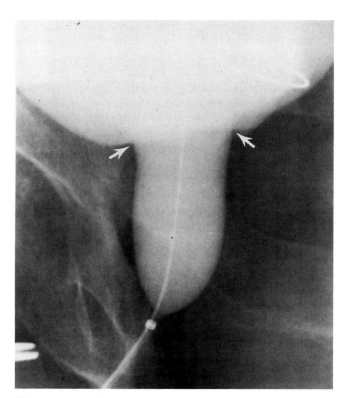

Figure 10–6. Prostatic urethroplasty balloon is fully inflated across the prostatic urethra, including the bladder neck (arrows).

good forceful injection to distend the anterior and posterior urethra adequately.) A good retrograde urethrogram is performed in an oblique projection to evaluate the prostatic urethra (Fig. 10–8). If no significant dilation has been obtained, repeat dilation would be necessary. We have not seen an increased incidence of hematuria or complications because of repeat dilations. Again, a voiding cystourethrogram can be obtained on the table (Fig. 10–9), although this is not mandatory.

To verify that the prostatic commissures have been disrupted, the retrograde urethrogram is repeated in a straight anteroposterior projection. The radiographic impression here would be one of a much narrower prostatic urethra as compared with the oblique projection. This is due to the fact that the anterior and posterior commissures have been disrupted, allowing an increase in the anteroposterior caliber but not in the transverse diameter because of the opposing prostatic lobes. The increase in the anteroposterior caliber by disruption of the prostatic commissures, plus the stretching of the prostatic capsule, is enough to allow the creation of a larger lumen so that the bladder outlet resistance decreases.

If the dilation is adequate, the partially inflated Councill catheter balloon is deflated and removed to be advanced later *over* the guidewire into the bladder. At this point the guidewire is removed, and the 5-mL Councill catheter balloon is inflated with 20 mL of very dilute contrast material or saline. The balloon usually will not rupture at this volume, since it is made of latex, which is very distensible. Tension on the catheter from the inflated balloon will prevent it from falling into the traumatized prostatic fossa, which might produce significant discomfort and bleeding once the local anesthesia has worn off.

The bladder is irrigated vigorously, and all blood and clots

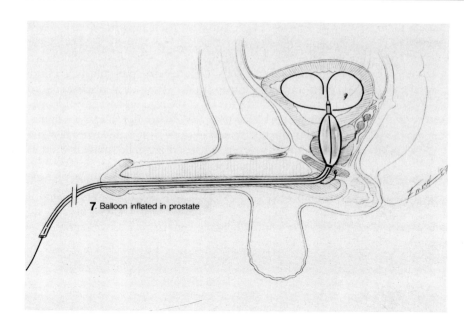

Figure 10–7. Diagram shows the anatomic relationships for an adequate procedure and results.

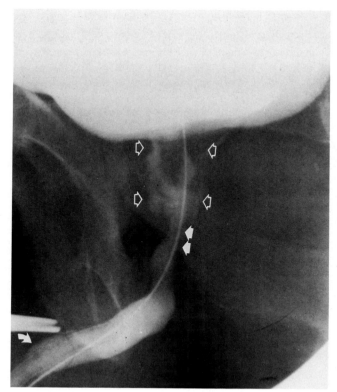

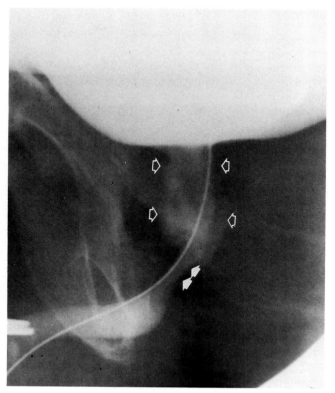

Figure 10–8. Retrograde urethrogram obtained immediately after dilation shows significant widening of the prostatic urethra (open arrows) extending from the base to the apex of the prostate. The location of the external sphincter is shown by the white arrows. Note that the Councill catheter has been advanced alongside the guidewire, and its balloon (curved arrow) is partially inflated to obtain an adequate urethrogram.

Figure 10–9. Voiding cystourethrogram obtained to document in a different way the increase in the prostatic urethral caliber (open arrows) and the adequate function of the external sphincter (white arrows).

are removed. The catheter should be left in place, with slight tension applied to the end to decrease the amount of subsequent hematuria. Most of the hematuria occurs during catheter manipulations, especially during balloon inflation. The hematuria may seem excessive, but once the bladder has been well irrigated and the clots have been removed, the urine will have only a light red tint in most cases. If the hematuria remains significant, the 20 F to 22 F Councill catheter should be exchanged over a guidewire for a larger one, perhaps 26 F to 30 F, so that the small capillary bleeding is tamponaded. Also, continuous tension at the end of the catheter should help to decrease the hematuria, which should be minimal by 24 h.

The patient is instructed to be relatively sedentary the rest of the day so that the hematuria does not recur or continue. In most instances, the Councill catheter is removed the following morning. The patient's bladder is fully filled before catheter removal. The patient is instructed to void after removal to ensure that he can void and will not go into retention at home. There have been a few instances in which the patient has developed delayed retention and required recatheterization. This has occurred in patients with very large prostates, in whom the superimposed edema has resulted in retention. If this situation seems likely, the drainage catheter should be left for longer periods of time (48–72 h).

SUMMARY

Although this is a simple interventional uroradiographic procedure, certain technical guidelines should be followed carefully to minimize its risks and maximize its success.

First, precise localization of the external sphincter will prevent injury to this structure and thereby avoid causing incontinence. Second, dilation of the prostatic urethra must include the bladder neck, the site where prostatic hyperplasia most significantly impairs urinary flow, as well as the apex of the prostate, in order to extend the commissurotomy throughout the length of the prostate. Third, all catheter manipulations after dilation should be done over a guidewire to avoid further injury to the traumatized prostatic urethra. Mild to moderate hematuria and dysuria are routine and are presumed to arise from tears in the prostatic urethra and the surrounding tissues. They usually stop or subside significantly in 24 h and are rarely of sufficient severity to necessitate admission of the patient for close observation.

REFERENCES

1. Castañeda F, Lund G, Larson BW, et al. Prostatic urethra: experimental dilation in dogs. *Radiology* 1987;163:649–654
2. Castañeda F, Johnson S, Hulbert J, et al. Urethroplasty with balloon catheter in prostatic hypertrophy. *AJR* 1987;149:313–314
3. Castañeda F, Reddy P, Wasserman N, et al. Benign prostatic hypertrophy: retrograde transurethral dilation of the prostatic urethra in humans: works in progress. *Radiology* 1987;163:649–654
4. Castañeda F, Reddy P, Hulbert J, et al. Retrograde prostatic urethroplasty with balloon catheter. *Semin Intervent Radiol* 1987;4:115–121
5. Castañeda F, Isorna S, Hulbert J, et al. The importance of separation of prostatic lobes in relief of prostatic obstruction by balloon catheter urethroplasty: studies in dogs and humans. *AJR* 1989;153:1301–1304

11

Balloon Urethroplasty Under Cystoscopic Guidance: Transcystoscopic Urethroplasty

Ramon Perez-Marrero, S. Larry Goldenberg, Laurel E. Emerson

Mechanical dilatation of the prostate was first attempted in the midnineteenth century. In 1956, Deisting reported his results in 324 patients dilated with an instrument resembling a reverse action forcep.[1] In 1984, Burhenne et al. applied the coaxial balloon dilatation system of Gruntzig and Hopf[2] to the prostate, demonstrating its use in 10 cadavers and 1 living patient.[3] Several animal and human trials followed,[4-10] and in most, placement of the balloon was controlled by fluoroscopic means. In 1988, Klein and Leeming reported on a cystoscopic method of balloon placement.[5] We have adopted this method because of its accuracy in balloon placement and its use of techniques familiar to all urologists.[11]

The balloon dilation kit (ASI Uroplasty Catheter, Advanced Surgical Intervention, Inc., San Clemente, CA) includes a calibration catheter for exact measurement of the prostatic urethral length, a high-pressure balloon dilation catheter with its own disposable sheath and obturator, and a high-pressure inflation device (Fig. 11–1). The balloon catheter is designed for easy use and accurate placement and permits easy withdrawal after dilation. It is a triple-lumen catheter with a Foley balloon at its tip for fixation to the bladder neck and a high-pressure dilation balloon that is available in several lengths (15–45 mm in 5-mm increments) and has 70-degree shoulders at both ends, providing for accurate dilation and nonmigration. It has a distinct blue band 5 mm distal to the balloon that allows for accurate endoscopic placement at the level of the urethral sphincter (Fig. 11–2). Several markings in its shaft indicate to the operator the position of the Foley balloon and the dilating balloon with respect to the sheath. A third lumen provides a channel for continuous irrigation. The dilating balloon distends to 75 F (25 mm) and is capable of sustaining pressures of up to 5 atm.

The introducing sheath is disposable and accommodates both the dilating catheter and a standard 0-degree or 30-degree cystoscopic lens. It is 26 F in diameter and has a soft rim at its tip that permits easy retraction of the deflated balloon and smooth withdrawal from the urethra.

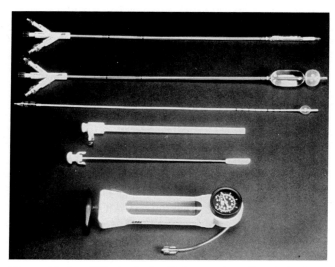

Figure 11–1. ASI uroplasty dilating system. Top to bottom: dilating catheter with balloons deflated and inflated, graduated catheter with Foley balloon, introducing sheath, high-pressure inflation device with gauge.

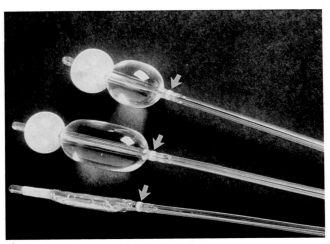

Figure 11–2.   ASI uroplasty catheter. Note 70-degree shoulders at both ends and blue band (arrow) 5 mm distal to the balloon.

TECHNIQUE

After suitable anesthesia, cystoscopy is performed with a standard 21 F cystoscope fitted with an operating channel. The calibration catheter is introduced into the bladder, where its Foley balloon is inflated with 10 mL of sterile water. The cystoscope is withdrawn to the bulbomembranous urethra, and the graduated catheter is retracted until its balloon is seated against the bladder neck. The distance from bladder neck to the external sphincter is determined by counting the centimeter markings (Fig. 11–3). A dilation balloon corresponding to the distance from bladder neck to sphincter is selected. This measurement is rounded off to the nearest 0.5 cm.

The cystoscope is withdrawn, and the introducing sheath is inserted. The dilating catheter is passed through the sheath and advanced until the marking that indicates that the Foley balloon is protruding from the sheath is at the septum (Fig. 11–4). Once the Foley balloon is inflated to 15 mL, the sheath and catheter are withdrawn until the Foley balloon is seated against the bladder neck. This allows retraction of the sheath over the catheter until the second set of markings rests against the septum. This indicates that the dilation balloon is now exposed to the prostatic urethra. The position is now checked cystoscopically by introducing a standard 0-degree or 30-degree lens and lining up the blue band of the catheter with the external sphincter (Fig. 11–5). This ensures that the balloon is positioned within the full length of the prostatic urethra. Under visual control, the balloon is inflated to a pressure of 3 atm for 10 min. The position of the blue band is checked intermittently to ensure that proximal migration into the bladder has not occurred (Fig. 11–6).

Once dilation has been completed, both the Foley balloon and the dilation balloon are deflated and retracted into the sheath. When both shaft markings protrude from the septum,

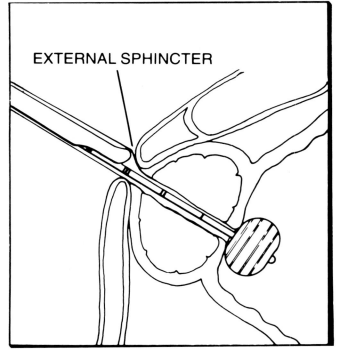

Figure 11–3.   Measurement of prostatic urethra from bladder neck to external sphincter using graduated catheter.

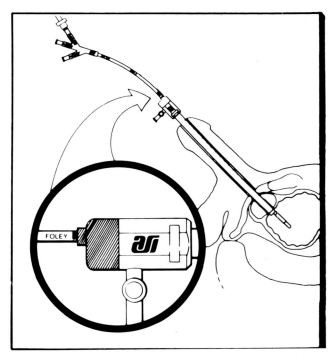

Figure 11–4.   Dilating catheter introduced through the sheath. (Inset) Details of catheter shaft with the Foley mark at the septum.

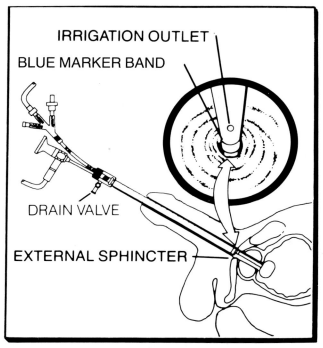

Figure 11–5. Sheath withdrawn over catheter, exposing dilating balloon to prostatic urethra. (Inset) Cystoscopic view of blue marker band at the level of the external sphincter.

the balloons are in the sheath, and the entire system can be removed easily and atraumatically (Fig. 11–7). Cystoscopy is repeated to confirm dilation of the prostatic urethra. We now believe that the hallmark of a good dilation is some amount of bleeding and a tear at the 12 o'clock position. Continuous bladder irrigation rarely is necessary after evacuating bladder clots through the cystoscope. An 18 F double-lumen catheter is left in situ.

ANESTHESIA

This technique lends itself to the outpatient surgery setting and can be performed under several forms of anesthesia. We use either a short spinal anesthetic or a periprostatic block, as described in Chapter 12. This block shortens the postoperative observation period and can be used in patients with significant medical problems that would make regional or general anesthetic risky.

PATIENT SELECTION

Experience has taught us that the single most important determinant of a good response to dilation is patient selection. The best possible candidate for transcystoscopic urethroplasty (TCU) is a patient with moderate symptoms of

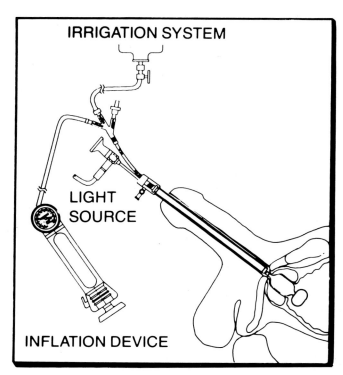

Figure 11–6. Under cystoscopic control, the dilating balloon is inflated to 3 atm (45 psi). Note that the balloon dilates the entire prostatic urethra from bladder neck to apex.

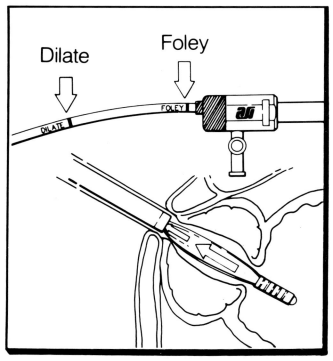

Figure 11–7. Both Foley balloon and dilating balloon are deflated and withdrawn into sheath until the two markings in the catheter shaft protrude from the septum. Removal of the entire system is now safe.

Table 11–1. Best Candidate for Balloon Dilation

Bilobar prostatic enlargement
Prostatic size less than 50 g
Prostatic urethral length between 2.5 and 4.5 cm
Moderate symptoms of prostatism
Adequate detrusor function

Table 11–2. Contraindications to Balloon Dilation

ABSOLUTE CONTRAINDICATIONS	RELATIVE CONTRAINDICATIONS
Localized prostatic malignancy	Multiple large prostatic calculi
Obstructing median lobe	Chronic bacterial prostatitis
Decompensated detrusor	High residual urine (>50% of total bladder capacity)
Very large prostate (>60–70 g)	Urethral strictures

prostatism, a moderate size prostate as estimated by digital rectal and cystoscopic assessment, and adequate detrusor function (Table 11–1).

We believe that an obstructing median lobe, untreated localized prostatic malignancy, multiple prostatic calculi, and severe urethral stricture disease are contraindications to dilation. Patients in chronic urinary retention or with high residual urines and those with very large prostates do not respond as well as others to dilation. We do not dilate prostates with a urethral length longer than 4.5 cm. Patients with a documented history of chronic prostatitis present a special problem. Their prostatic secretions should be cultured several times to rule out an ongoing bacterial infection. In our series, one such patient developed significant septicemia postdilation even after what seemed to be adequate treatment of his prostatitis.

Prostatic calculi are common in this patient population, but if they are multiple, large, and located near the center of the gland, they can present problems after dilation. One such patient developed urethral colic from the passage of these calculi after dilation of his prostate. This proved to be so disabling it forced us to perform a transurethral resection of the prostate (TURP) to evacuate these calculi. Adequate detrusor function is necessary for TCU. In our series, patients in chronic urinary retention have not responded at all

to dilation, and those with large residual urine (>50% total bladder capacity) tended to show less improvement than those with lower residuals. (Table 11–2).

CLINICAL EXPERIENCE

There have been more than 2000 TCUs performed worldwide, and to date there have been no reports of incontinence or retrograde ejaculation as a result of the procedure. In our personal series, we have evaluated 60 patients clinically (using the Boyarsky symptom score[12]), cystoscopically, and urodynamically. Our report is based on a minimum 3-month follow-up.

Our patients were young (median age 61 years), had relatively small prostates (median weight 30 gs), and had moderate prostatic symptoms (mean symptom score of 13.6). Table 11–3 shows our results up to 12 months of follow-up. Mean symptom score values were significantly lowered at each follow-up interval compared to pretreatment values ($p < 0.05$). Peak flow rates ($\dot{Q}max$), expressed as a percentage of the expected peak flow rate for voided volume (corrected $\dot{Q}max$, Corr $\dot{Q}max$), increased from 40% to 55% of expected values by 1 year ($p < 0.05$). Residual urine values decreased, but these changes were not statistically significant. Thus, there seemed to be a measurable and sustained improvement after dilation at least over the first 12 months. The most improved parameters were symptom score and Corr $\dot{Q}max$. Of 39 patients evaluated at 6 months, 32 had shown a significant improvement in one or both of these parameters (82%). This improvement was sustained over the subsequent 6 months (Table 11–4).

Forty-seven of our patients reported normal potency and antegrade ejaculation preoperatively and retained them after dilation. We have not noted any incontinence postoperatively. Bleeding tended to be moderate and temporary and was easily controlled by an indwelling catheter. In our series, only 4 patients required continuous bladder irrigation and hospitalization for bleeding, and only 1 required a blood transfusion. Dilation of the prostate produces a significant amount of edema, and we believe that 48 h of catheterization is necessary to prevent urinary retention. We have noted that voiding symptoms persist for 1–2 weeks. Thus, we warn our patients not to expect improvement sooner than 3–4 weeks postoperatively.

We found that the great majority of our failures occurred in

Table 11–3. Mean Improvement in Symptom Score, Corrected $\dot{Q}$max, and Residual Urine after Balloon Dilation of Prostate

VARIABLE	PREOPERATIVE MEAN (n)	3 MONTHS MEAN (n)	6 MONTHS MEAN (n)	12 MONTHS MEAN (n)
Symptom score	14 (60)[a]	4 (54)[a]	5 (43)[a]	5 (25)[a]
Corr Qmax	40 (57)[a]	53 (48)[a]	53 (41)[a]	55 (25)[a]
Postvoid residual in mL	50 (66)	40 (28)	35 (29)	25 (25)

[a]Differences are statistically significant ($p < 0.05$).

Table 11–4. Patients Showing Improvement in Either Symptom Score or Corrected Peak Flow Rate or Both at 6 and 12 Month Follow-up

IMPROVEMENT	FOLLOW-UP	
	6 Months (n = 39)	*12 Months* (n = 25)
>50% in both	11 (28%)	7 (28%)
>25% in both	17 (44%)	8 (32%)
>25% in symptom score	29 (74%)	20 (80%)
>25% in Corr Qmax	21 (54%)	11 (44%)
>25% in one or both	32 (82%)	23 (92%)

the first 6 months of our experience. These were primarily due to improper patient selection and not to errors in technique. Since endoscopic skills are familiar to all urologists, the learning curve should be rather steep. If a patient derives temporary benefit from TCU, it is likely that a second dilation will be effective. We have redilated 4 of our patients, with excellent response.

CONCLUSION

It is unlikely that TCU will replace TURP in the treatment of BPH, but there is a subgroup of patients in whom balloon dilation may be a reasonable alternative. The advantages of balloon dilation are that it can be performed under regional block on an outpatient basis, it is associated with minimal morbidity, and it preserves antegrade ejaculation in sexually active males. It is an attractive alternative for those patients who are unwilling or unable to undergo general or spinal anesthetic.

We prefer the cystoscopic method of prostatic dilation (transcystoscopic urethroplasty) for its accuracy and simplicity. It uses skills already familiar to all urologists and provides for monitoring of the balloon location in relation to the urethral sphincter at all times. There is no radiation exposure and no need for ultrasound equipment. The ASI system, with its unique balloon design and variable balloon length, provides for a specific prostatic dilation and minimizes proximal migration. The accuracy that this system has

in delivering dilating forces to the prostatic urethra obviates the need for larger size balloons and higher dilating pressures.

We have to keep in mind that proper patient selection is the most important factor in ensuring good response to dilation regardless of the technique used.

REFERENCES

1. Deisting W. Transurethral dilatation of the prostate: a new method in the treatment of prostatic hypertrophy. *Urol Int* 1956;2:158–171
2. Gruntzig A, Hopff H. Perkutane Rekanilsation chronischer arterieller Verschlusse mit einem neuen Dilatation skatheter. Modification der Dotter-Technik. *Deutsch Med Wochenscher* 1974;99:2502–2502
3. Burhenne HJ, Chisholm RJ, Quenville NF. Prostatic hyperplasia. Radiological intervention. *Radiology* 1984;152:655–657
4. Quinn SF, Dryer R, Smathers R, et al. Balloon dilatation of the prostatic urethra. *Radiology* 1985;157:57–58
5. Klein LA, Leeming B. Balloon dilatation for prostatic obstruction: long-term follow-up. Presented at the 83rd Annual Meeting of the American Urological Association, Boston, MA, 1988; abstract 444
6. Castañeda F, Julbert J, Maynar M, et al. Nonsurgical approach for benign prostatic hypertrophy: prostatic urethroplasty with balloon catheter: long-term results. Presented at the 74th Scientific Assembly and Annual Meeting of RSNA, Chicago, 1988; abstract 881
7. Oravisto KJ. Indications for Deisting's prostatic dilatation in the treatment of prostatic hypertrophy. *Urol Intervent* 1961;11:202–206
8. Backman KA. Dilatation of the prostate according to Deisting: results of follow-up one and two years after the operation. *Acta Chir Scand* 1963;126:266–274
9. Sandberg I, Sandstrom B. Dilatation according to Deisting for prostatic hyperplasia. *Scand J Urol Nephrol* 1967;1:225–226
10. Reddy PK, Wasserman N, Castañeda F, Castañeda-Zuniga WR. Transurethral balloon dilatation of prostate for prostatism: preliminary report of nonsurgical technique. *J Endourol* 1987;1:269–273
11. Goldenberg SL, Perez-Marrero RA, Lee LM, Emerson L. Endoscopic balloon dilatation of the prostate: early experience. 1990;144:83–88
12. Boyarsky S, Jones G, Paulson DF, Prout GR Jr. A new look at bladder neck obstruction by the Food and Drug Administration. Regulators Guidelines for investigation of benign prostatic hypertrophy. *Trans Am Assoc Genitourin Surg* 1977; 68:29

12

Balloon Urethroplasty Using Digital Guidance

Deepak A. Kapoor, Pratap K. Reddy

Transurethral balloon dilation of the prostate (TUDP) is a nonsurgical procedure for the treatment of benign prostatic hypertrophy (BPH). Although the concept is not new,[1,2] TUDP has been gaining in popularity recently in the United States and abroad.[3-5] There are currently a number of different techniques used to perform this procedure, and the purpose of this chapter is to illustrate the technique of TUDP under transrectal digital guidance.

PREOPERATIVE EVALUATION

The complete preoperative evaluation of patients for balloon dilation of the prostate is covered in detail elsewhere in the text. In short, it is important to remember that proper patient selection results in better success when using TUDP to treat BPH. All patients should undergo a thorough history and physical examination, with particular attention to voiding symptoms. We use a symptom score to facilitate patient evaluation.[6] The nature and consistency of the prostate gland also are important. A baseline cystoscopic examination should be performed to assess the anatomy of the prostate (it has been shown that patients with significant median lobe hypertrophy do not respond as well to TUDP). Any suggestion of prostate neoplasia should be investigated aggressively to determine if an alternative method to relieve the bladder outlet obstruction as well as treat the carcinoma of the prostate is indicated. A basic laboratory evaluation consisting of serum creatinine, prostate-specific antigen, urinalysis, and urine culture is mandatory.

ANESTHETIC TECHNIQUE

TUDP is inherently a painful procedure. Although the glandular tissue of the prostate itself is not richly innervated,

the prostatic capsule does contain many sensory fibers. Stretching of the prostatic capsule during dilation causes significant discomfort often associated with an intense urge to void. Some form of anesthesia is essential to enable the patient to tolerate the procedure comfortably.

Initially, TUDP was performed under regional or general anesthesia. It seems logical that if one is to utilize a procedure that obviates the need for surgery with its associated morbidity, minimizing the risk associated with the anesthetic also would be of value. We have utilized a prostate block with a high degree of success to completely anesthetize the prostate during this procedure.[7]

The patient is placed in the dorsal lithotomy position and prepared and draped in the usual sterile manner for balloon dilation. Anatomic landmarks for this technique are illustrated in Figure 12–1. Initially, a skin wheal is raised utilizing a 25 gauge needle to instill 1% lidocaine (Xylocaine) solution. After the skin is adequately anesthetized, a 22 gauge, 5-inch spinal needle is advanced gently along the lateral border of the prostate gland until the junction of the prostate and the seminal vesicles (Fig. 12–2). The procedure is guided with the surgeon's finger in the rectum. Once the correct region at the base of the prostate is reached, 15–20 mL of 1% lidocaine solution is infiltrated. During withdrawal of the anesthetic needle, approximately 5 mL of lidocaine solution is instilled along the tract. The same procedure is carried out for the opposite side of the prostate. It is important not to advance the spinal needle in too anterior or lateral a direction, since if this occurs, the pubic ramus will block needle passage. If this technique is performed correctly, it is possible to perform TUDP with no ancillary anesthetic agent. A minimal amount of IV sedation can be utilized as adjunctive anesthesia in the occasional patient in whom the block is incomplete or who may be experiencing an inordinate amount of anxiety.

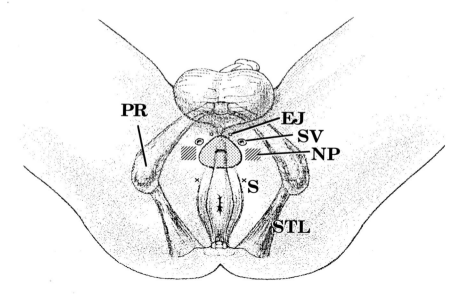

Figure 12–1. Perineal view illustrating landmarks for administration of prostate block. PR, pubic ramus; EJ, ejaculatory duct; SV, seminal vesicle; NP, area of anesthetic infiltration; S, site of needle insertion 1 cm lateral and anterior to the anus; STL, sacrotuberous ligament.

SURGICAL PROCEDURE

In order to facilitate TUDP it is important to select the proper catheter system for each patient. There are currently a number of balloon catheters that are available commercially, but not all of them are ideally suited for the digitally guided approach. We believe that the best catheter for this purpose is the Optilume catheter (Fig. 12–3) (American Medical Systems, Minnetonka, MN). This catheter has been designed specifically for facilitating localization with digital guidance. The catheter measures 10 F in diameter and is 50 cm in

length. It has a wire lumen that will accommodate 0.038 gauge guidewire. The dilating balloon itself is 4 cm long and inflates to 90 F while exerting 4 atm of pressure on the enlarged prostate. There is an easily palpable collar on the distal margin of the dilating balloon called the locator. However, the unique feature of this catheter is the presence of a second balloon (called the fixation balloon), which is 1.5 cm distal to the locator. The fixation balloon dilates to 40 F. The Optilume catheter has radiopaque markers situated at the proximal and distal aspects of the dilating balloon as well as a radiopaque marker at the proximal aspect of the fixation

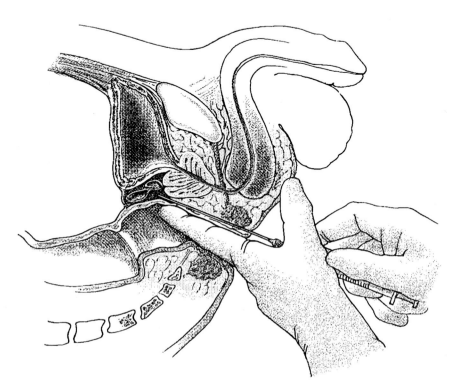

Figure 12–2. Sagittal view depicting administration of local anesthetic to the base of the prostate gland.

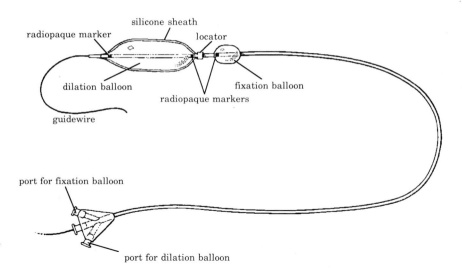

radiopaque marker

silicone sheath

locator

dilation balloon

radiopaque markers

fixation balloon

guidewire

port for fixation balloon

Figure 12–3. The AMS Optilume balloon dilating catheter.

port for dilation balloon

balloon. When the catheter is positioned correctly, the fixation balloon will lie in the bulbous urethra, and the dilating balloon will be in the prostatic urethra. The external sphincter will be situated between these two balloons, which preserves sphincter integrity during the dilation procedure.

After a satisfactory prostate block has been achieved, local anesthesia in the urethra is obtained utilizing 2% lidocaine jelly. A Councill tipped catheter is then advanced into the bladder. It facilitates the rest of the procedure if the bladder is partially distended with water or saline solution. The Councill catheter is then exchanged for a 0.038 gauge guidewire. The Optilume catheter is then advanced over the guidewire while the surgeon places a finger in the rectum (Fig. 12–4).

The catheter is easily palpable as it traverses the soft tissue immediately distal to the prostate gland. The operator completely passes the catheter into the bladder. The Optilume catheter is slowly withdrawn until the uninflated fixation balloon is palpated. This has a distinctive texture that is easily distinguishable from the surface of the catheter. If necessary, the balloon can be inflated and deflated for better identification (Fig. 12–5). The Optilume catheter is further withdrawn until the locator at the distal margin of the dilating balloon is palpable.

Once the locator is in the correct position at the apex of the prostate, the fixation balloon is inflated with no more than 1.3 mL of water or saline (contrast material may be utilized if

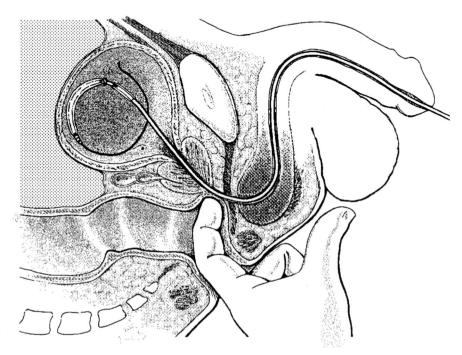

Figure 12–4. Sagittal view of balloon catheter in the bladder. Initially, a 0.038 guidewire is placed into the bladder via a Councill catheter. This is then exchanged for the balloon catheter.

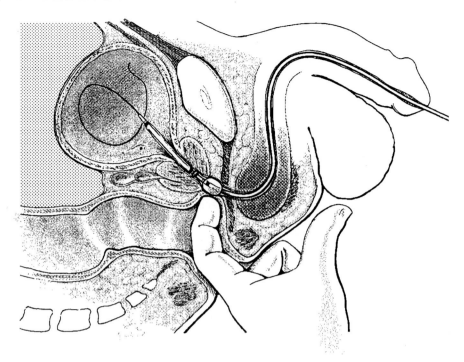

Figure 12–5. Sagittal view illustrating verification of dilating balloon location via palpation of fixation balloon. The balloon catheter is positioned initially by withdrawing the catheter until the locating ring is palpable at the apex of the prostate. The fixation balloon is inflated and palpated in the bulbous urethra.

fluoroscopic visualization is desired). Once the balloon is situated in the correct location, it is possible to proceed with dilation of the prostate. The fixation balloon is left inflated during the procedure to stabilize the catheter. Although this second balloon helps hold the balloon catheter in place, it is important to recognize that there still will be a tendency for proximal migration of the balloon and that very gentle traction on the balloon catheter will still be necessary. The

dilating balloon is inflated until a total of 4 atm of pressure is exerted on the prostate (Fig. 12–6). This pressure is maintained for a period of 10 min. The operator will find that as dilation of the prostate proceeds, there will be less traction required on the balloon catheter to hold it in place. It is important to note that as the dilating balloon is inflated, it may no longer be possible to feel the locator. There is an O ring provided with the Optilume catheter that is placed at the

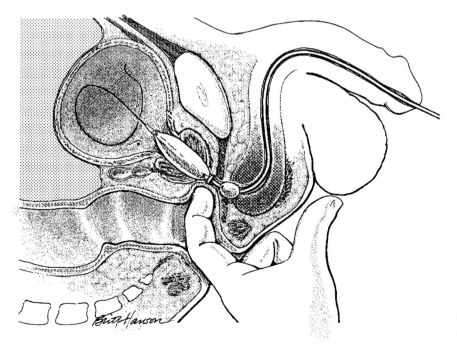

Figure 12–6. Sagittal view depicting inflation of dilating balloon under digital guidance.

urethral meatus and indicates if there is any migration of the catheter. After completing the dilation, both the fixation and dilation balloons are deflated, and the Optilume catheter is withdrawn. A Councill catheter is advanced over the wire and placed in the bladder for gravity drainage. The catheter generally is removed on the first postoperative day.

It generally is unnecessary to utilize any form of localization beyond digital guidance. With this catheter, however, it is possible to utilize fluoroscopic or endoscopic localization techniques as well. For operators who have used either of those techniques, it may be prudent initially to use radiographic visualization by instilling contrast material into both the fixation and dilating balloons. It also is possible to visualize the correct location of the fixation balloon in the bulbous urethra by passing a cystoscope alongside the catheter. With relatively little experience, it is possible to localize the catheter accurately using digital guidance exclusively.

RESULTS

We have performed this procedure on over 90 patients. All of the patients tolerated the procedure well, with minimal morbidity. In 93% of patients, the Foley catheter was removed the day after the procedure. No patient required blood transfusion. Relief of symptoms was obtained in over 65% of unselected patients, with mean follow-up now approaching 2 years. No patient is incontinent after the procedure. To date, only 17 patients have required TURP.

DISCUSSION

As time progresses, there is likely to be increasing pressure on urologists to utilize less invasive methods to manage bladder outlet obstruction.[9] Balloon dilation of the prostate is still in its infancy, but it shows promise as a potential trend

for the future. The technique of balloon dilation utilizing digital guidance is the only one that obviates the need for any radiologic accessories (such as fluoroscopy or ultrasonography) as well as eliminates the need for an adjunctive intraoperative procedure (endoscopy). Digital guidance is thus the simplest and least expensive technique to perform balloon dilation of the prostate. Digitally guided balloon dilation of the prostate under local anesthesia would seem to be the ideal choice for a procedure whose main purpose is to relieve bladder outlet obstruction in a simpler and more cost-effective way.

REFERENCES

1. Aalkjaer V. Transurethral resection versus dilatation treatment in hypertrophy of the prostate. *Urol Int* 1962;14:119–124
2. Aboulker P, Steg A. La divulsion de la prostate a'apres 218 observations personnelles. *J Urol Nephrol* 1964;70:338–364
3. Machan L, Gill KP, Abel P, Jager HR, Williams G, Allison DJ. Prostatic urethroplasty. Results at the Royal postgraduate medical school. *Semin Intervent Radiol* 1989;6:65–71
4. Reddy PK. Role of balloon dilation in the treatment of benign prostatic hyperplasia. *Prostate Suppl* 1990;3:39–48
5. Reddy PK, Wasserman N, Sidi AA. Balloon dilation of the prostate: can it help the patient with BPH? *Contemp Urol* 1989; Feb/Mar:44–53
6. Madsen P, Iverson P. A point system for selecting operative candidates. In: Hinman F (ed). *Benign Prostatic Hypertrophy.* New York: Springer Verlag, 1983:763–765
7. Reddy PK. New technique to anesthetize the prostate for transurethral balloon dilation. *Urol Clin North Am* 1990; 17:55–56
8. Reddy PK, Hulbert JC, Lightner DJ, Wasserman N, Castañeda F, Castañeda-Zuniga W. Transurethral balloon dilatation of the prostate for benign prostatic hyperplasia. *Curr Surg Tech Urol* 1989;2:1–8
9. Wennberg J, Roos N, Sola L, Schori A, Jaffe R. Use of claims data systems to evaluate health care outcomes. Mortality and reoperation following prostatectomy. *JAMA* 1987;257:933–936

13

Prostatic Urethroplasty Under Transrectal Ultrasound Guidance

Flavio Castañeda, Wilfrido R. Castañeda-Zúñiga

Transrectal ultrasound (TRUS) has advanced significantly since its beginning with the experimental work of Watanabe et al. in the late 1960s.[1] The current high-resolution axial and sagittal images of the prostate obtained with state-of-the-art technology have placed this technique in the forefront of early prostatic cancer detection and staging.[2,3] Because of its high-resolution and real time imaging capabilities, TRUS is the ideal imaging modality for prostatic urethroplasty with balloon catheter.[4]

IMAGING

TRUS not only offers the advantage of real time monitoriza-tion throughout the procedure but also helps to assess for the presence or absence of an enlarged median bar (Fig. 13–1A, B), which has been shown to be a relative contraindica-tion.[5–9] It also screens for malignancy and determines the exact anatomic landmarks, such as the position of the external sphincter and bladder neck, as well as the length of the prostatic urethra.

PATIENT AND METHODS

Patients are selected for the procedure after a thorough clinical history and physical examination and confirmation of prostatic obstructive uropathy. Patients with significant median bar hyperplasia and carcinoma of the prostate are excluded because of poor results and the theoretical risk of tumor spread, respectively. However, these two relative contraindications have been waived by some because of the lack of other options or for palliative purposes.

After a rectal enema to reduce stool or air artifacts, the patients are placed in an oblique-supine position, and the penis and genitals are prepared and draped in the usual sterile fashion. An intravenous line is started for sedation purposes, and a generous instillation of 2% viscous lidocaine is admin-istered through the urethra for local anesthesia as well as for lubrication purposes.

A 20 F to 22 F Councill catheter is advanced into the bladder. Once in position, an 0.038 inch stiff guidewire is advanced through the Councill catheter and curled in the bladder. At this point, TRUS imaging is initiated with a high-frequency (5–7 MHz) sagittal or biplane transducer. Once the probe has been positioned adequately and all the landmarks have been identified (external sphincter, prostatic urethra, and bladder) (Fig. 13–2A), the Councill catheter is exchanged for the prostatic urethroplasty balloon catheter.

Once the balloon catheter is in position, it is inflated to its maximum diameter and pressure for 10–15 min (Fig. 13–2B). Strong tension on the balloon is required to prevent migration into the bladder, but the operator must ensure that the proximal portion of the balloon is always just proximal to the external sphincter to avoid damage to this structure. This is relatively easy because of the excellent determination of pelvic structures and real time possibilities that ultrasound provides.

Once the dilation has been accomplished, the balloon is deflated and removed over the guidewire. A 20 F to 22 F Councill catheter is once more advanced into the bladder over the guidewire and then removed (Fig. 13–2C). The Councill catheter retention balloon is overdistended with 20–25 mL of fluid to avoid lodging in the traumatized prostatic fossa and causing more discomfort and is left to gravity drainage.

The postprocedure care is the same as described through-out this book.

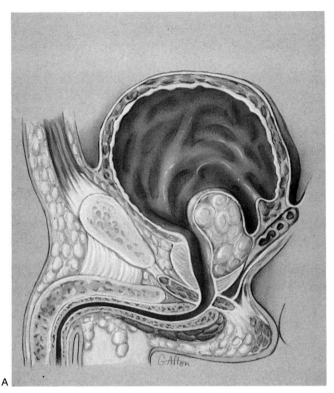
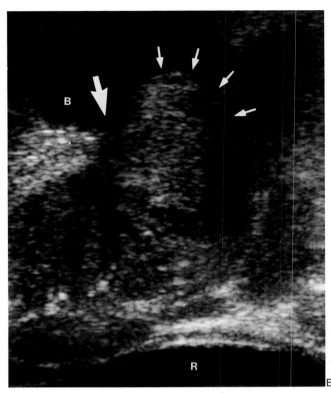

Figure 13–1. **A.** Schematic appearance of enlarged median prostatic lobe in lateral view extrinsically indenting the bladder floor posterior to the neck. This flap of tissue acts as a ball valve at the bladder neck, which makes dilation of the bladder neck obsolete. **B.** Lateral transrectal ultrasound view of the hypertrophied median lobe (small arrows) indenting the bladder base at the neck region (large arrow). R, rectum; B, bladder.

DISCUSSION

TRUS guidance for prostatic urethroplasty has several advantages over the other modalities used for this procedure. Rectal guidance alone is inaccurate, risky, and difficult. During a rectal examination, the key landmark is the prostatic apex (Fig. 13–3), and the location of the external sphincter is inferred from this. During balloon inflation, the expansion deforms the prostate and perineal tissues, and the balloon catheter may seem close to the prostatic apex when in reality it could have migrated into the more proximal prostatic urethra (Fig. 13–4). The operator may feel that the prostatic apex is being dilated, but what is being felt is distention and displacement of the prostate and perineal structures, which are very mobile because of the lax attachments of the perineal structures that are only tendinous and muscular. Also, because of the strong tension required on the catheter, it is difficult to maintain the rectal finger in position while pulling on the urethral dilation catheter.

Cystoscopic guidance is very accurate in identifying the position of the external sphincter as well as facilitating the precise initial placement of the balloon catheter. Once the cystoscope is removed and inflation is initiated however, the same tendency to migrate occurs. Therefore, fluoroscopy

usually is required for adequate continuous monitoring. In an attempt to avoid this problem, shorter balloons have been developed to fit exactly in the prostatic fossa. With this type of balloon, however, the base of the prostate may not be dilated adequately where most of the prostatic bulk is located, thereby precluding the best chance for an adequate result.

Fluoroscopic guidance requires adequate imaging equipment as well as knowledge and expertise in radiologic anatomy and handling catheters and guidewires. Most of this is available to the majority of practicing urologists and interventional radiologists.

The radiation dose is minimal, and since in most instances fluoroscopy is still used at one time or another regardless of the guidance used initially, this should not be a deterrent.

The only disadvantage of TRUS as a guiding modality for prostatic urethroplasty is that it is more uncomfortable for the patient, since besides the urethral catheter, it requires the insertion of a large rectal probe, which must remain in place throughout the procedure (Fig. 13–5). If this is not a concern, we think that TRUS has more advantages than all other modalities, since it actually shows the relationship between the external sphincter and proximal end of the balloon catheter in real time throughout the procedure and assures the

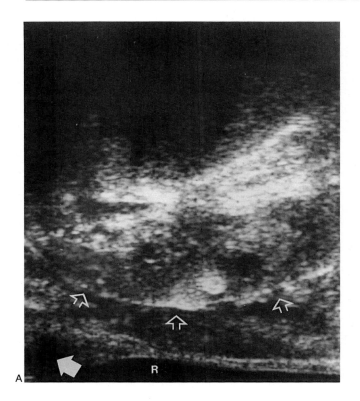

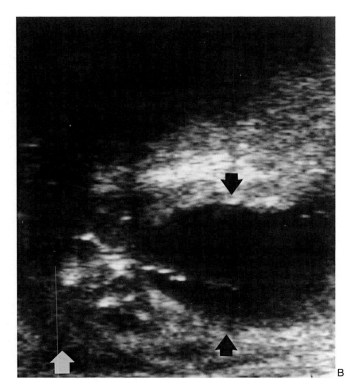

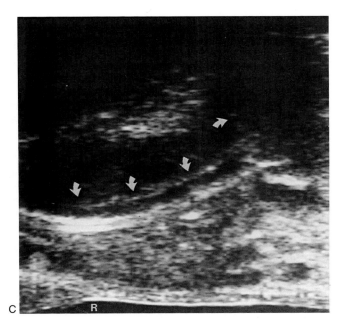

Figure 13–2.   A. Lateral view of transrectal ultrasound of the prostate showing guidewire already in place coursing through the urethra (open arrows). The position of the external sphincter is noted (large white arrow) by its characteristic hypoechoic appearance in the prostatic apical region. R, rectum. **B.** Lateral transrectal ultrasound view showing the balloon catheter fully inflated in the prostatic urethra (black arrows). Note correct relationship between the prostatic apex and external sphincter (white arrow). **C.** Lateral transrectal ultrasound view showing the Councill catheter (white curved arrows) coursing through the prostatic urethra, with its balloon overdistended in the bladder after the procedure. R, rectum.

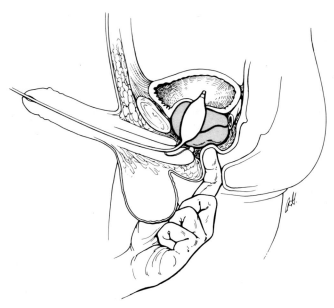

Figure 13–3. Diagram showing the desired relationships (external sphincter, prostate apex, and inflated balloon catheter) during the performance of transrectal digital-guided balloon dilation of the prostate, assuming optimal circumstances.

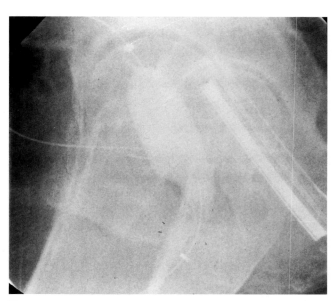

Figure 13–5. Radiographic image in lateral position showing the balloon catheter fully inflated and the transrectal ultrasound probe in place simultaneously. Note that there is still residual waste in the balloon along the distal prostatic urethra.

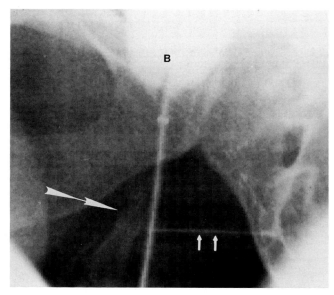

Figure 13–4. Radiographic image showing needle (small arrows) and finger (large arrow) marking the position of the prostate apex and external sphincter, whereas balloon catheter (B) has migrated into the proximal prostatic urethra, missing the distal two thirds.

operator that the entire prostatic urethra, including the bladder neck, is being dilated. As with the other modalities, this is inferred from direct or indirect visualization of the urethra or by palpation of the prostatic apex.

REFERENCES

1. Watanabe H, Kato H, Kato T, et al. Diagnostic application of the ultrasonotomography to the prostate. *Jpn J Urol* 1968; 59:273–279
2. Lee F, Littrup PJ, Torp-Pedersen S, et al. Prostate cancer: comparison of transrectal ultrasound and the digital rectal examination for screening. *Radiology* 1988;169:351–354
3. Lee F, Torp-Pedersen S, Littrup PJ, et al. Hypoechoic lesions of the prostate: clinical relevance of tumor size, digital rectal examination, and prostate-specific antigen. *Radiology* 1989; 170:29–32
4. Littrup PJ, Lee F, Borlaza G, Solomon MH. Prostatic urethroplasty: guidance by transrectal sonography. *Semin Int Radiol* 1989;6:42–45
5. Castañeda F, Reddy P, Wasserman N, et al. Benign prostatic hypertrophy: retrograde transurethral dilation of the prostatic urethra in humans. Works in progress. *Radiology* 1987; 163:649–654
6. Castañeda F, Reddy P, Hulbert J, et al. Retrograde prostatic urethroplasty with balloon catheter. *Semin Intervent Radiol* 1987;4:115–121
7. Galdenberg LS, Perez-Marrero RA, Lee LM, Emerson L. Endoscopic balloon dilation of the prostate: early experience. *J Urol* 1990;144:83–88
8. Dowd J, Smith JJ. Balloon dilation of the prostate. *Benign Prostatic Hyperplasia* 1990;17:671–677
9. Doughtry J, Rodan B, Bean W. Balloon dilation of prostatic urethra. *Urology* 1990;36:203–209

14

Mechanism of Prostatic Balloon Dilation

S. Larry Goldenberg, Ramon Perez-Marrero

The exact mechanism by which balloon dilation of the prostate gland improves voiding is not yet well understood. The acute compression of tissue and distention of capsule may decrease resistance to flow directly or do so indirectly by disrupting alpha-adrenergic receptors and smooth muscle tone. Creation of an anterior commissurotomy reflects the mechanical effect on the prostatic urethra. Many questions need to be answered. Why is the clinical response so variable? Does the bladder neck need to be included in the dilation? Why do very large glands and those with middle lobes not respond as well? Do patients with more fibrous glands fare better than those with a lower stroma/epithelium ratio? Is there a difference between single length balloons and variable length (made to measure) balloons? Investigators currently are pondering these questions while clinically applying balloon dilation of the prostate as an alternative to transurethral resection.

MECHANICAL EFFECTS

Canine Studies

The dog is the only readily available laboratory animal known to develop prostatic hypertrophy. Unfortunately, the histology of canine prostatic enlargement differs from that of humans in that there is an excess of adenomatous tissue as compared to the predominantly stromal hyperplasia in man. The capsule around the dog's prostate is quite weak compared to the strong capsule that surrounds the human prostate.

Quinn et al.[1] dilated six dog prostates up to a diameter of 20 mm in an antegrade fashion through an open cystotomy. Postdilation voiding urethrograms showed definite widening of the prostatic urethra in five of the six dogs. This change persisted for up to 23 weeks. Histologic examination of these prostates showed periurethral hemorrhage and a patulous urethra immediately postdilation, with chronic inflammatory changes on later examinations. Castaneda et al.[2] applied a number of different balloon sizes to dog prostates. They were able to achieve adequate dilation in all dogs with balloons of greater than 20 mm in diameter and with inflation pressures of 4–6 atm. Under these conditions, they demonstrated an increase in urethral diameter from an upper limit of 4.1 mm before dilation to 18.5 mm immediately postdilation. They noted very minimal congestion and hemorrhage in the subepithelial tissue following dilation. These two canine studies suggested that balloon dilation can be accomplished quite safely, and they set the stage for subsequent clinical trials.

Experimental Human Studies

In 1984, Burhenne et al.[3] studied balloon dilation in 10 human cadavers. They demonstrated increased radiographic caliber of the prostatic urethra following dilation to 24 F diameter. Denstedt et al.[4] have performed balloon dilation (75 F) on 12 cadavers, 2 cystoprostatectomy specimens, and 2 radical retropubic prostatectomy specimens. They have not observed disruption of the bladder neck or capsule in any of the in situ specimens. However, 4 of the 7 that were dilated ex vivo split at the 12 o'clock apical position from urethra to capsule.

We have applied the ASI dilation system (Uroplasty catheter, Advanced Surgical Intervention, Inc., San Clemente, CA) to the prostates of transplant organ donors. Our first patient was a 47-year-old with early BPH. Immediately after completion of transplant organ retrieval, the prostatic fossa was dilated with a 75 F diameter balloon for 10 min at

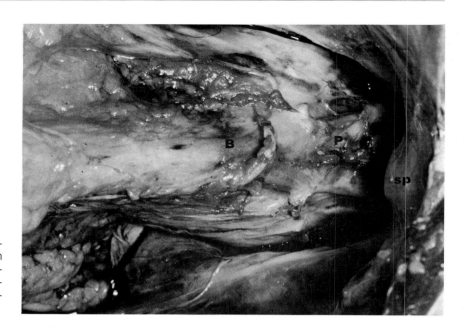

Figure 14–1. Superior view of bladder and prostate (in situ dilation) with balloon inflated to 25 mm (75 F) diameter at 3 atm of pressure. B, bladder; P, prostate; sp, symphysis pubis.

3 atm (44 psi). The 15-mm long balloon did not pass through the bladder neck, and on inflation, there was no gross disruption of the capsule (Fig. 14–1). The bladder and prostate were then removed en bloc, fixed in formalin, embedded, step-sectioned, and stained with H & E. The dilation created an anterior commissurotomy that extended from urethra to but not through capsule (Fig. 14–2). In Figure 14–3, we illustrate the tear approaching the fibers of the capsule (H & E). We also examined all specimens with elastin and smooth muscle stains and did not observe any histologic abnormalities in these tissues. We noted that the

bladder neck remained intact grossly and histologically during the dilation (Fig. 14–4).

In a second living organ donor (28 years old), in vivo dilation of a small prostate to 75 F created a large anterior divulsion between the lateral lobes (Fig. 14–5). The corre-

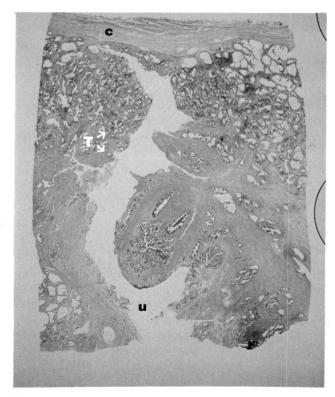

Figure 14–2. Whole mount, transverse section illustrating the anterior tear (T), which extends from the urethra (u) to but not through the capsule (c).

Figure 14–3. Corresponding photomicrograph showing the tear (T) extending from the urethra (u) to the fibers of the capsule (c). H & E.

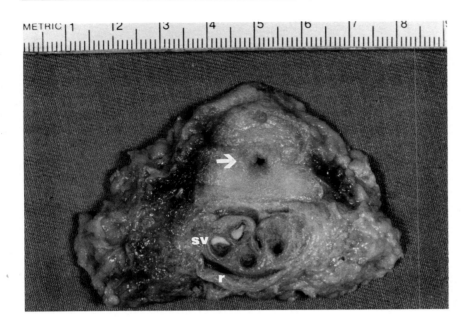

Figure 14–4.   Bladder neck (arrow) has remained intact following dilation. sv, seminal vesicles; r, rectum.

sponding photomicrograph (Fig. 14–6) shows the tear extending to but not through the capsule. The bladder neck also remained intact in this case.

Our third case involved another small gland (38 years old) that was removed from the donor before dilation and tacked down as securely as was possible to a dissecting board. Unlike the in vivo situation, the tear that was created in this gland extended all the way through the anterior capsule (Figs. 14–7, 14–8). This is probably a *false exaggeration* of the effect of dilation, due to a lack of buttressing tissue. Once

again we observed that even with this extreme degree of divulsion, the bladder neck remained intact.

To place the dilation of living organ donor prostates in perspective with respect to the other cadaveric studies, we also dilated 4 cadaver prostates in vivo using the same

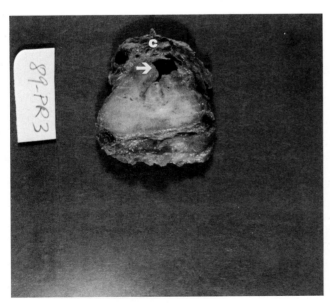

Figure 14–5.   Whole mount, transverse section illustrating a large anterior divulsion (arrow) of the lateral lobes of the small gland. c, capsule.

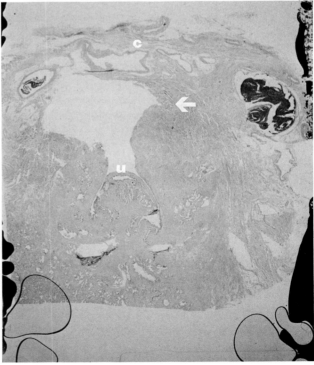

Figure 14–6.   Corresponding photomicrograph of divulsion and tear (arrow) extending from urethra (u) to but not through the fibers of the capsule (c). H & E.

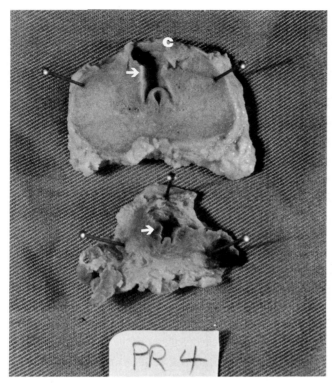

Figure 14–7. Whole mount, transverse section illustrating an anterior tear (arrow) extending through the capsule (c) in upper section. Lower section illustrates intact bladder neck (arrow).

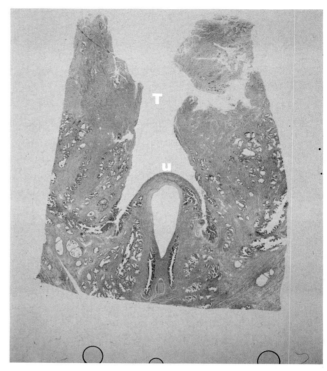

Figure 14–8. Corresponding photomicrograph showing a complete disruption of the gland. u, urethra; T, tear.

techniques. Unlike the organ donor glands, these did not tear significantly (Fig. 14–9). This may be due to a loss of compliance in the postmortem state, suggesting a *false minimization* of the true clinical situation and thus not representing an adequate model.

In vivo balloon dilation of the living donor organ prostate with a 75 F catheter most closely approximates the clinical situation. We have demonstrated that the balloon leads to a mechanical anterior commissurotomy with significant tissue trauma. When a made to measure balloon is positioned only within the confines of the prostatic urethra, the bladder neck

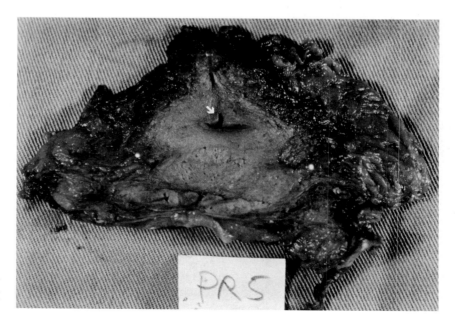

Figure 14–9. Whole mount, transverse section illustrating a minor anterior tear (arrow).

is spared. This may explain the preservation of antegrade ejaculation in the clinical setting.

Clinical Studies

In 1956, Deisting[5] emphasized the importance of exhausting the elasticity of the prostate capsule during dilation as well as of disrupting the anterior and posterior commissures. He utilized an instrument that resembled a reverse-action forcep to dilate the prostate in a single plane. In clinical experience, the balloon often requires additional fluid to maintain the applied 3–4 atm of pressure, implying that the prostate capsule is indeed distending and losing elasticity.

Following dilation of the prostate to 75 F or 90 F, most authors have visualized an anterior tear (commissurotomy, divulsion) between the lobes of the gland. Whether this in itself leads to improved voiding is questionable. We believe that it is important to observe this tear cystoscopically as an indicator of adequate dilation.

In our clinical studies, we measured serum prostate-specific antigen (PSA) levels before and after dilation.[6] We found that serum PSA increased by greater than 1.5 ng/mL in 16 of 22 patients and in all cases returned to predilation levels within 3 months. This observation also supports the concept of mechanical disruption of the prostate by balloon dilation.

EFFECT OF CAPSULAR STRETCH ON NEURORECEPTORS

Alpha-neuroreceptors are distributed throughout the bladder neck and prostatic adenoma, particularly within the prostatic capsule.[7] These are predominantly of alpha$_1$ type, though alpha$_2$-adrenoreceptors are present as well. The contractility of the prostatic urethral smooth muscle is mediated primarily by alpha$_1$-adrenoreceptors and plays a significant role in the dynamic component of bladder outlet obstruction, as defined by Caine.[8] Pharmacologic therapy with alpha-blockers has been used in multiple clinical trials to decrease the tone of the prostate smooth muscle and the resistance to outflow, with improvement in urinary symptoms.

Our clinical studies have shown that prostate dilation with a 75 F measured balloon is most effective in smaller glands. The made to measure multiple length balloon maximally dilates the prostate capsule from bladder neck to apex. The single length balloon may not stretch the prostate capsule as much, since the bladder neck musculature limits the degree of circular expansion. We carried out intraoperative transrectal ultrasound (TRUS) to measure the circumference of the midprostate during dilation with the ASI measured balloon. On transverse scanning, the circumference increased from a mean of 12.1 cm to a mean of 13.3 cm (+10%). Comparable increases were noted at the apex and base of the gland.

The full-length compression of the prostate adenoma with expansile stretching of the capsule may alter neuroreceptor distribution or function or both. This concept, which remains to be proven, would explain the remarkable reduction of irritative voiding symptoms in patients who have undergone balloon dilation.

DISCUSSION

There is much to be learned about the mechanism of prostatic balloon dilation. The concentration of extremely high pressures (3–4 atm) by a noncompliant balloon within the posterior urethra leads to compression of prostatic tissue and creation of an anterior commissurotomy that may or may not be involved in the resolution of symptoms. During dilation, the downward drifting of the applied inflation pressure suggests that the capsule yields to the expansion. It seems important to visualize the anterior divulsion, since this implies an adequate mechanical dilation. The fact that the split does not extend through bladder neck when using the made to measure balloon explains why antegrade ejaculation is maintained, a most important factor in the young, sexually active patient. It is unlikely that the bladder neck needs to be dilated or split. This is supported by a group of our patients with primary bladder neck hyperplasia (and minimal lateral lobe enlargement), who responded well to dilation without endoscopic or radiologic disruption of the bladder neck.[6] Their resolution of symptoms can be explained by capsular distention and an alteration or disruption of neuroreceptor activity.

The differences between clinical trials may be attributed to the different types of balloons and the variability of their effect on the capsule. Undoubtedly, any balloon that can distend to 75 F or 90 F will lead to a mechanical disruption. What may be more important is achieving an adequate stretch of the entire prostatic capsule, including the apical region. This may not occur with a single length or a radiographically placed balloon.

It is not necessarily true that bigger is better. A 90 F balloon in a very small prostate may be too traumatic for the gland. On the other hand, a 75 F balloon in a very large prostate is unlikely to be effective in achieving capsular stretch. Finally, selection of patients is important, and the means of longitudinal study is vital in assessment of this technique.

Future studies will examine the possible role of submucosal ischemia, neuroreceptor alterations, and smooth muscle tone in the mechanism of balloon dilation of the prostate.

REFERENCES

1. Quinn SF, Dyer R, Smathers R, et al. Balloon dilatation of the prostatic urethra. *Radiology* 1985;157:57–58
2. Castañeda F, Lund G, Larson BW, et al. Prostatic urethra: experimental dilation in dogs. *Radiology* 1987;163:645–648
3. Burhenne HJ, Chisholm RJ, Quenville NF. Prostatic hyperplasia: radiological intervention. *Radiology* 1984;152:655–657
4. Denstedt JD, Chin JL, Grignon DJ, Garcia B. Histopathologic

study of changes induced by extensive balloon dilatation of the prostate to 75 F. Presented at the 85th Annual Meeting of the American Urological Association, New Orleans, Louisiana, 1990; abstract 376

5. Deisting W. Transurethral dilatation of the prostate: a new method in the treatment of prostatic hypertrophy. *Urol Intervent* 1956;2:158–171

6. Goldenberg SL, Perez-Marrero R, Lee LM, Emerson L. Endoscopic balloon dilatation of the prostate: early experience. *J Urol* 1990;144:83–88

7. Lepor H. Nonoperative management of benign prostatic hyperplasia. *J Urol* 1989;141:1283–1289

8. Caine M. The present role of alpha-adrenergic blockers in the treatment of benign prostatic hypertrophy. *J Urol* 1986;136:1–4

15

Endoscopic Findings After Balloon Prostatic Divulsion

Santiago Isorna, Manuel Maynar, J. A. Belon

The prostate, one of the largest glands in the body, is the organ where neoplastic growth is most common.[1] This pathologic growth, benign prostatic hyperplasia (BPH), presents a problem because of its anatomic situation surrounding the urethra, and it may produce an obstruction of the lower urinary tract. The degree of such obstructive uropathy does not correlate with the size or with the time of evolution of the prostatic growth, but when it reaches a significant intensity, it must be relieved. This need has a lot to do with the development of urology since the earliest times in medical practice.

Several instrumental methods have been described to relieve prostatic obstruction through a transurethral approach, thus avoiding surgical removal of the adenoma. Later, the development and continuous advances in the safety and efficacy of prostatic surgery, especially in transurethral resection of the prostate (TURP), forced those early methods to be abandoned.

In 1984, Burhenne revived the idea of applying a dilation balloon, and in 1986, Castañeda et al. at the University of Minnesota reported a method to safely dilate the prostatic urethra by using a large dilation balloon in animals.[2] Later, they began to treat humans, with no complications and with good initial results, except in patients with predominance of the middle prostatic lobe, where because of anatomic characteristics, a valvular mechanism precluded improvement in micturition after the procedure.[3] Castañeda was concerned about the mechanism of action by which the balloon, maximally distended in the prostatic urethra, would cause diminution or disappearance of the obstructive uropathy caused by BPH and how this effect could become permanent.

In their experience with dogs,[2] Casteñeda et al. determined that to be effective in dilation of the prostate, the balloon must measure 20 mm in diameter at maximal distention and be dilated for 10 min. When using balloon dilation in humans, they deduced that since the human urethra is larger, the balloon must have a larger diameter. The limit of this diameter was established according to the appearance of intense pain, which was the result of stretching of the prostatic capsule and the internal sphincter. Casteñeda et al. then designed a trifoil 25 mm in diameter balloon catheter, which they later enlarged to 30 mm in monofoil balloons. The length of the balloon was 10 cm, to include the entire length of the prostatic urethra, even in very large prostates. They stated that a second dilation could be performed after repositioning to ensure that the dilation would include the bladder neck in those cases where the prostatic urethra is significantly elongated, as it is in patients with a significant enlargement of the gland.[3]

Castañeda et al. warn that the pressure of balloon distention must not exceed 3–4 atm because if it reaches values close to 6 atm in the 10 min of dilatation, restenosis at the level of the adenoma by tissue ischemia and secondary fibrosis might occur. They stated also that the hemorrhage observed immediately after dilation in secondary to small lacerations of the urethra and adjacent tissues, which in most instances has healed by 2 weeks, showed complete reepithelialization by this time.[2]

These findings led Castañeda initially to elaborate a hypothesis that the fundamental mechanism of dilation in prostatic urethroplasty with a balloon catheter is the compression or flattening of the hyperplastic glandular tissue

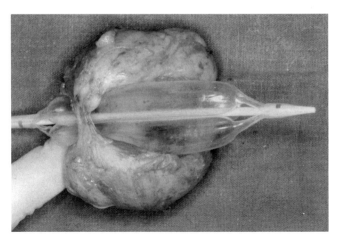

Figure 15–1. Trifoil balloon dilating a surgical prostate specimen. Note disruption of anterior commissure.

against its own capsule, which could produce ischemic atrophy of the glandular tissue with subsequent atrophy, decrease of volume, and, therefore, diminution of compression on the urethral lumen at that level. This hypothesis seemed to be confirmed by ultrasonic and MRI studies performed before and after the procedure[4] but could not be confirmed histologically by prostatic biopsies because the invasiveness of biopsy could not be justified for research purposes.

In a later publication in which we were co-workers,[5] Castañeda et al. rectified those initial suppositions and consider that the main mechanism of action of prostatic dilatation is the anterior and posterior commissures disruption thus allowing the separation of the two prostatic lobes during micturition (Fig. 15–1).

Bearing in mind the precedents of this technique with the metallic instrument by Deisting,[6] the physiopathologic explanation given by Aboulker and Steg[7] is the following. The forceful separation of the two metallic branches of the dilator in an anteroposterior sagittal direction causes rupture of the anterior and posterior commissures of adenoma of the prostate, and prolonged dilation causes a change in elasticity of the prostatic capsule (or true prostate), producing stretching or distention (Fig. 15–2). Thereafter, during micturition, the two prostatic lobes, which are no longer fixed to each other, can separate within a looser capsule. The authors consider that in order to obtain maximal efficacy with this procedure, separation of the branches of the metallic divulsor must approach at least double the distance of the separation existing when the operator starts to notice resistance during divulsor progressive opening, which is around 7–8 cm.

We initiated the procedure by Castañeda almost 3 years ago, and although our series is short, as it has been used only in carefully chosen cases, follow-up of our patients has been very close. With a longer follow-up than that described in a preliminary work,[8] we have performed endoscopy of the prostatic urethra before and after the procedure. We have done this in an effort to clarify the effects produced by dilation of the catheter balloon in the prostatic urethra and with the intention of providing a new point of view about its mechanism of action.

MATERIAL AND METHODS

The procedure was applied in 26 patients from 56 to 80 years of age (mean 69.1 years), all of whom had a definitive diagnosis of BPH (Fig. 15–3). In the study were included detailed history and urologic exploration, complete blood

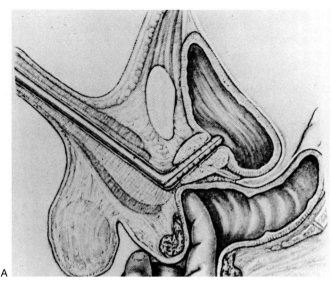

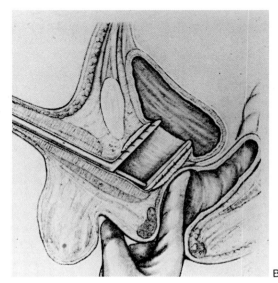

Figure 15–2. Prostatic divulsion with Deisting dilator. **A.** Dilator with arms closed. Rectal palpation reveals the position of the external sphincter. **B.** Arms have been separated as far as possible.

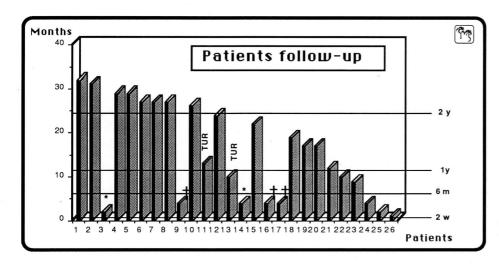

Figure 15–3. Patients in the series and follow-up period. †, dead; TUR, operated for BPH by transurethral resection; *, lost.

count and blood chemistries, including phosphatase, urinalysis with sediment examination and cultures, retrograde and voiding cystourethrograms, uroflow studies, measurements of postvoiding residuals, and urethrocystoscopy in all the cases and, occasionally, suprapubic echography. All of these studies, including urethrocystoscopy, were repeated in the subsequent evaluation, the uroflow and residual measurements repeated at 2 weeks, 6 months, and 1 and 2 years after dilation.

Once the possibility of an associated adenocarcinoma of the prostate was excluded, the patients' were chosen according to the following criteria: patients with a high surgical risk because of cardiopulmonary pathology or concurrent systemicic disease or advanced age, a high degree of reluctance to undergo surgery, and religious beliefs that precluded the use of blood transfusions during surgery.

The size of the BPH, as judged by clinical methods, was grade 1 in 6 cases (<25 g), grade II in 15 cases (25–50 g), grade III in 5 cases (50–80 g), and no cases of grade IV (>80 g). According to the prostatic morphology observed during cystoscopy, 2 patients had lobular enlargement and only showed a bladder neck obstruction, 18 had pure bilobular enlargement, and 4 had trilobular enlargement. We deliberately excluded all those cases with a clear predominance of the middle lobe.

The procedure was performed according to Castañeda's description.[3] One-half hour before the procedure, an analgesic (Nolotil) and a sedative (diazepam 5 mg IM) were administered, and local intraurethral anesthesia (tetracaine 10 mg) was used during the procedure. Urinary antiseptics (norfloxacin) were administered from the day before to 2 days after the dilation, and a single dose of antibiotic (tobramycin 100 mg IM) was given before the procedure. During the procedure, the patient was monitored, and an intravenous line was in place for immediate administration of medication.

All the maneuvers were performed under fluoroscopic

control on a radiologic table. Once the correct placement of the catheter was checked by fluoroscopy, dilation was maintained for 10 min at a pressure of 2–3 atm. During that time, traction had to be exerted to maintain the correct position of the balloon and prevent its emigration to the bladder. In the first 10 patients, a 25 mm in diameter trifoil balloon catheter (Medi-tech, Watertown, MA) was used, and a 30 mm in diameter monofoil balloon catheter was used in the next 16. In the last 6 cases, the time of dilation was increased to 20 min.

With regard to the endoscopic study, we carried out a urethrocystoscopy before the procedure in all patients, as required by the protocol, with the intention of excluding those in whom prostate morphology showed a predominance of the middle lobe. Among them, we obtained graphic endoscopic documentation in 10 patients (in 8 patients, photographic series, and in 2 patients, video). After the procedure, we carried out endoscopic assessment in 8 patients (in 6, photographs, and in the 2 others, video). In 1 of the 8 patients, the study was performed at 6 months and 2 years after the procedure, and in the rest at 48 h after the dilation, immediately after the uroflow control. Two of these patients (Cases 11 and 13) were reassessed endoscopically at about 1 year after the dilation, with the purpose of performing a TURP, since they had not improved with this method. All the images were obtained through a Storz Hopkins II type cystourethroscope (O °). In all of them, antibiotic prophylaxis was used.

RESULTS

All the patients showed, despite local anesthesia, an instantaneous pain at maximal distention of the balloon, which immediately became tolerable, and no further measures were required.

There were no important complications. The hematuria that usually appears on ending the dilation subsided spontaneously with withdrawal of the bladder drainage catheter 24 h postprocedure. Only 2 patients had infectious episodes, which were not significant, an epididymitis and a urinary infection coinciding with the expulsion of a previously known ureteral calculus.

Three patients died of causes that were not related to the procedure or to the underlying prostatic pathology. Two died of cardiac failure 4 and 6 months after dilation, and 1 died of lung cancer 4 months after dilation. Two more patients have been lost to follow-up, although we know that 1 patient's subjective opinion is that he urinates well. In 2 other patients, the obstructive syndrome did not improve, and they had to be operated for their BPH by TUR. These patients are included only for follow-up purposes until their last visit before death, loss, or TUR (Fig. 15–3).

The clinical evolution of micturitional function, demonstrating the difference before and after application of the procedure with regard to difficulty and frequency, is shown in Figure 15–4.

To determine changes in dysuria or micturitional difficulty (Fig. 15–4A), we established four grades: 0, normal micturition without any feeling of difficulty; 1, mild micturitional difficulty; 2, severe micturitional difficulty; 3, complete retention. All the patients showed improvement in degree of dysuria, except that 2 patients who had been grade 1 reverted to grade 0 (normal micturition). Except for the 2 patients mentioned previously who underwent a TURP, the rest of the 17 patients (65.3%) with grade 2 dysuria improved as follows: 11 reverted to mild difficulty (grade 1) and 4 to complete normality (grade 0). The 6 patients (23%) who were in complete retention (grade 3) before the procedure improved to different grades, all of them overcoming the situation of urine retention. With regard to pollakiuria, or increase in the urinary frequency (Fig. 15–4 B), we also established a grading system: grade 0, normal micturitional frequency; grade 1, nocturnal urinary frequency one or two times; grade 2, nocturia two to four times; grade 3, nocturia more than four times. All the patients, except 3 who showed no changes, improved their nocturnal urinary frequency. All 20 patients who originally had grade 3 frequency showed an improvement. Five of them reverted to completely normal micturitional frequency in the last follow-up.

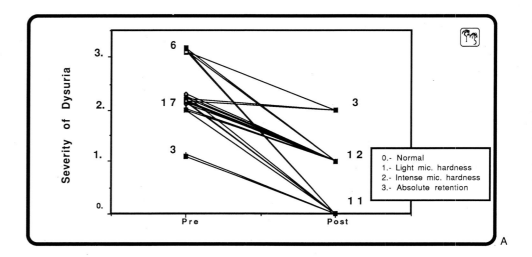

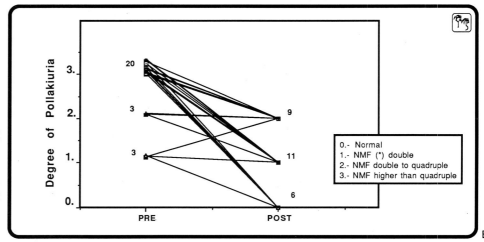

Figure 15–4. Effect of procedure on urinary symptoms. **A.** Difficulty of urination; 0, none; 1, slight difficulty; 2, intense difficulty; 3, retention. **B.** Changes in nocturnal urinary frequency. O, usually no arising at night; 1, one or two times per night; 2, two to four times per night; 3, more than four times per night.

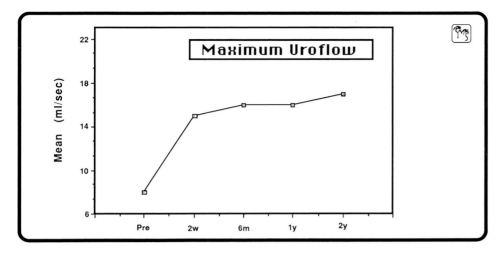

Figure 15–5. Average peak uroflow in relation to time since the procedure.

The uroflow and residual volume, objective clinical measures of micturition determined before treatment and in subsequent follow-up, are shown in Figures 15–5 and 15–6. To quantify them, we used peak flow rates ($\dot{Q}$ max), giving a value of 0 in cases of complete urinary retention. Likewise, to analyze the results of bladder residual volume determinations, we arbitrarily established a value of 300 mL of urine (the approximate capacity of the normal bladder) if the patients required an indwelling bladder catheter for complete urinary retention.

As Figure 15–5 shows, the baseline uroflow showed severe obstruction (8 mL/sec) in the control before the procedure, but a significant improvement was noted, which persisted and remained stabilized from the second week to the second year follow-up.

Average postvoiding residual volumes in subsequent controls show a clear tendency to diminish (Fig. 15–6), which also remained stabilized until the second year follow-up.

In assessing the final clinical situation at the time of the last follow-up in each patient and taking into account not only the evolution of the symptoms and clinical measures described but also the urgency, daily micturitional frequency, and, above all, the patient's subjective feeling of improvement, we have found the following results (Fig. 15–7): 63.3% were significantly improved, 23.0% manifested an appreciable improvement, only 11.5% did not experience a noticeable change, and no patient suffered a deterioration of micturition function as a result of balloon prostatic dilation.

The first postprocedural endoscopic study was performed six months after the procedure in our first patient. It showed a curious image at the level of the bladder neck that looked very wide, with alterations in its margins that we attributed to tears that had reepithelialized caused by the balloon dilation. Among the morphologic changes that could be appreciated at the neck, a deep fissure was highlighted at around 11 o'clock and a lesser one at about 2 o'clock (Fig. 15–8A). When withdrawing the cystoscope, we observed that the deep fissure continued distally to the point where we were able to see both lateral lobes (Fig. 15–8B) and disappeared more distally at the level of the maximum prominence of the

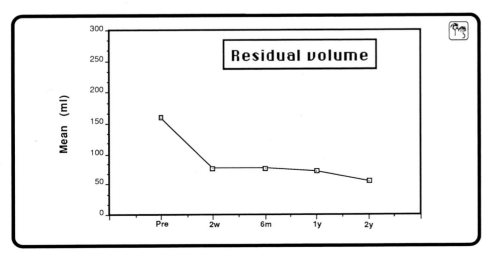

Figure 15–6. Average residual volume in relation to time since the procedure.

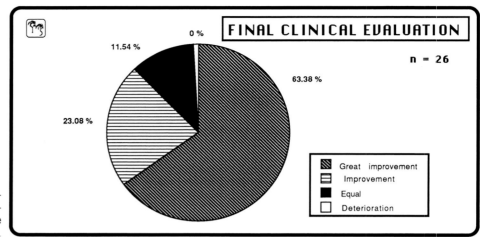

Figure 15–7. Final clinical evaluation, considering objective parameters and subjective sensations at the time of last follow-up in each patient.

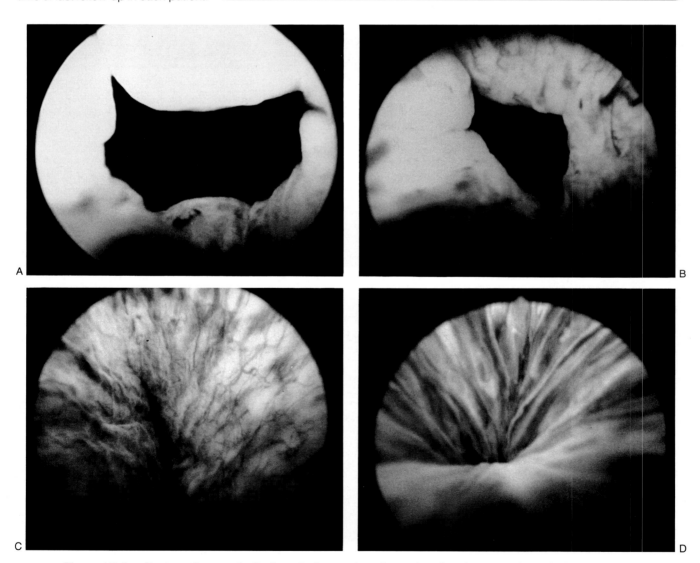

Figure 15–8. Cystourethroscopic findings in first patient 6 months after the procedure. **A.** Bladder neck region. **B.** View more distally in prostatic urethra. **C.** View even more distally in prostatic urethra: lateral fissures are no longer visible. **D.** Complete closure at the membranous urethra, proving intact function of the external sphincter.

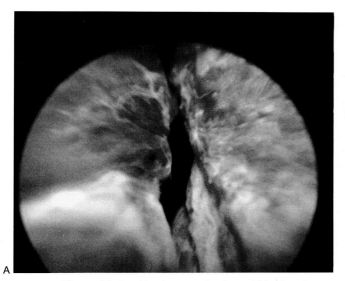
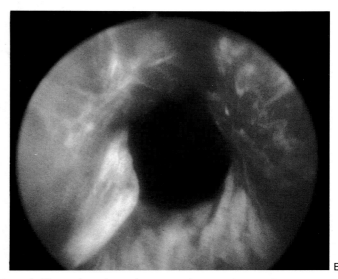

A   B

Figure 15–9. Urethroscopic views 48 h after the procedure. **A.** Disruption of anterior prostatic commissure. **B.** Another patient shows disruption of anterior commissure as well as significant increase in the caliber of the prostatic urethra.

prostatic lateral lobes (Fig. 15–8C). The lateral lobes did not show any changes relative to the preprocedure appearance except that they appeared to be easily separated by the pressure of the irrigating fluid. Finally, at the level of the membranous urethra, we could see perfect closure of the external sphincter without any kind of postdilation effect (Fig. 15–8D). We have noted the persistence of those same endoscopic findings 2 years after the procedure.

In the rest of the patients, when all images were obtained 48 h after the procedure, the finding was, in all cases, disruption of the anterior prostatic commissure (at 12 o'clock H), especially proximal to the neck (Fig. 15–9A, B). In 2 cases, we observed that the posterior prostatic commissure was also disrupted at 6 o'clock (Fig. 15–10). As we were withdrawing the urethroscope so that we could completely examine the prostatic lateral lobes, we observed that at this level, we could note almost no difference between the predilation and postdilation images (Fig. 15–11A, B) except for an extremely small erosion in the anterior commissures and the impression of a separation of the lobes with infusion of the irrigating fluid. The verumontanum showed no alterations (Fig. 15–11C).

The lacerations of the anterior interlobular commissures were much deeper in 2 cases, constituting true tears (case 6, Fig. 15–12, and case 12, Fig. 15–13A, B). In both patients, the results were very good. The bleeding at 48 h was minimal, as demonstrated by the excellent images obtained in almost all cases. Occasionally, a vessel with active bleeding at the level of the tear could be seen (Fig. 15–14).

In no case did performance of the endoscopic study increase the hemorrhage or cause urinary infection. In the 2 patients who had to undergo a TURP of the adenoma, since they did not manifest any improvement after the procedure,

endoscopic observation during surgery did not show any difference with respect to the previous endoscopic control, performed approximately 1 year earlier.

DISCUSSION

When comparing the surgical modalities for BPH, either open surgery or TURP, with any other alternative treatment, we have to be very cautious. No other present method can, with the safety and efficacy of the current surgical modalities, completely and definitively resolve the obstructive

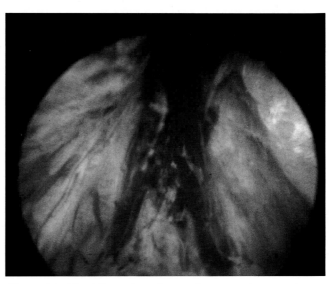

Figure 15–10. Disruption of posterior prostatic commissure seen 48 h after procedure.

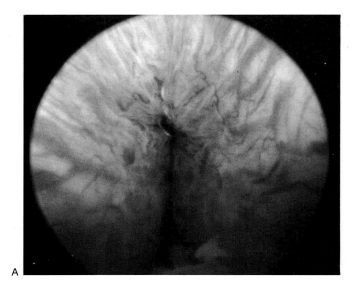

A

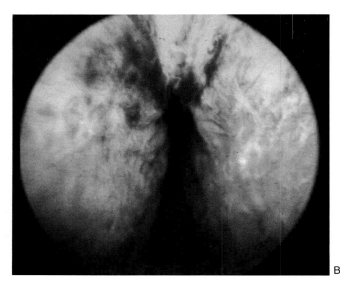

B

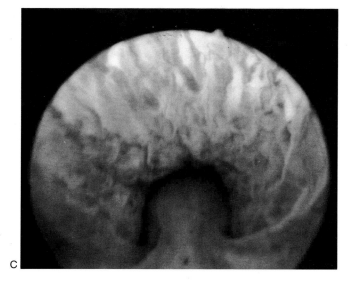

C

Figure 15–11. Urethroscopic views before and after procedure in tenth patient in our series. **A.** Preprocedural view shows moderate obstruction secondary to benign prostatic hyperplasia. **B.** View 48 h after the procedure shows no appreciable change. **C.** View at the level of the verumontanum also shows no alterations.

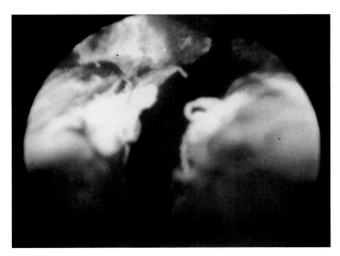

Figure 15–12.   Very deep tears seen 48 h after procedure in sixth patient in our series. Clinically, the patient did extremely well.

lower tract uropathy by removing the pathologic tissue while respecting the nearby anatomic structures and the sphincteric mechanisms.

This is probably the reason why very old methods, such as the prostatic incision of Bottini[9] or the prostatic dilation of Deisting,[6] in spite of their demostable efficacy and low risk, fell into disuse rapidly. This was so especially after 1950, when TURP was developed and spread rapidly as the surgical modality of choice in patients with BPH, even those with a

risky general physical condition. On the basis of our limited experience, the results obtained allow us to make the following points.

In the first place, no deaths were encountered with this procedure, whereas the mortality rate is around 2% for open surgery[10] and around 1% for the best TURP statistics.[11]

All patients tolerated the procedure well with local anesthesia, and there were no complications. Of importance is the degree of hematuria, which can be of concern at the time of withdrawal of the dilation catheter but which diminishes significantly in intensity, stopping completely in a few hours in the majority of cases. This good tolerance of the procedure reduces the trauma of treatment and allows this technique to be considered for use in an ambulatory setting.

It is important to mention that in the 2 patients in whom infection developed subsequently, only the epididymitis was attributable to the procedure, and this subsided easily without sequelae. Epididymitis is a frequent complication of prostatic surgery, 6%–19% of the cases in the absence of prophylactic vasectomy.[10] Curiously, Castañeda does not mention any case of epididymitis in his review of the 150 cases treated in the University of Minnesota with this procedure.[12]

Of all the possible complications associated with prostatic surgery, such as hemorrhage with systemic repercussion, phlebitis, incontinence, or delayed urethral stenosis or sclerosis of the vesical neck, none has been detected up to the present in the current series. A much longer follow-up, as well as a larger number of procedures, is necessary to document that no bladder neck stenosis will occur. This

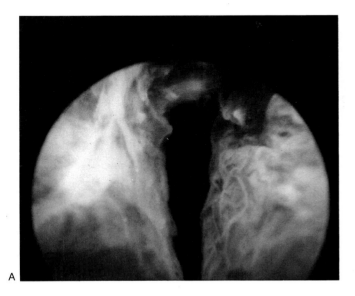

A

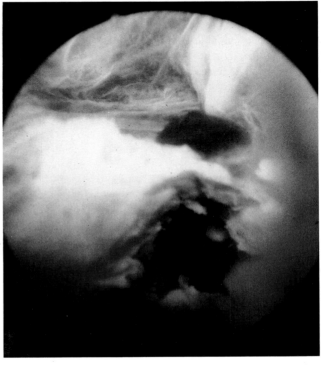

B

Figure 15–13.   The twelfth patient in the series, with extensive tears. **A.** Both commissures are affected. **B.** Areas of prostatic tissue laceration with deep tears in other areas. The clinical results were excellent.

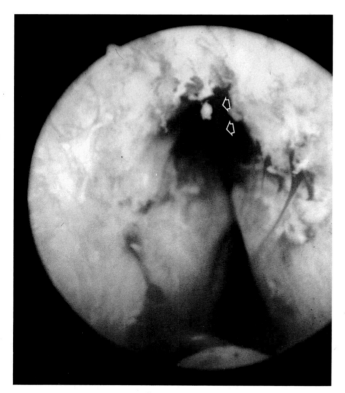

Figure 15–14. Immediately after the procedure, active bleeding (arrows) is visible at the site of the tear. Bleeding subsided after placement of a drainage catheter.

complication, although not very frequent in surgery (1.3%[10]), is important because of its tendency to recur independent of the method used for its resolution. The absence of urethral stenosis, present in other surgical methods,[7] can be explained by the softness of the modern materials utilized in the balloon catheter of Castañeda, by the cleanliness of the technique, always performed under radiologic control, and also by withdrawal of the indwelling bladder catheter in the first 24 h.

The ease with which the technique is executed and the absence of complications encourage us to consider repeating this method as many times as we would determine it to be necessary.

With regard to the efficacy of this procedure to resolve obstructive uropathy, the results are sufficiently significant to encourage further use. In all cases except 3, there was an improvement in dysuria and pollakiuria (Fig. 15–4). The mean peak flows in all patients stabilized within normal limits, and there was a significant and clear tendency to resolution of the bladder residual volume. Above all, we can confirm that these improvements persist in the second year follow-up (Fig. 15–5, 15–6). In the final clinical evaluation obtained from each patient during the last follow-up and, therefore, with different times of follow-up (Fig. 15–3), where we considered both objective clinical measures and

the subjective opinion of the patient, we observed that 63.3% of the patients manifested a significant improvement in micturition function, and in no instance was a detriment found (Fig. 15–7). However, we must not forget that this does not mean that no obstruction persists, which is the case in the majority because the BPH tissue remains. This is not the case in surgery, and only a longer follow-up will tell us how long it will take for recurrence of symptomatology.

More in favor of the procedure is the fact that it was performed in the majority of cases as a palliative alternative because of the significant surgical risk to the patients due to their age or associated pathologic conditions.

If we compare this technique with other palliative methods for the treatment of BPH, such as cryosurgery[13] or the spiral endoprosthesis of Fabian,[14] we can postulate a much superior advantage with this procedure. Cryosurgery has a mortality rate of 3%.[15] Patients are subjected to an indwelling catheter for 15–21 days after the procedure, and there is a high incidence of infections that are difficult to eradicate because of the presence of prostatic necrotic tissue. The Fabian prothesis is a foreign body lodged in the prostatic urethra, and there are great possibilities of dislodgment, calcific incrustation, smoldering infections, and urethral erosion.

After analyzing the endoscopic findings obtained after balloon dilation of the prostatic urethra, it is possible to make several statements about the mechanism of action of this procedure that are closely related to the reasoning explained in the introduction.

First, we have not found any sign suggesting that the mechanism is related to a possible tissue ischemia and subsequent atrophy of the tissue against its capsule during maximal distention of the balloon for a long period of time, as suggested by preliminary ultrasound and MRI studies.[4] On the contrary, the endoscopic picture of the hyperplastic prostatic tissue is the same at 48 h as at 6 months after dilation. The only alterations observed are those already described and acute inflammatory changes of the mucosa that covers the BPH secondary to any instrument manipulations. Neither the rectal examination nor our own ultrasound observations indicated changes that would support an ischemic/atrophic physiopathologic mechanism. The anatomopathologic result in the 2 patients who had TURP approximately 1 year after the procedure did not show any lesion or histologic alteration different from any other sample of BPH. Therefore, we consider that the supposed histologic signs of vascular thrombosis and subsequent fibrous retractions, as we had already assumed, do not occur in the prostate after application of the dilation balloon.

We have not observed endoscopically any changes that might be judged as the permanent consequences of an axial dilation of the prostatic obstruction. The great elasticity of the prostatic tissue permits its morphologic restoration once strong compression of the tissue by the balloon ceases. It is possible, however, that a sufficiently ample dilation, in regard to caliber and pressure, could cause a stretching and loosening of the external prostatic capsule (or true prostate). We think that this could be a very important mechanism to explain the efficacy of the procedure. In essence, the endoscopic findings show the following mechanism.

1. Disruption or laceration of the prostatic commissures, especially the anterior, in the sagittal plane, particularly at the proximal aspect of the vesical neck. With this rupture, the opening of the bladder neck is accomplished, and there is a breakage of the fibers that join the prostatic lobes.
2. Distention of the prostatic capsule, producing stretching that is more or less permanent. This permits the lateral prostatic lobes, already freed from one another by rupture of the interlobular fibers during the increase in the interbladder pressures, to separate to a greater extent because they are contained in a less restrictive space by the loosening of the prostatic capsule.
3. Maintenance of the external sphincter intact.

In fact, these findings correspond exactly to the mechanism of action reported by Aboulker and Steg[7] for prostatic dilation by transurethral metal instruments, such as the very old one described by Mercier and later modified by Deisting. However, in spite of this great similarity in the mechanism of action, at present we see advantages to the Castañeda procedure, based on the fact that this method shows an absence of morbidity and mortality in Castañeda's results and our own results in this series.

In contrast, the complications reported in the literature with Deisting's instrument are not so benign. The hemorrhages are significant, requiring transfusion. Some patients developed permanent urinary incontinence, and there was a significant mortality rate. We attribute the absence of complications with the Castañeda procedure in the first place to the design of the instrument, which permits dilation of the entire prostatic urethra while preserving the urethral caliber at the level of external sphincter, and to the added safety provided by maintaining the correct position of the balloon throughout the procedure by means of radiographic control. Second, the tissues receive better treatment with a flexible instrument made of plastic, which is much softer than the metal instruments.

Accepting these mechanisms as the explanation for the endoscopic findings and the clinical results obtained using Castañeda's balloon catheter, we suggest some simple modifications in the design of the balloon and in the procedure itself. (1) Increasing the diameter of the balloon up to 45–50 mm to create deeper disruptions of the prostatic commissures, which achieved good clinical results when viewed endoscopically. This balloon diameter means a circumference of approximately 14–16 cm, corresponding more or less to the capsular perimeter obtained with the Deisting divulsor at maximal distention, with the metal branches 7–8 cm apart. (2) Increasing the length of the balloon by approximately 2

cm to avoid the need to repeat the dilation in very large prostates and to be able to cover the entire cervicoprostatic length. (3) Developing a balloon catheter that could withstand higher pressures (6 atm or more) without bursting. (4) Dilating for longer periods of time, with progressive sequential increases in the pressure (for instance, increase the time of distention to 20 min, starting with 3 atm and slowly increase by 1 atm each 5 min until reaching maximum distention). We believe that we were able to achieve greater stretching of the prostatic capsule using these variations of the procedure because one of the most important mechanisms for reducing obstruction is allowing the prostatic lobes to spread out in a larger space.

The mechanism of action of the Castañeda balloon catheter suggests that its use could be expanded to other types of obstructive pathologies at the level of cervicoprostatic urethra, such as stenosis or hypertrophy of the bladder neck, postsurgical diaphragmatic sclerosis of the bladder neck, and postsurgical sclerosis of the prostatic compartment. This method could be tried in patients with functional dysuria, in whom it could be speculated that prostatic capsular distention might cause some change in the sensitive nerve fibers, perhaps producing some benefit in a condition that can be very difficult to interpret and treat. It is interesting that improvement in polyuria has been proportionally much more evident than improvement in any other symptom. This observation has been more obvious as we work with more patients. Almost as a rule, they insist on pointing out this aspect of their clinical improvement. This suggests to us that we can include possible changes at the level of the nerve endings related to the prostatic capsule as another mechanism of action accompanying disruption of the BPH commissures and the distention of the prostatic capsule. We hope these results can be confirmed in larger series, with longer follow-ups.

It will be necessary to corroborate the effects of this technique in large BPHs, which up to now we have avoided, and confirm whether in cases of predominant middle lobe enlargement results can always be expected to be poor.

In the intense search for alternative methods to prostatic surgery, both old and innovative ones, this method of balloon prostatic divulsion will always deserve consideration. It can be offered as a first step, if not permanent, to most of the patients with obstructive prostatic syndrome.

TERMINOLOGY

Throughout this and another works,[8,16,17] we have used indiscriminately the terms *prostatic dilation, prostatic urethroplasty,* and *prostatic divulsion* or *prostatodivulsion*. We have even read somewhere the word *avulsion* referring to this technique. However, *avulsion* signifies extraction or removal of a part of an organ, which means it does not fit here, since no extraction of tissue takes place. *Dilation* can be instrumentation to increase or reestablish the caliber of an aperture or conduit, and in a sense, it could be used here, but then we should say, *prostatic urethral dilation,* because *prostatic dilation* would not be understood in this context. The suffix—*plasty* indicates artificial neoformation. Therefore, *prostatic urethroplasty* would be equivalent of plastic surgery of the prostatic urethra, which is not the case. Finally, *divulsion* translates the idea of separation or forceful and violent dilation. After having seen the images of the tears of the prostatic commissures, silently and violently caused by balloon distention, we think that the most proper term for this technique is *prostatic divulsion* or *prostatodivulsion* with balloon catheter, which we will use from now on. This is why we use this term in the chapter title and think it should be applied to denominate this type of technique.

REFERENCES

1. Walsh PC. Benign prostatic hyperplasia. In: *Campbell's Urology.* Philadelphia: W.B. Saunders Co., 1978;2:949–964
2. Castañeda F, Lund G, Larson BW, et al. Prostatic urethra: experimental dilatation in dogs. *Radiology* 1987;163:645–648
3. Castañeda F, Reddy P, Wasserman N, et al. Benign prostatic hypertrophy: retrograde transurethral dilatation of the prostatic urethra in humans. Work in progress. *Radiology* 1987;163:649–653
4. Johnson SD, Kuni CC, Castañeda F, Castañeda-Zúñiga WR, Hunter DW, Amplatz K. Magnetic resonance imaging of patients undergoing prostatic balloon dilatation. Paper presented at annual meeting of Radiological Society of North America, Chicago, 1987
5. Castañeda F, Isorna S, Hulbert JC, et al. The importance of separation of prostatic lobes in relief of prostatic obstruction by balloon catheter urethroplasty: studies in dogs and humans. *AJR* 1989;153:1301–1304
6. Deisting W. Transurethral dilatation of the prostate. A new method in the treatment of prostatic hypertrophy. *Urol Int.* 1956;2:158–171
7. Aboulker P, Steg A. La divulsion de la prostate. D'après 218 observations personnelles. *J Urol Nephrol* 1964;70:337–364
8. Isorna S, Maynar M, Belón JL, Pulido JM, Martell R, Nogueira JAF, Castañeda F. Prostatic urethroplasty. Endoscopic findings. *Semin Intervent Radiol* 1989;6:46–56
9. Bottini, noted by Legueu. In: *Tratado Médico Quirúrgico de las vías urinarias.* Barcelona: Salvat Editores, 1927;2:345–348
10. Whitehead ED, Leiter E. Surgical treatment of benign prostatic hypertrophy. In: *Current Operative Urology.* Philadelphia: Harper & Row, 1984
11. Reuter HJ. Urologische Operatioslehre. Transurethrale Operationen. In: Heise GW, Hienzsche, Mebel M, Krebs W (eds) *Allemeine and Spezielle Urologie.* Leipzig: VEB Thieme, 1977, Vol. 6
12. Castañeda F. Prostatic urethroplasty. Complications. *Semin Intervent Radiol* 1989;6:79–81
13. Reuter HJ. Endoscopic cryosurgery of prostate and bladder tumors. *J Urol* 1972;107:389
14. Garbit JL, Blitz M. La prothèse endoprostathique spirale de Fabian. *J Urol* 1988;94:5–6
15. Soanes WA, Gonder MJ. Cryosurgery in benign and malignant diseases of the prostate. In: Whitehead ED, Leiter E (eds). *Current Operative Urology,* 2nd ed. Philadelphia: Harper and Row, 1984
16. Maynar M, Isorna S, Reyes R, Pulido JM, Belón J, Baldó C, Pérez MA, Castaneda F. Nueva técnica de uretroplastia prostática con catéter de Balón. Estudio preliminar. *Radiología* 1988;30:345–349
17. Isorna S, Maynar M, Belón J, Pulido-Duque JM, Déniz F, Reyes R, Nogueira JAF. Prostatic urethroplasty results. Spanish experience. *Semin Intervent Radio* 1989;6:72–79

16

Transurethral Balloon Dilation: University of Iowa Experience

*Howard N. Winfield, Flavio Castañeda,
Kathy Richardson*

Based on preliminary work performed by interventional radiologists, transurethral balloon dilation of the prostate has been employed since 1987 for the management of clinically obstructive benign prostatic hyperplasia (BPH).[1-3] It has captured the interest of all urologic surgeons and has engendered considerable debate on its effectiveness in treating symptomatic BPH. Recent American Urological Association national meetings have held symposiums questioning the true value of balloon dilation as well as the long-term effects of the procedure. To date, there have been a minimal number of articles discussing the subject of balloon dilation of the prostate that have been accepted by reputable peer review journals.[4,5] The reason for this paucity of studies is the fact that the number of patients in these reports is limited, and the postoperative follow-up has been short. The studies have not been randomized and never had a control arm. An interesting double-blind randomized study on 30 men was reported by Sypherd et al., comparing balloon dilation of the prostate to simple placement of the balloon without inflation. There apparently was no difference in objective or subjective results.[6]

One fact that has become clear in evaluating the effectiveness of balloon dilation of the prostate is how little we understand about the natural history of BPH. Furthermore, we also realize that the investigator is somewhat limited in the degree to which prostatic obstruction and treatment results can be objectively evaluated. Considerable data accumulated on BPH are very subjective on the part of both the patient and the surgeon. It also appears that what may be most important as a determinant of success or failure following balloon dilation is how the patient thinks he feels. All clinicians who have performed balloon dilation of the prostate are aware of patients who objectively show no significant improvement in flow rates, postvoid residual urine measurements, or other urodynamic parameters. However, subjectively, they emphasize that there is a marked improvement. This certainly could be a placebo effect. It has been shown in double-blind clinical investigations evaluating the effectiveness of pharmacotherapy that the placebo effect may account for up to 35%–50% improvement.[7] Therefore, until the literature has clarified these issues and our own results demonstrate that balloon dilation is truly effective in treating symptomatic BPH, we will continue to view this procedure as investigational. The objective of this chapter is to discuss our approach to and results following balloon dilation of the prostate and to draw some final conclusions.

MATERIALS AND METHODS

Since balloon dilation of the prostate is still considered an investigational procedure, our evaluation of the potential candidate is more extensive than what would be required for a routine BPH patient undergoing transurethral resection.

All patients undergo a complete history and physical examination. A symptom questionnaire is obtained to quantify the degree of obstructive and irritative components of the prostatism (Table 16–1). Patients with marked irritative symptoms would most likely undergo urodynamic evaluation, and urine is obtained for cytologic studies. A rectal examination suggestive of cancer of the prostate would require full investigation in the form of transrectal ultrasound, biopsy and blood prostatic enzymes (prostate-specific antigen and prostatic acid phosphatase).

Urinalysis and culture are routine before any instrumentation. The presence of microhematuria would require more

Table 16–1. Symptom Score Analysis of Prostatism

OBSTRUCTIVE SYMPTOMS	SCORE (MAXIMUM 18)	IRRITATIVE SYMPTOMS	SCORE (MAXIMUM 10)
Size of urinary stream		Urge	
Normal	0	None	0
Variable	1	Mild	1
Weak	3	Moderate	2
Dribbling	4	Severe	3
Force of urinary stream		Diuria	
No strain to void	0	Once every 3–4 h	0
Occasional strain to void	1	Once every 2–3 h	1
Always strain to void	2	Once every 1–2 h	2
Hesitancy of urination		Every hour	3
No	0	Nocturia	
Yes	3	0–1	0
Bladder emptying		2	1
Complete	0	3–4	2
Variable	1	>4	3
Incomplete	2	Dysuria	
Retention	3	No	0
Postvoid dribbling		Yes	1
No	0		
Moderate	2		
Severe	3		
Intermittency			
No	0		
Yes	3		

extensive investigation of the upper urinary tracts, and glucosuria may suggest diabetes mellitus.

Uroflowmetry is performed on all patients. It is necessary that the voided volume be greater than 125 mL in order to obtain an interpretable result. Mean and peak uroflow and the shape of the voiding curve are analyzed. Peak urinary flow greater than 15 mL/sec would suggest that prostatic obstruction is not the problem.[8] Following the uroflowmetry, residual urine is measured by means of Foley catheterization or transabdominal ultrasound. Patients who persistently carry a residual urine greater than 400–500 mL require further urodynamic evaluation to rule out a hypotonic bladder. Obviously, patients with significant detrusor muscle insufficiency will not benefit greatly by any form of corrective bladder outlet surgery.

Upper tract imaging in the form of intravenous pyelography or renal ultrasound is performed in patients with a history of urinary tract infections, urolithiasis, or other urologic abnormalities. The presence of microhematuria or pyuria also warrants these tests. In the otherwise healthy male, upper tract radiologic studies are not performed, since the chance of finding a significant abnormality is low and does not justify the cost of screening all men with BPH.[9]

Cystourethroscopy is a key test in evaluating candidates for balloon dilation of the prostate. Patients with urethral strictures that will not accept a 17 F cystoscope are not eligible for dilation of the prostate. Those with a significant median or subcervical lobe of the prostate are also ineligible.

These patients are not expected to have successful dilation. Bladder calculi or tumors require other forms of treatment. Patients with predominantly lateral lobes of the prostate are good candidates. The length of the prostatic urethra is measured as a means of assessing the prostate size.

Since the effect of transurethral balloon dilation of the prostate that may harbor carcinoma is unknown and that tissue is not obtained with this procedure, we feel that all methods to rule out malignancy should be incorporated. Therefore, prostatic enzymes (PSA and PAP) are obtained, as well as transrectal ultrasound of the prostate on all patients. The latter procedure also allows another volume measurement of the prostate in addition to the rectal and cystoscopic examinations. Prostatic biopsies are obtained only if there is suggestion of cancer of the prostate.

As a general rule, complete urodynamic evaluation in the form of cystometrogram, urethral pressure profile, pressure–flow studies, and video urodynamics is not performed unless there is a significant irritative component to the symptomatology or a suggestion of a neurogenic bladder disorder or if the patient is less than 55 years of age.

If the patient with BPH has the tests as described and is still a candidate for balloon dilation of the prostate, he undergoes the usual preoperative evaluation that is required for all operative patients. General blood tests, prothrombin and partial thrombin clotting times, electrocardiogram, and chest x-ray are obtained. All patients are seen by an anesthesiologist before the operative date. Patients are fully informed about the potential risks and complications of this new procedure.

The procedure is performed under intravenous sedation, with fentanyl citrate supplemented with midazolam or meperidine administered by an anesthesiologist. A broad-spectrum cephalosporin is administered intravenously 1 h before the procedure. The patient is placed in the dorsolithotomy position, and 2% lidocaine jelly is instilled into the urethra for local anesthesia. The balloon catheter is positioned by either a cystoscopic or a fluoroscopic technique.

FLUOROSCOPIC TECHNIQUE

With the patient in the dorsolithotomy position with a 30-degree tilt of the pelvis, a cystoscope is passed into the anterior urethra up to the level of the external urethral sphincter. It is then advanced through the external sphincter, stopping just distal to the verumontanum. A 22 gauge spinal needle is placed under the skin in the suprapubic region so that fluoroscopically it would superimpose over the tip of the cystoscope. The cystoscope is advanced through the prostatic urethra and then positioned at the bladder neck region. Fluoroscopy allows an assessment of the prostatic urethral length from the needle positioned almost at the level of the external sphincter to the tip of the cystoscope situated at the bladder neck. One must be aware of the expected 10% magnification that occurs with radiologic measurements. A 0.038 inch Amplatz super stiff guidewire is passed through the cystoscope into the bladder. The cystoscope is then removed.

A retrograde urethrogram is performed confirming the position of the external urethral sphincter that previously had been located cystoscopically. The high-pressure inflation balloon catheter (Microvasive Inc., Watertown, MA, and Cook Inc.) is passed over the previously placed guidewire and positioned in the prostatic urethra. The catheter's distal radiopaque marker should superimpose fluoroscopically over the needle positioned just proximal to the external sphincter. The balloon is slowly inflated with half-strength contrast media to 4 atm of pressure and held here for 10 min. The balloon has a tendency to migrate into the bladder, and, thus, the operator must hold constant tension, pulling outward to maintain the correct position. Once the balloon is fully inflated, it tends to seat itself well into the prostatic fossa, and little or no backpull is required. With the dilation, an initial waist is visualized fluoroscopically in the prostatic urethra, which should disappear with full inflation. Depending on the size of balloon utilized, the prostatic urethra may be stretched to 75 F (25 mm) or 90 F (30 mm).

After 10 min of full balloon dilation, the balloon is deflated and removed using a twisting maneuver. Unfortunately, the balloons utilized in this study by the fluoroscopic technique did not collapse smoothly and may have caused some tearing of the urethra on removal. A retrograde urethro-

gram is repeated, which hopefully will demonstrate significant dilation and widening of the prostatic urethra. Repeat cystourethroscopy is performed to visually identify the prostatic dilation and any tearing or splitting of the anterior or posterior prostatic commissures. A 20 F Foley catheter is placed for overnight drainage. All blood clots are irrigated out of the bladder prior to leaving the operating room.

CYSTOSCOPIC TECHNIQUE

In the last 13 patients, we have utilized the cystoscopic approach to placement of the balloon catheter. This technique was designed by Advanced Surgical Intervention, Inc., San Clemente, CA. This technique utilizes a specific measuring catheter that determines the length of the prostatic urethra from the bladder neck to the external sphincter. Then a chosen balloon catheter length (25–45 mm) is positioned cystoscopically in the prostatic urethra. The balloon is inflated to 3 atm of pressure (45 psi) for 10 min. Radiologic monitoring is not required. The catheter is removed through a sheath, thus eliminating the risk of urethral tearing. Cystoscopy is repeated to determine the degree of dilation and tearing of the commissures. A 20 F Foley catheter is again placed.

If the patient is feeling well and bleeding is not significant, he is discharged the same day and told to report back the following morning to remove the Foley catheter. All patients receive 3 days of an oral antibiotic known to be effective against typical urinary pathogens. The follow-up schedule is at 1, 3, 6, 12, 18, and 24 months. At these visits, repeat symptom score questionnaires are obtained, and rectal examinations are performed. A uroflow is performed, and a postvoid residual is measured by either Foley catheterization or transabdominal ultrasound. Prostatic enzymes (PSA and PAP) are obtained.

RESULTS

Transurethral balloon dilation of the prostate was initiated at the University of Iowa in June 1988. Since that time, this procedure has been performed on 50 patients. The average age is 68 years (range 50–84 years), and associated medical or surgical problems are listed in Table 16–2. As can be seen, these were not the healthiest patients but perhaps were more reflective of the age group affected by symptoms of prostatism. It was our belief that the vast majority of these patients would be capable of undergoing a TURP should this have been chosen and that they would be expected to live for longer than 1 year.

The average size of the prostate was 27.9 g (range 15–75 g) based on digital rectal examination and transrectal ultrasound examination. Based on cystourethroscopy, the average prostatic urethral length was 3.7 cm (range 2–6 cm). There were 11 patients in urinary retention prior to balloon

Table 16–2. Patient Medical & Surgical Problems

PROBLEM	PATIENTS
Coronary artery disease	20
Hypertension	14
Coronary artery bypass	11
Chronic obstructive pulmonary disease	11
Lung cancer	1
Peripheral vascular disease	10
Diabetes mellitus	11
Gastrointestinal disorders	6
Ca colon	2
Alcoholism	3
Myelodysplasia	1
Polycythemia vera	1
Pancreatitis	1
Seizure disorder	1
Gout	1

dilation. Of the patients not in retention, the predilation average and peak uroflow results were 4.5 mL/sec and 8.0 mL/sec, respectively. The average urine voided was 236 mL, and the postvoid residual was 266 mL.

Following dilation, patients were reevaluated with uroflowmetry and residual urine at 1, 3, 6, 12, 18, and 24 months. As can be seen in Figures 16–1 and 16–2, of the patients not in retention preoperatively, there was improvement in average and peak uroflow rates up to 6 months following dilation. However, by 12 months postdilation, the uroflow results were drifting back to the preoperative state. Average volume voided demonstrated no significant change from the predilation state (Fig. 16–3). Postvoid residual urine showed a favorable decrease for the first 6 months following dilation but then manifested an increase by 12 months (Fig. 16–4).

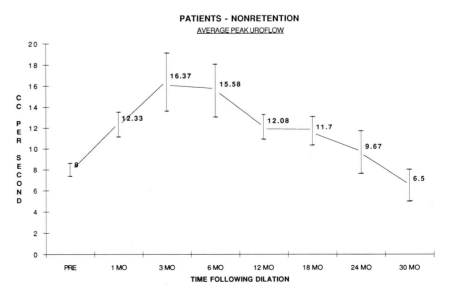

Figure 16–1.   Average uroflow rate of patients not in retention.

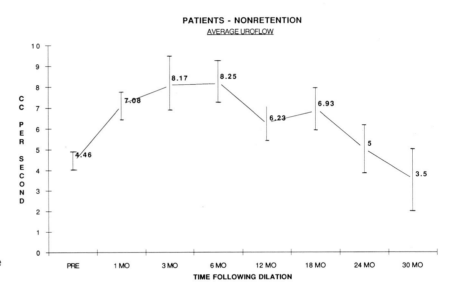

Figure 16–2.   Average peak uroflow rate of patients not in retention.

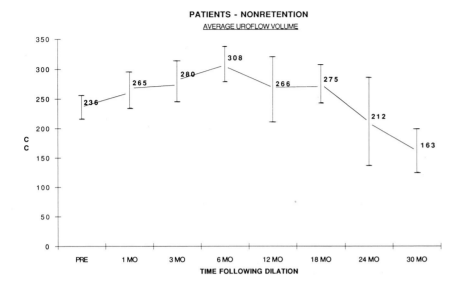

Figure 16–3. Average volume of urine voided in patients not in retention.

Of the patients in retention prior to dilation, there was a very good response in uroflow seen at 1 month, which fell off by 1 year (Figs. 16–5, 16–6). Despite the apparent improvement in uroflowmetry within the retention group, postvoid residual urine volumes showed an unacceptably high level. The result at 18 months is skewed by the small number of patients (Fig. 16–7). The voided volume (Fig. 16–8) combined with the postvoid residual urine volume (Fig. 16–7) would suggest that the patients in retention prior to dilation had large capacity bladders.

As described earlier, symptoms were separated into obstructive and irritative scores (Table 16–1). As can be seen in Figures 16–9 and 16–10, obstructive and irritative symptomatology diminished considerably in the first 6 months but began to increase as the 1 year point was obtained. It is difficult to establish significant differences on symptoms alone.

Patients were asked to fill out a global assessment of their urinary status following balloon dilation on a scale from 0 to 10. Those patients claiming 7–10 out of 10 were considered symptomatically "much better." Those reporting 3–6 out of 10 were "mildly better," whereas a score below 3 probably represented "no improvement or failure." As can be seen from Figure 16–11, more than 80% of the patients thought there had been "some improvement" up to 6 months following balloon dilation. By 12 months, the failure rate or return to predilation state appears to be increasing.

When one examines the characteristics of the 16 patients who failed initially, a few important findings become apparent. Of the 8 patients who subsequently underwent transurethral resection of the prostate, the average gland size was estimated to be 37 g, which is larger than the overall average. Cystoscopically, these men had significant prostatic obstruction and bladder trabeculation. Although it is solely our

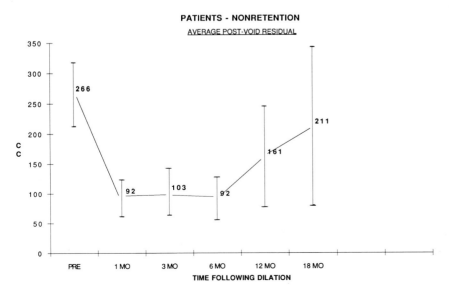

Figure 16–4. Average postvoid residual urine of patients not in retention.

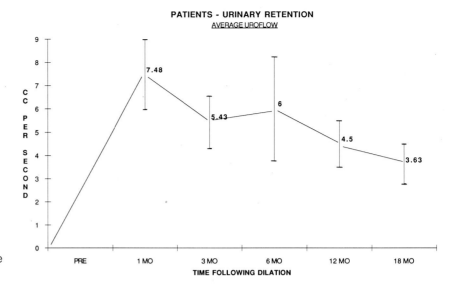

Figure 16–5. Average uroflow rate of patients in retention.

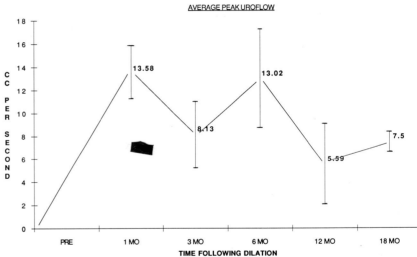

Figure 16–6. Average peak uroflow rate of patients in retention.

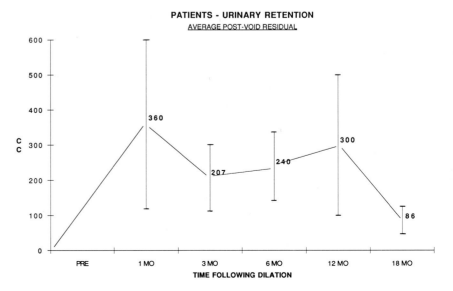

Figure 16–7. Average postvoid residual urine of patients in retention before dilation.

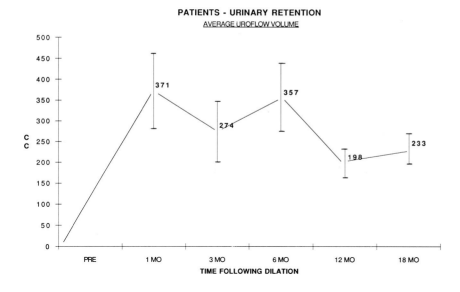

Figure 16–8. Average volume of urine voided in patients in retention.

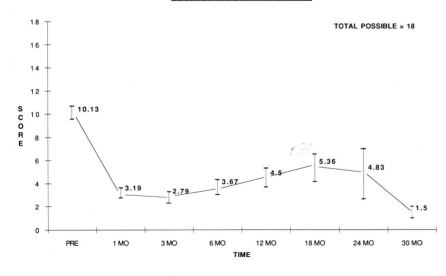

Figure 16–9. Obstructive symptom scores of patients undergoing balloon dilation of the prostate.

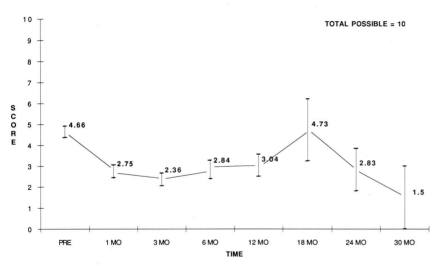

Figure 16–10. Irritative symptom scores of patients undergoing balloon dilation of the prostate.

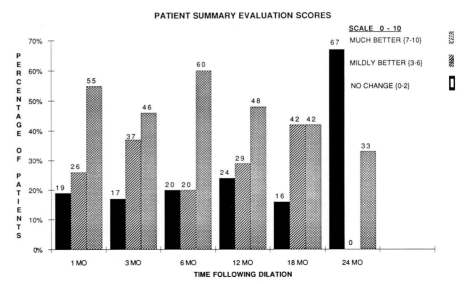

Figure 16–11. Patient summary evaluation scores—assessment of level of improvement.

impression, these prostates appeared more compliant and resilient to balloon dilation, suggesting a higher epithelial (glandular) component. Following dilation, there was very little or no widening of the prostatic urethra, with no evidence of splitting at the prostatic commissures. It is our impression that smaller prostates, with perhaps higher fibromuscular (stromal) component, tear more easily with dilation, resulting in improved results. Again, this is all theoretical and not based on scientific data at the present time.

There were 4 patients who failed and were managed by intermittent catheterization. These patients appeared to have more significant medical problems, and 2 had long-standing diabetes mellitus. There were 4 patients who subjectively claimed to have no improvement. It is unclear why these patients were not improved, since the procedure appeared technically successful. There was a question that perhaps there was a greater irritative component to their symptoms of prostatism, which was not borne out.

There were no significant long-term complications. One of the patients early in our series had stress incontinence and perineal discomfort, which lasted for 3 weeks and subsequently resolved. This was most likely a result of incorrect placement of the balloon across the external sphincter. Significant bleeding following dilation necessitated admission in 2 patients. These patients were found to have poorly controlled hypertension, and 1 had been on aspirin-containing medication up to 1 week prior to the procedure. They did not require any further surgical intervention other than continuous bladder irrigation. No blood transfusions were required. Two further patients required admission, 1 for postoperative nausea and vomiting and the other for significant tearing of the posterior prostatic urethra and bladder neck, with uplifting of the trigone. A Foley catheter was directed into the bladder and left in place for 5 days. This latter patient had been in urinary retention predilation and had a markedly improved uroflow even at 12 months follow-

ing the procedure. All other patients have been managed on an outpatient basis and generally have been able to have the Foley catheter removed within 24 h of the procedure.

Many of the patients who underwent transurethral balloon dilation of the prostate were impotent or had absence of ejaculation prior to the procedure. Of the patients who were potent or had ejaculatory ability prior to the procedure, all maintained these functions following dilation.

Prostatic enzymes were not evaluated immediately following balloon dilation. These values were not changed significantly at subsequent monthly follow-ups, as listed previously.

DISCUSSION

Transurethral balloon dilation of the prostate appears to be a very safe outpatient procedure tolerated well under intravenous sedation with local urethral anesthetic. These factors make it very attractive as a minimally invasive procedure, with potential financial advantages to both the patient and society. It appears to be a viable option for the younger patient who wishes to preserve his ejaculatory ability, and the frail patient with significant medical problems may be able to tolerate balloon dilation of the prostate but not transurethral resection.

On the negative side, however, transurethral balloon dilation does not work for everyone. It does not yield good results for a prostate size much greater than 30 g or if there is significant median lobe enlargement. There is a strong suggestion that the initial favorable results of balloon dilation diminish over ensuing months, only to return to baseline by 1 year. Obviously, if the patient requires a repeat dilation or proceeds to transurethral resection of the prostate, the savings in hospitalization days, convalescence period, and monetary costs may be negated and in fact greater than TURP alone. However, these negative statements should be tempered by the fact that there are patients who continue to show excellent improvement and are delighted with their voiding ability beyond 12 months. The challenge has been to consistently identify these patients preoperatively. In addition, patients who require temporary relief from urinary obstruction and bladder catheterization in order to recover from an orthopedic procedure or cardiopulmonary event may benefit significantly and be given sufficient time to tide them over until the time when a TURP may be feasible.

Results from other centers have been limited to date but seem to indicate similar trends of success or failure to ours.[4,5,10] Unfortunately, to date, no investigator has undertaken a large, randomized, double-blind study comparing balloon dilation to cystoscopy or transurethral resection. In addition, follow-up is less than 24 months in most studies, and a wide variety of balloon catheter sizes and configurations have been employed, with variations in placement techniques.

It is our belief that transurethral balloon dilation is a viable alternative option for the management of clinically significant BPH. However, it should be employed selectively, and it is the obligation of the urologist to fully inform the patient of the potential for failure and subsequent requirement of other forms of treatment.

REFERENCES

1. Burhenne HJ, Chisholm RJ, Quenville NF. Prostatic hyperplasia: radiologic intervention. *Radiology* 1984;152:655–657
2. Quinn SF, Dyer R, Smathers R, et al. Balloon dilation of the prostate urethra. *Radiology* 1985;157:57–58
3. Castañeda F, Lund G, Larson BW, et al. Prostatic urethra: experimental dilation in dogs. *Radiology* 1987;163:645–648
4. Klein L, Perez-Marrero RA, Bowers GW, et al. Transurethral cystoscopic balloon dilation of the prostate. *J Endourol* 1990;4:115–123
5. Goldenberg SL, Perez-Marrero RA, Lee LM, et al. Endoscopic balloon dilation of the prostate: early experience. *J Urol* 1990;144:83–88
6. Sypherd D, Derus J, Remynse L, Lepor H. A double-blind randomized study comparing the effectiveness of cystoscopy vs transurethral dilation of the prostate (TUDP). In: Proceedings of the 64th Annual Meeting of the North Central Urological Section. Colorado Springs, Colorado, October 21–27, 1990
7. Benson H, Epstein MD. The placebo effect. *JAMA* 1976;232:1225
8. Abrams PH. Prostatism and prostatectomy: the value of urine flow rate measurement in the preoperative assessment for operation. *J Urol* 1977;117:70–71
9. Bauer DL, Garrison RW, McRoberts JW. The health and cost implications of routine excretory urography before transurethral prostatectomy. *J Urol* 1980;123:386–389
10. Reddy PK, Wasserman N, Castañeda F, et al. Balloon dilation of the prostate for treatment of benign prostatic hyperplasia. *Urol Clin North Am* 1988;15:529–535

New Trends in Benign Prostatic Hypertrophy Treatment

17

Hyperthermia of Prostatic Diseases

M. Vandenbossche, C. C. Schulman

The first effect of heating tissue was described on cancer by Busch in 1866.[1] He related a case of a histologically proven sarcoma that disappeared completely following a febrile attack caused by erysipelas infection.[1] Tumor cells are more sensitive to heating than are normal cells when the temperature ranges between 42°C and 44°C. This is why hyperthermia may induce irreversible damage to malignant cells while leaving normal cells intact. It has been demonstrated that hyperthermia has a synergistic effect with radiotherapy and with various chemotherapeutic medications. The S-phase of the cell cycle is the most heat sensitive.[2–5] Probably the most important factor is defective heat dissipation by neoplastic tissue due to poor blood supply and a decreased vasodilation capacity of the neovascular bed in response to thermal load.[6] Hyperplastic prostatic elements probably react to overheating in the same way as neoplastic tissues, and the thermal damage induced is time and temperature dependent.[7,8] A dense, round cell mononuclear infiltration with macrophages, eosinophils, and leukocytes usually is seen, which is the indicator of an immune response.[9]

There are three methods of clinical hyperthermia: local, regional, and whole body hyperthermia, with a wide use of radiowaves and microwave frequencies. For the prostate, only local hyperthermia is suitable, with temperatures ranging from 42°C to 45°C. In some cases, cellular necrosis was described. Thermotherapy uses temperatures between 45°C and 55°C, causing necrosis of benign prostatic tissue.

DESCRIPTION OF AVAILABLE DEVICES

Several hyperthermia or thermotherapy devices are now available, and the majority uses microwaves to heat the prostate with either a transrectal or a transurethral probe. One device uses radiofrequency waves (Tables 17–1, 17–2).

Transrectal Devices

The first hyperthermia devices used a transrectal probe. The prostathermer (Biodan Medical Systems, Rehovot, Israel) heats the prostate using a transrectal applicator with a microwave emission of 915 MHz. There is a cooling system for the rectal wall, and a urethral catheter is placed during each treatment to monitor the temperature in the prostatic urethra. Multiple sessions are mandatory (e.g., six 1-h treatments given at weekly intervals[10]).

The Primus machine (Tecnomatix Medical, Antwerp, Belgium) consists of a transrectal 915 MHz microwave generator and a water-cooling system to cool the rectal wall. With this device, temperatures are estimated by computer and there is no urethral catheter to measure the temperature in the urethra. Multiple sessions are mandatory (10 sessions for 1 h each for 5 weeks[11]).

Transurethral Devices

The Thermex-II device (Direx, Technorex LTD, Petah-Tikva, Israel) is applied transurethrally. The generator is a microcomputer-controlled heating system that delivers a mixture of radiofrequency waves creating temperatures of 44.5°C–47°C in the urethra.

A 16 F Foley catheter is equipped with an antenna just beneath the balloon. This catheter is used for both heating and temperature measurement and also enables drainage of the bladder during treatment. Temperature measurements in the prostate were made in some cases using a thermosensor pushed transrectally in the prostate through a fine biopsy needle. It has been shown that when the temperature in the prostatic urethra is raised to 44°C, a temperature of 43°C can be registered as far as 20 mm from the urethra. The end of the

Table 17–1. BPH: Transurethral Hyperthermia Devices

	THERMEX-II/DIREX	BSD	PROSTATRON/TECHNOMED
Single session	Yes	No	Yes
Rectal probe	No	No	Yes
Simultaneous treatment	Yes	No	No
Cooling system	No	No	Yes
Wavelength	Radiofrequency Mixture of waves	915 MHz	1296 MHz

hyperthermic zone (42°C) was 22 mm from the urethra. The rectal temperature measured 38°C during treatment.[12] With this device, two patients can be treated simultaneously in one session of 3 h.

The BSD machine is a transurethral microwave hyperthermic device (BSD Medical Corporation, Salt Lake City, UT). The microwaves (915 MHz) are delivered by a computerized generator that also allows intraurethral temperature measurements. The transurethral applicator consists of a helical antenna wound on a 14 F Foley catheter. Temperatures to 45 ± 2°C were confirmed by thermal mapping. Intrarectal temperatures were measured during some treatments and never exceeded 38°C.[13,14] A study of interstitial temperature measurements has demonstrated symmetrical heating around the prostatic urethra. Multiple sessions are mandatory. The duration of each session was fixed arbitrarily at 1 h (5–10 treatment sessions separated by 72–96 h[14]).

The Prostatron (Technomed International, Lyon, France) is also a transurethral microwave device (1296 MHz). It allows thermotherapy (temperatures in the prostate ranging from 45°C to 55°C). A single treatment session of 55 min is delivered. Temperature was monitored in real time inside the urethra and inside the rectum. The 20 F catheter passed transurethrally does not allow passage of urine and is equipped with a cooling system at 20°C to protect the urethral mucosa and to permit a deeper penetration of microwaves into the prostate. A rectal probe measures the temperature during treatment. After a phase of 5 min to cool the urethra, there is a progressive increase of temperature in the urethra to enlarge the heat field backward from the periphery of the gland in the direction of the urethra. During treatment, rectal and urethral temperatures were maintained below 42°C and 45°C, respectively.[15]

Two devices work either transurethrally or transrectally,

the Bruker and the Microfocus BPH from Breakthrough. No clinical data are available with these two machines.

The clinical results are expressed differently from one study to another, and there are various treatment regimens.

RESULTS OF TREATMENT

Transrectal Devices

The first clinical experience was published by Yerushalmi et al. in 1985. Patients benefited from the treatment, with a decrease in score ratios for each urinary symptom.[16] Servadio et al., Leib et al., and Lindner et al. also used this method and have the largest series of transrectal treatments.[17–19] In contrast to these encouraging data, Strohmaier et al. reported poor results with transurethral hyperthermia for BPH with the Prostathermer device,[20] as did Saranga et al.[21] Zerbib et al. reported a controlled study comparing the transrectal Prostathermer treatment with a sham procedure. They showed a significantly greater improvement in the treated group as compared with the sham group.[22,23] The results of transrectal treatment with the Primus device by Van Erps et al. also were encouraging.[11] However, Fabricius performed a placebo-controlled randomized study with the same machine, and there was no change in objective criteria in both groups.[24]

Watson and Perlmutter did a comparative study of two transrectal devices (prostathermer and Primus) and a transurethral device (Thermex-II),[10,25] but statistical comparison is difficult because patients and follow-up are different from one study to another.

Test results with transrectal devices are summarized in Table 17–3.

Table 17–2. BPH: Transrectal Hyperthermia Devices

	PROSTATHERMER/ BIODAN	PRIMUS/ TECNOMATIX
Single session	No	No
Rectal probe	Yes	Yes
Simultaneous treatment	No	No
Cooling system	Yes	Yes
Wavelength	915 MHz	915 MHz

Table 17–3.   Results with Transrectal Devices

PROSTATHERMER (BIODAN)

Author	Result
Yerushalmi et al., 1985	"All the patients benefited from the treatment" ↓ Of score ratios for each urinary symptom
Servadio, 1988	70% objective improvement 90% subjective improvement
Servadio, Leib, Lindner, 1990	51% improved subjectively and objectively
Saranga, 1990	25% objective 50% subjective
Strohmaier, Bichler, 1990	7% objective 54% subjective
Zerbib, 1989	45% objective 58% subjective Controlled study with sham procedure ↑ improvement in the treated group
Perlmutter, Watson, (AUA, June 1991)	Flow 7.3–10.5 Residue 160–50 Score 11–7.5

PRIMUS (TECNOMATIX)

Author	Result
Van Erps (AUA, June 1991)	35% objective Flow 8.1–15.7 68% subjective
Fabricius (AUA, June 1991)	Placebo-controlled randomized study No objective improvement in both groups Subjective 32% placebo group ← 53%–61% Treated → (Obstructive symptoms) (Irritative symptoms)

Transurethral Devices

Subjective improvement is obtained in 60%–70% in accordance with the series, and the increase of peak flow is the main criterion for objective improvement.[10,12,14,15,25,26] Differences are especially marked if selection of patients is performed. We showed a better objective improvement in a selected group with a peak flow of less than 10 mL/sec. In a group of patients in retention in our series, 47% were catheter free 2 weeks after treatment, with an acceptable flow and minimal residue.[12] Nissenkorn and Rotbard obtained 66% of patients catheter free in a similar patient group.

The results with the Prostatron are given for a selected group with strict inclusion criteria. With this machine, the results differ in accordance with the software of the machine, the first giving a low thermal dose and the second one a higher thermal dose (Tables 17–4, 17–5).[15] Carter et al., in a comparative study from five centers using the Prostatron, showed very different results from one center to another.[29] The increase in peak flow ranged from +1.5 to +7 (Table 17–6).

Results of studies with transurethral devices are summarized in Table 17–7.

Histologic Studies

Animals studies were published first by Leib et al.[18] In order to determine pathologic modifications after hyperthermia treatment of BPH, histologic studies were performed, and results are summarized in Table 17–8. Using the Prostathermer in the transrectal approach, Strohmaier et al. showed interstitial inflammation.[20] Necrosis was never demonstrated, and this is in accordance with the fact that no modifications were found in PSA levels after transrectal treatment.[30] On the other hand, with the transurethral BSD

Table 17–4.   Prostatron—Low Thermal Dose (n = 49)

	D 7	D 21	D 90	D 180	D 270
Boyarsky score % change	−5	−29	−30	−30	−39
Qmax before 8.5 mL/sec % change	+5	+7	+21	+20	+22
Voided volume	193	238	245	249	271
PSA % change	+277	+0.05	−0.03	+0.09	+0.1
Prostatic volume % change	+2	−4	−2	−2	+6

From Devonec et al.[28]

Table 17–5.   Prostatron–High Thermal Dose (n = 20)

	SYMPTOMS SCORE	FLOW	RESIDUE	PROSTATIC VOLUME	PSA	PSA D 7
Average before	11	11	58	44	5.7	5.8
Average after	5.5	14.5	45	40	4.1	57.4
% change	50%	32%	−22%	−9%	−28%	890%

From Devonec et al.[28]

Table 17–6. TUMT—Prostatron Selection Inclusion Criteria

	GOTEBORG	LONDON	NIJMEGEN	ROME	LYON
Flow	+7	+4.2	+1.5	+3.3	+3.3
Residue	NS	−20%	NS	—	NS
Symptoms score	−8.3	−6.2	−5	−4.7	−5

From Carter et al.[29]

device, Sapozink et al. described moderate desiccation,[14] and Baert et al. reported coagulative necrosis and fibrosis.[26] We have demonstrated this with the Thermex-II, where we found inflammatory edema, hemorrhagic vascular lesions with coagulative necrosis, glandular necrosis with ghost cells, and preservation of glands in malpighian metaplasia. In some areas, the urethra is preserved at a temperature of 44.5°C because there is a different sensitivity to heat in the urothelium (malpighian) and the glands in malpighian metaplasia. A disorganization and a necrosis of smooth muscle fibers of the stroma were encountered (at a distance 21 min from the urethra).[12]

PSA levels increase 2- to 30-fold the day after the treatment, which indicates glandular necrosis. There is a return to the initial value at 1 month. There was no correlation between PSA increase and prostatic volume and no correlation between PSA increase and success.[31] The most impressive pathologic lesions were described by Devonec et al. using the Prostatron.[28] The urethral mucosa and the periurethral tissue were preserved within a distance of 2–4 mm from the urethral lumen. Beyond that, necrosis of adenomatous tissue was observed up to a depth of 15 mm from the urethra and was roughly symmetrical on both lobes. The transition between the treated and nontreated area was sharp. Smooth muscle cells were found to be more sensitive to heat than were acinar cells. After 2 months, the treated area was replaced by a retractile fibrosis comparable to the ischemic

fibrosis observed after infarction. Also, PSA levels increased dramatically at day 7 after the treatment, with a 28% decrease in the initial value after 3 months. This diminution in the PSA could be related to the slight decrease (9%) of prostatic volume at 3 months that is obtained with the high thermal dose protocol.[15] Nobody knows if the volume of the prostate has to be reduced with this technique to be effective, since the size of the prostate is not necessarily related to obstruction or to the symptoms of prostatism.

COMPLICATIONS

With the transrectal approach, the most severe complications reported to date are two rectoprostatic fistulas in 2 patients. One had a history of a prostatic abscess that was drained through the rectum, and the other had chronic proctitis. A history of or a current rectal pathologic condition is a contraindication to transrectal treatment. Most of the complications occurred during or after the first treatment session, and half of the complications were either infection, hematoma, or epididymitis. These conditions all can be attributed to the insertion of a catheter and not to the hyperthermia treatment itself. Of 435 patients treated, the overall complication rate was of 6.6%.[32] The transurethral approach causes some urethral pain, slight transient hematoma in the majority of patients, and rare urinary tract infection. There is a temporary deterioration of urinary performance and about 10% of transient retention after treatment.[12]

CONCLUSIONS

This new approach to the treatment of obstructive BPH is still controversial. All the results presented are preliminary.

Table 17–7. Results with Transurethral Devices

THERMEX-II (DIREX-TECHNOREX)

Author	Result
Vandenbossche, Schulman, 1991	Subjective: 51%–60% (nonselected group) (selected group)
	Flow 11.9–13.9 NSG 7.3–10.7 SG
	Residue 166–122

BSD (BSD-MED-CORP)

Author	Result
Sapozink, 1990	81% objective response 71% subjective response Flow 11–15.9 Residue 177–91
Baert, 1990	Flow 6.25–12.49 Residue 269–50 Score 14.7–5.1

Table 17–8. Histology

TRANSURETHRAL

Sapozink[20] (BSD)	Moderate Dessicative Effects
Baert[2] (BSD)	Coagulative Necrosis and Fibrosis
Vandenbossche, Schulman[28] (Thermex-II)	Glandular and Muscular Necrosis
Devonec[7] (Prostatron)	Glandular and Muscular Necrosis and Fibrosis

TRANSRECTAL

No Histologic Changes

Results are expressed in different ways: overage peak flow rates, difference of flow rate, residual urine, nocturia, different subjective symptoms scores, and, therefore, these studies are not comparable with each other. Moreover, results are different with the same device from one study to another, probably because of different patient selection. A standardization of evaluation criteria is mandatory in order to assess the efficacy, the maintenance of effects, the patient's acceptability, and the cost–efficacy ratio. Comparative studies must be performed, such as hyperthermia vs drugs, hyperthermia vs hyperthermia and drugs, hyperthermia vs drugs followed by hyperthermia. The patients' hopes remain subjective criteria and the urologists's goal is to obtain objective measures of improvement.

The clinical results certainly showed subjective improvement from clinical prostatism to silent prostatism, since less than 30% of the patients treated still wish an operation. The good results are based more on an absence of symptoms than on a lack of demonstrated obstruction. Even if pathologic lesions are the indicators of the action of heating of cells, they do not correlate with the effectiveness of the treatment, and they cannot explain the definite mechanism of hyperthermia in BPH. A hypothetical mode of action could be neuromuscular lesions on alpha-receptors, with a reduction of irritative symptoms. Tissue necrosis could lead to a urethral decompression and subsequent flow improvement, but this has to be demonstrated.

The exact efficacy of treatment of BPH with hyperthermia or thermotherapy is unknown, but it definitely is lower than the efficacy of surgical treatment. Hyperthermia or thermotherapy should be viewed as a possible treatment option in selected patients with symptomatic BPH, but longer follow-up periods and randomized trials are mandatory to select which patient will respond and to determine if these new techniques will become part of the standard armamentarium of therapy.

REFERENCES

1. Busch W. Uber den Einflusse welchen heltigere Erysipeln zuweiten auf organisierte neubildungen. _Verh Naturheid Preuss_ 1866;23:28–30
2. Cavaliere R, Ciocatto EC, Clovanelle BC, et al. Selective heat sensitivity of cancer cells: biochemical and clinical studies. _Cancer_ 1967;20:1351–1381
3. Hahn GM. Hyperthermia and drugs: potential for therapy. _Cancer Res_ 1979;39:2263–2268
4. Hahn GM, Straude D. Cytotoxic effect of Adriamycin on chinese hamster cells. _J Natl Cancer Inst_ 1976;57:1063
5. Kim SH, Kim JH, Hahn EW. The radiosensitization of hypoxic tumor cells by hyperthermia. _Radiat Res_ 1976;66:337
6. Song CW. Effect of hyperthermia on vascular functions of normal tissues and experimental tumors. _J Natl Cancer Inst_ 1978;60:711–713
7. Mendecki J, Friedenthal E, Botstein C. Microwave applica-

tiors for localized hyperthermia treatment of cancer of the prostate. _Int J Radiat Oncol Biol Physics_ 1980;6:1583–1588
8. Sterzer F. Microwave apparatus for the treatment of cancer by hyperthermia. _Microwave J_ 1980;23:39–45
9. Leveen H. Radiofrequency in the treatment of malignant tumours. In: _Topical Reviews in Radiotherapy and Oncology_. Great Britain: John Wright, 1982:192
10. Watson GM, Perlmutter AP, Shah TK, Barnes DG. Heat treatment for severe, symptomatic prostatic outflow obstruction. _World J Urol_ 1991;9:7–11
11. Van Erps PM, Dourcy B, Denis LJ. Transrectal hyperthermia in benign prostatic hyperplasia. _J Urol_ 1991;145:Abstract 203
12. Vanden Bossche M, Noël JC, Schulman CC. Transurethral hyperthermia for benign prostatic hypertrophy. _World J Urol_ 1991;9:2–6
13. Astrahan MA, Ameye F, Oyen R, Willemen P, Baert L, Petrovich Z. Interstitial temperature measurements during transurethral microwave hyperthermia. _J Urol_ 1991;145:304–308
14. Sapozink MD, Boyd S, Astrahan MA, Jozsef G, Petrovich Z. Transurethral hyperthermia for benign prostatic hyperplasia: preliminary clinical results. _J Urol_ 1990;143:944–950
15. Devonec M, Berger N, Bringeon G, Carter S, Perrin P. Long-term results of transurethral microwave therapy (TUMT) in patients with benign prostatic hypertrophy. _J Urol_ 1991;145:Abstract 709
16. Yerushalmi A, Fishelovitz Y, Singer D, et al. Localized deep microwave hyperthermia in the treatment of poor operative risk patients with benign prostatic hyperplasia. _J Urol_ 1985;133:873–876
17. Servadio C, Lindner A, Lev A, Leib Z, Siegel Y, Braf Z. Further observations on the effect of local hyperthermia on benign enlargement of the prostate. _World J Urol_ 1989;6:204–208
18. Leib Z, Rothem A, Lev A, Servadio C. Histopathological observation in the canine prostate treated by local microwave hyperthermia. _Prostate_ 1986;8:93–102
19. Lindner A, Braf Z, Lev A, Golomb J, Leib Z, Siegel Y, Servadio C. Local hyperthermia of the prostate gland for the treatment of benign prostatic hypertrophy and urinary retention. _Br J Urol_ 1990;65:201–203
20. Strohmaier WL, Bichler KH, Flüchter SH, Wilbert DM. Local microwave hyperthermia of benign prostatic hyperplasia. _J Urol_ 1990;144:919–917
21. Saranga R, Matzkin H, Braf Z. Local microwave hyperthermia in the treatment of benign prostatic hyperthrophy. _Br J Urol_ 1990;65:349–353
22. Zerbib M, Steg A, Conquy S, Maugenest JP. Hypertrophie benigne de la prostate. Traitement pour hyperthermie localisée. _Presse Med_ 1989;18:1379–1382
23. Zerbib M, Steg A, Conquy S. A prospective randomized study of localized hyperthermia versus placebo in obstructive benign hypertrophy of the prostate. _J Urol_ 1990;143 (suppl):Abstract 284
24. Fabricius PG, Schäfer J, Schmeller N, Chaussy C. Efficacy of transrectal hyperthermia for benign prostatic hyperplasia: a placebo-controlled study. _J Urol_ 1991;145:Abstract 602
25. Perlmutter AP, Shah TK, Watson GM. Prostatic microwave hyperthermia for the treatment of urinary outflow obstruction. _J Urol_ 1991;145:Abstract 604
26. Baert L, Ameye F, Willemen P, Vandenhove J, Lauweryns J, Astrahan M, Petrovich Z. Transurethral microwave hyperthermia for benign prostatic hyperplasia: preliminary clinical and pathological results. _J Urol_ 1990;144:1383–1387

27. Nissenkorn I, Rotbard M. Transurethral hyperthermia for benign prostatic hyperplasia (BPH) using the Thermex-II. *J Endourol* 1991;5 (Suppl 1):5

28. Devonec M, Berger N, Bringeon G, Carter S, Perrin P. Long-term histological effects of transurethral microwave therapy (TUMT) on benign prostatic hypertrophy. *J Urol* 1991;145:Abstract 603

29. Carter S, et al. First Symposium on Prostatron Thermotherapy. Toronto, June 4, 1991

30. Lindner A, Siegel YI, Korczak D. Serum prostatic-specific antigen levels during hyperthermia treatment of benign prostatic hyperplasia. *J Urol* 1990;144:1388–1389

31. Schulman CC, Vandenbossche M. Transurethral hyperthermia and PSA markers. *J Endourol* 1991;5 (suppl 1):Abstract 588

32. Lindner A, Siegel YI, Saranga R, Korczak D, Matzkin H, Braf Z. Complications in hyperthermia treatment of benign prostatic hyperplasia. *J Urol* 1990;141:1390–1392

18

Transrectal Local Hyperthermia Treatment for BPH

Arie Lindner

Resection of the adenomatous tissue is the accepted method for treating BPH. However, for many patients, this surgical procedure involves additional risks due to associated health problems common at such an advanced age, and other patients may refuse surgery because they fear incontinence, retrograde ejaculation, impotence, and other anesthetic-associated complications.[1] As a result, the search for an alternative to surgery in the treatment of BPH has never stopped.

The application of hyperthermia in the treatment of cancer is based on the observation that many types of tumor cells are more sensitive to elevated temperatures than are normal cells. Several biologic facts support this hypothesis.[2] This selective thermosensitivity makes it possible to destroy malignant tumors without injuring normal tissue. The mechanism by which hyperthermia affects BPH is different from the one for cancer, and a theoretical explanation has yet to be proved.

WHY TRANSRECTAL?

The prostate gland is traversed by the urethra and is in contact with the rectal wall. When considering how to heat the prostate, it is fairly obvious that the heating element should be placed in one of these cavities.

Heating of the tissue, which occurs after applying microwave energy, results from the absorption of radiation by the tissue. The temperature increase is a direct function of several parameters, the most significant of which is the absorption coefficient of the tissue, which in turn mostly depends on the water content of the tissue and is proportional to the microwave frequency. The prostate gland is a relatively homogeneous organ, and accordingly, its absorption coefficient can be assumed as a constant value.

The heating pattern in a medium with a constant absorption coefficient is shown in Figure 18–1. At a short distance from the source of the microwave energy, the temperature gradient is high, on the order of 1.5°C/mm. Therefore, if the maximum temperature is limited to 44°C, which is the upper limit of temperature before massive normal cell destruction occurs, only about 2 mm of tissue around the urethra will be heated to 42°C or more if the heating element is placed in the urethra. This means that only a small percentage of the volume of an average prostate gland will be heated to the hyperthermic range.

It is similarly obvious that when applying microwave energy from the rectal cavity, only the rectal wall will be heated, unless it is cooled. Cooling by conduction alone is illustrated in Figure 18–2. If the graphs for heating by energy absorption and the cooling effect by conduction are com-

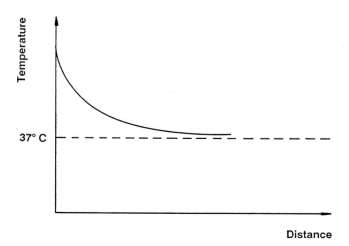

Figure 18–1. Heating pattern by an RF source.

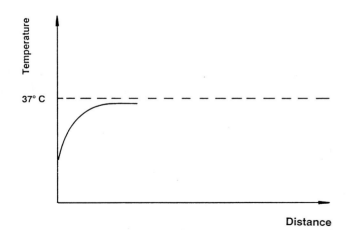

Figure 18–2. Cooling of tissue by conduction.

bined, a shift of the maximum temperature occurs (Fig. 18–3). The combination of heating by radiation absorption and cooling by cold water conduction produces a shift of the heating profile into the prostate without overheating the rectal wall.

Furthermore, the temperature profile in the prostate corresponds to a part of the curve that is considerably flatter than the area near the energy source, and a substantially larger portion of the prostate is heated to the hyperthermic range without exceeding at any point the 44°C limit.

The same cooling effect can be applied to transurethral systems, thus moving the maximum temperature point away from the urethra and into the prostate. However, it becomes extremely difficult to control the maximum temperature and the magnitude of the affected area.

WHAT DEVICE IS USED TO ACCOMPLISH TRANSRECTAL HEATING?

The Prostathermer, manufactured by Biodan Israel, is an example of a transrectal system. It is one of the first devices

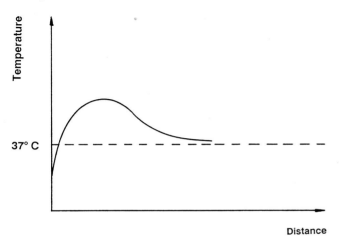

Figure 18–3. Heating pattern by an RF source with surface cooling.

developed and is the most widely used today (Fig. 18–4). The Prostathermer is an integrated hardware and software system for applying, monitoring, and controlling the delivery of microwave energy by a radiofrequency (RF) power unit through a rectal applicator. A urethral catheter contains a probe that serves to properly direct the microwave energy to the prostate, and there is a separate cooling system for controlling the rectal wall temperature. The software contains carefully constructed safety provisions.

The physicians operating the system enter their instructions on a flat keyboard, and there is a color graphic display of the RF transmitted and the temperature in the urethra and the prostate throughout the course of the treatment. Treatment preparation and posttreatment procedures also are displayed on the monitor, as are appropriate messages and menus for changing the treatment parameters at the physician's discretion. Each of the main components of the Prostathermer system is described in more detail in the following paragraphs.

The **computer system** is built around a standard off-the-shelf microcomputer configured with standard disk drives, monitor, and expansion slot cards.

The **catheter system** (Fig. 18–5) is comprised of a catheter and a temperature measurement probe. The catheter used is a Tiemann balloon catheter. The largest lumen is used for urine outflow, and the smallest is used to inflate the balloon tip of the catheter. The third lumen is used for

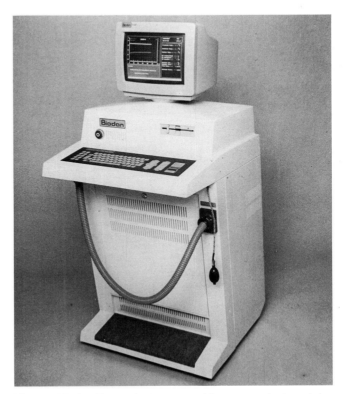

Figure 18–4. Prostathermer machine, manufactured by Biodan Israel.

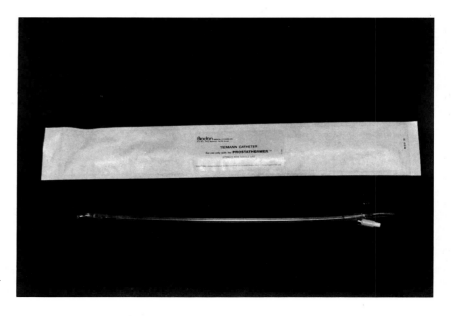

Figure 18–5. Transurethral catheter and temperature sensing probe.

insertion of the probe. The probe is inserted to a specific depth within the catheter. As a result of this configuration, the probe can be positioned reliably within the prostatic urethra. Temperatures in the prostatic urethra are measured by three copper–constantan thermocouples. An RF locator enables the operator to optimize applicator alignment in the rectum, directly opposite the prostate gland.

The **applicator system** (Fig. 18–6) consists of the applicator, the disposable balloon sleeve, and the alignment clamp. Inside the applicator is a skirt-type dipole antenna made up of a coaxial cable and cylindrical reflector, operating at 915 MHz. To heat the prostate, the RF source drives the antenna, and the RF energy is transmitted directionally toward the prostate gland. Three high-performance copper–constantan thermocouples affixed to the surface of the

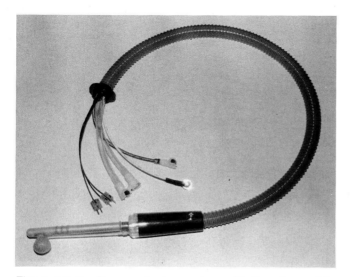

Figure 18–6. The applicator system with the disposable balloon sleeve.

applicator measure temperatures in the rectal cavity. To cool the rectal wall, forced coolant (deionized water) flows inside the applicator, and a circulating bath device maintains the specified coolant temperature.

A disposable latex balloon sleeve fits tightly around the applicator. The balloon sleeve has an inflatable protuberance on one side, which when inflated by the operator, pushes the front side of the applicator against the rectal wall. Since the balloon sleeve is very thin, it does not hinder efficient cooling of the rectal wall or significantly influence RF transmission. Additionally, the disposable balloon sleeve maintains the cleanliness of the applicator. An alignment clamp is used to set the applicator properly in place and maintain its position in the patient's rectum during the treatment session. The base of the alignment clamp is affixed magnetically to the metal extension shelf of the treatment chair, and its flexible arm is attached to the applicator handle.

The **RF microwave unit** consists of an RF source and an RF matching unit. The RF source is a 0–80 W power generator (limited to 60 W by the software), which delivers continuous wave (CW) at a fixed frequency of 915 MHz ± 0.045 MHz. The operator can set the output wattage for the treatment session within these limits. Forward and reflected RF are monitored continuously during the treatment session by a bidirectional coupler. The RF matching unit accomplishes matching to 50 ohms with a double stub tuner located beneath the computer keyboard.

IS THIS TREATMENT SAFE?

The first question that has to be answered when introducing a new treatment modality is how safe is the treatment. In one of the earliest reports on transrectal hyperthermia treatment of prostatic diseases, Servadio et al.[3] reported that in two patients a fistula was noted between the rectal cavity and the prostatic urethra. This was very alarming and even more so because it occurred in a small series of patients. Since then, however, thousands of hyperthermia treatments have been delivered, and not a single case of such a fistula has been reported. It is possible that the complication was a result of poor patient selection at a time when the very clear exclusion criteria currently in use, such as rectal pathology or previous rectal surgery, were not applied, and the treatment was performed using both a technique that was not refined and first generation equipment.

In a recent study dealing specifically with the complication rate,[4] it was found to be 6.6% per patients, or 1.1% per treatment session, for 435 patients treated with a total of 2630 treatment sessions. Most of the complications can be attributed to the insertion of the catheter, including urinary tract infection (1.6% of all patients) and epididymitis (0.4% of all patients). Other complications may be related directly to the treatment, such as rectal pain (0.9% of all patients), chest pain and cold sweats (1.8% of all patients), hematuria (1.4% of all patients), and urinary retention (0.4% of all patients). Cold sweats and chest pain occurred only in the first session of treatment and may be a result of anxiety. Reassurance and a mild tranquilizer may reduce these side effects. Nine of the 27 patients who developed a complication continued the treatment despite the complication. For the other 18 patients, the treatment was discontinued.

In other reports using different machines and protocols, the complication rate was low, and no severe complications were noted.[5–9] It appears that transrectal local hyperthermia treatment to the prostate is a safe technique, with a very low immediate complication rate.

In the very few reports with a longer follow up-period, no severe late complications were mentioned. With the growing interest in this treatment modality, attention should be directed to this point. A substantial number of patients who failed to respond to local hyperthermia treatment or patients with a temporary response underwent resection of the prostate. The surgery was performed using transurethral, transvesical, or retropubic techniques.

Whether the hyperthermia treatment has had any influence on the course of surgery or its final outcome is an interesting question that has neither been asked nor responded to in the present literature. My personal impression is that bleeding is somewhat more pronounced during transurethral resection of the prostate but has no effect on the final result, the number of blood transfusions needed, or the hospitalization time. There seems to be no adverse effect on open prostatectomy.

IS TRANSRECTAL LOCAL HYPERTHERMIA TREATMENT EFFECTIVE FOR BPH?

It is very difficult to assess the effectiveness of a treatment in a disease with such heterogeneous subjective symptoms, with large rhythmic changes, and where there may be great variability in consecutive measurements of the objective parameters, such as uroflowmetry.[10] The very high rate of placebo effect also should be kept in mind.[11,12]

Zerbib et al.[8] randomized 100 patients with BPH into two groups: 50 patients were treated by local hyperthermia using the Prostathermer, and 50 underwent the same manipulation but without hyperthermia. The objective evaluation consisted of peak flow rate, urinary volume, and postvoiding urinary volume. At 3-month follow-up, a 50% objective response was recorded in the treatment group compared to 13% in the control group, and this difference is statistically significant.

This prospective, randomized, carefully designed and performed study provides the most convincing evidence that treatment of BPH with transrectal local hyperthermia is effective.

Patients with an indwelling catheter due to chronic urinary retention caused by BPH are a very special group for evaluation of the efficacy of hyperthermia. For these patients, the otherwise very unclear definitions of objective response and success rate of treatment become relatively simpler.

Seventy-two patients with an indwelling catheter were treated with the Prostathermer.[13] Thirty-six patients (50%) were able to dispense with the catheter 1 month after treatment, and 1 year later, 29 patients (40%) remained catheter free with no need for further treatment. In the same study, one group of patients was treated with a high thermal dose, and another group of patients was treated with a low thermal dose. There was a statistically significant difference in the results between the two groups in favor of the high thermal dose group, thus further refuting the placebo effect of this treatment. In several reports from different centers, the response rate was 50%–70%.[3,5–9,13–15,18,19] All of these results strongly suggest that treatment of BPH by transrectal microwave hyperthermia when carefully carried out has a real beneficial effect. The question remains: Is it a long-lasting cure in the responding patients or merely a palliative modality? Since this is a newly developed technique, there are no long-term follow-up studies. Recently, the results for 72 patients followed up for 40 months with a minimal follow-up of 3 years were reported.[16] Twenty-two patients with a good response are still being followed up and responding. Eight patients died during the follow-up period of unrelated causes while still responding, so that for 30 patients (41.5%), hyperthermia was the only treatment required. Forty months cannot be considered as long-term follow-up when evaluating the results in treating BPH, but a pattern is emerging.

In a large prospective study conducted in three medical centers in Israel (data not published), 302 patients with BPH and a clear indication for surgery were treated with transrectal local hyperthermia. During the first year of follow-up, 25% were diagnosed as treatment failures, during the second year of follow-up, another 10% of the patients were redesignated for surgery, and after this, stabilization was noted. During the third year, the same 65% of the patients were not considered to be candidates for prostatic surgery. One hundred seventeen patients from this group were followed up for 4 years, and in the fourth year, the same trend was maintained—for 65% of the patients, prostate surgery was avoided.

Different treatment regimens were used, with six main variables.

1. The maximal temperature: high (41–43°C) or low (39–41°C)
2. The number of sessions per treatment (5–10)
3. The length of each session (30 or 60 min)
4. Sessions delivered once or twice a week
5. Adjuvant treatment with cyproterone acetate, 50 mg three times daily, during the course of the treatment or without such treatment
6. Continuous measurement of the temperature in the prostatic urethra, which requires insertion of a urethral catheter, or without such measurement

This last point is extremely important. Not only is the insertion of the urethral catheter a major source of patient discomfort, but it is also a major contributor to the complication rate. Consequently, it is very tempting to perform treatment without it. In a study presented at the Eleventh Conference of the European Society for Hyperthermic Oncology, there was no statistically significant correlation between the temperature and the microwave energy (power delivered). The temperature depends on the power delivered, but the relationship is also a function of several other variables that have a significant effect. Thus, determination of tissue temperature based solely on the power delivered is speculative at best. Hyperthermia techniques result in considerable heterogeneity, and this means that multiple points at multiple times over the course of the treatment must be monitored in order to obtain enough information about the effectiveness of the heating.

So far, there are no clear recommendations regarding the preferred protocol, but it appears that the most cost-effective protocol has the following characteristics.

- High temperature sessions lasting for 60 min
- Two sessions per week
- A total of five sessions per treatment course
- No adjuvant antihormonal therapy
- Measurement of prostatic urethral temperature

WHAT IS THE MECHANISM OF ACTION?

In the canine prostate, hyperthermia caused a mononuclear inflammatory infiltration in the interstitium and polymorphonuclear infiltration in the glandular elements.[20]

In attempts to understand the tissue changes in the human prostate exposed to heat, light microscopy and electron microscopy of prostate specimens were not discriminative. A morphometric method[21] was applied to evaluate hyperplastic prostate tissue after treatment by local hyperthermia in comparison to untreated specimens. Prostate tissue was obtained from 13 patients who completed a full course of hyperthermia treatment and underwent prostectomy because of failure of the treatment.[22] A significant reduction in the volume fraction of the fibrous tissue was found in the study group as compared with the control group, and there was also a significant increase in the volume fraction occupied by muscle cells. There was no difference between the groups in the volume fractions of the vascular and glandular tissue. It is possible that a change in the fibrous elements that constrict the stromal supporting structure of the entire gland is responsible for a change in the tissue tone and in this way relieves the symptoms. It is not known whether this change in tone is caused by reabsorption of the interstitial edema, by a down regulation of adrenegic receptors in the prostatic capsule, or by a different mechanism.

In some reports, a decrease in the size of the prostate gland was observed,[7,23] but this was not confirmed in other studies.[14,17] In an attempt to better understand the mechanism of action of hyperthermia on the cells of the human prostate, PSA serum was used as a marker for trauma in the hyperthermia-treated prostate in 18 patients.[24] No significant difference was observed between pretreatment and posttreatment PSA levels, which means that no PSA leaks out of these cells as a result of the heating. Therefore, hyperthermia treatment apparently has no destructive effect on the epithelial cells.

CONCLUSIONS

The pioneering work with transrectal local hyperthermia of the prostate was performed in Israel a decade ago[25,26] and was directed at first to treatment of cancer. To date, the following is known about the treatment of BPH with transrectal local hyperthermia.

- It is a safe procedure.
- It is not a placebo.
- The efficacy is most probably in the range of 50%–70%, but this is still debatable.[17]
- In some patients, the effect lasts for at least 4–5 years.

Clinical studies have to be performed to establish the response rate and its duration beyond any doubt. Attention should be directed toward researching how the hyperthermia mechanism operates and for a better definition of the group of patients who will respond to the treatment based on prostatic size, configuration, morphometry, or biochemistry.

Transrectal local hyperthermia of the prostate is a viable alternative to surgery in patients suffering from BPH. This is true for patients who are poor risks for surgery and also for younger patients who are concerned about surgery and its adverse effects.

REFERENCES

1. Holtgrewe HL, Mebust WK, Dowd JB, Cockett ATK, Peters PC, Proctor C. Transurethral prostatectomy: practice aspects of the dominant operation in American urology. *J Urol* 1989;141:248–253
2. Dickson JA, Calderwood SK. Thermosensitivity of neoplastic tissues In vivo. In: Storm FK (ed). *Hyperthermia in Cancer Therapy*. G.K. Hall Medical Publishers, 1983
3. Servadio C, Leib Z, Lev A. Further observations on the use of local hyperthermia for the treatment of diseases of the prostate in man. *Eur J Urol* 1986;12:38–40
4. Lindner A, Siegel Y, Saranga R, Korczak D, Matzkin H, Braf Z. Complications in hyperthermia treatment of benign prostatic hyperplasia. *J Urol* (in press)
5. Yerushalmi A, Fishelovitz Y, Singer D, et al. Localized deep microwave hyperthermia in the treatment of poor operative risk patients with benign prostatic hyperplasia. *J Urol* 1985; 133:813–816
6. Rigatti P, Guazzoni G, Maffezzini M, Colombo R, Montorsi F, Consonni P. Local deep microwave hyperthermia in the treatment of prostatic diseases. *Arch Ital Urol, Nefrol Androl* 1989;61:179–181
7. Van Erps PM, Daurcy BZ, Dennis LJ. Local hyperthermia in BPH. *J Urol* 1990;143:902A
8. Zerbib M, Steg A, Conquy S, Debre B. A prospective randomized study of localized hyperthermia vs placebo in obstructive benign hypertrophy of the prostate. *J Urol* 1990;143:383A
9. Servadio C, Lindner A, Lev A, Leib Z, Siegel Y, Braf Z. Further observations on the effect of local hyperthermia on benign enlargement of the prostate. *World J Urol* 1989;6:204–208
10. Golomb J, Siegel Y, Korczak D, Lindner A. Circadian changes in home uroflowmetry in patients with benign prostatic hypertrophy. *Eur Urol.* 1990;18(Suppl 1):328
11. Resnick MI, Jackson JE, Watts LE, Boyce WH. Assessment of the antilypercholesteroleric drug probucol in BPH. *J Urol* 1983;129:206–209
12. Lindner A, Ramon J, Brooks ME. Controlled study of cimetidine in the treatment of BPH. *Br J Urol* 1990;66:55–57
13. Lindner A, Braf Z, Lev A, Golomb J, Leib Z, Siegel Y, Servadio C. Local hyperthermia of the prostate gland for the treatment of benign prostatic hypertrophy and urinary retention. *Br J Urol* 1990;65:201–203
14. Saranga R, Matzkin H, Braf Z. Local microwave hyperthermia in the treatment of benign prostatic hypertrophy. *Br J Urol* 1990;65:349–353
15. Lindner A, Siegel Y, Korczak D, Golomb J. The efficacy of hyperthermia treatment for BPH—a prospective study. *Strahlenther Oncol* 1990;166:523A
16. Lindner A, Siegel Y, Korczak D, Golomb J. Local hyperthermia for the treatment of BPH—long-term follow-up. *Strahlenther Oncol* 1990;166:522A
17. Strohmaier WL, Bichler KH, Flüchter SH, Wilbert DM. Local microwave hyperthermia in benign prostatic hyperplasia (BPH). *J Urol* 1990;144:913–917
18. Servadio C, Braf Z, Siegel Y, Leib Z, Saranga R, Lindner A. Local thermotherapy of the benign prostate: a 1-year follow-up. *Eur J Urol* (in press)
19. Watson GM. Experience with a transrectal microwave device for hyperthermia treatment of prostatic disease. *J Urol* 1990;143:382A
20. Leib Z, Rothem A, Lev A, Servadio C. Histopathological observations in the canine prostate treated by local microwave hyperthermia. *Prostate* 1986;8:93–102
21. Bartsch G, Frick J, Ruegg I, Bucher M, Holliger O, Oberholzer M, Rohr HP. Electron microscopic stereological analysis of the normal human prostate and of BPH. *J Urol* 1979;122:481–486
22. Siegel Y, Zaidel L, Lindner A, Braf Z, Servadio C. The histopathologic changes of benign prostatic hyperplasia after hyperthermia treatment failure—a controlled study. *Br J Urol* (in press)
23. Servadio C, Leib Z, Lev A. Diseases of the prostate treated by local microwave hyperthermia. *Urology* 1987;30:97–99
24. Lindner A, Siegel Y, Korczak D. Serum prostate-specific antigen levels during hyperthermia treatment of benign prostatic hyperplasia. *J Urol* (in press)
25. Yerushalmi A, Servadio C, Leib Z, Fishelovitz Y, Rokowsky E. Local hyperthermia for treatment of carcinoma of the prostate. *Prostate* 1982;3:623–630
26. Servadio C, Leib Z. Hyperthermia in treatment of prostate cancer. *Prostate* 1984;5:205–211

19

Experimental High-Dose Prostatic Hyperthermia for Debulking of the Central Adenoma

Flavio Castañeda, Wilfrido R. Castañeda-Zúñiga

Hyperthermia is the central elevation of tissue temperature. The concept that hyperthermia has some curative benefits has been known for millennia. This idea developed from the observation that after a high fever many ailments resolved or improved. Busch, in 1866, published the first scientific report of the complete regression of a histologically proven sarcoma after a bout of erysipelas with high fever.[1] Bruns, in 1877, reported the complete cure of a patient terminally ill with multiple recurrent melanomas after erysipelas.[2] In 1893, Coley reported a series of patients with advanced cancer who were either cured or significantly improved by accidental or deliberate exposure to erysipelas.[3] Many other reports followed, with similar results after natural exposure or injection of filtered extracts of highly pyrogenic toxins.[4,5] By the same principle, others reported cure or significant improvement after deliberate hyperthermia exposure locally or of the whole body.[4,6–15] It is well known that some bacteria and viruses adapted to body temperatures find it difficult to proliferate at temperatures only a few degrees higher.

In the past few years, there has been a revival of interest in the effects of hyperthermia on biologic systems, particularly for the treatment of cancer. Investigations have focused on hyperthermia as the sole treatment or combined with radiotherapy with or without cytotoxic drugs.

Hyperthermia alone has the capacity to kill cells selectively. Temperatures from 42°C to 45°C cause selective death of tumor cells.[16] One of the factors that make cancer cells more susceptible than normal cells is the defective heat dissipation by neoplastic tissue due to poor blood supply and decreased vasodilation capacity of the neovascular bed in response to the thermal load. Other factors known to influence tumor cell sensitivity to heat include nutritional factors,

pH, and O_2 concentration, all of which also are related to tumor perfusion.[17–19] These effects are potentiated by both radiation and chemotherapy.

Hyperthermia may be applied externally or interstitially. External techniques include radiofrequency current fields, ultrasound, and microwave. Interstitial techniques include radiofrequency current between implanted electrodes, microwave heating with needle-shaped implanted antennas, implanted ferromagnetic seeds or needles heated by radiofrequency magnetic induction, hot water circulated through implanted hollow tubes, and conductive heating catheters.[20–25] This expanding knowledge of hyperthermia benefits has motivated its use in almost every system and organ in the body, including the prostate. Hyperthermia has been used for both malignant tumors and benign prostatic hyperplasia (BPH).[26–33] There are two basic delivery methods: transrectally, as used by Servadio et al.,[24,30,32,34] Yerushalmi et al.,[26,31] and Mendecki et al.,[27] and transurethrally, as used by Astrahan et al.[33] All of these techniques have used temperatures in the range of 42–46°C and require a prolonged series of treatments ranging from 6 to 18. The preferred course for best results is 12–15 treatments. The treatments are 1 h each, one or two times a week. The reported early clinical results are encouraging, although most lack objective documentation, such as uroflow, urodynamic, and prostate volumetric data before and after treatments.

It is our opinion that this protracted course of treatments will not replace either completely or in specific instances the conventional mode of BPH therapy (transurethral resection of the prostate) and that they might merely provide a sitz bath effect (Fig. 19–1). To compete with transurethral resection, a procedure would have to be safer, less expensive, less

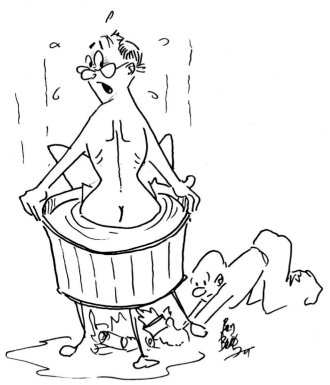

Figure 19–1. Probable sitz bath effect of current low temperature treatments.

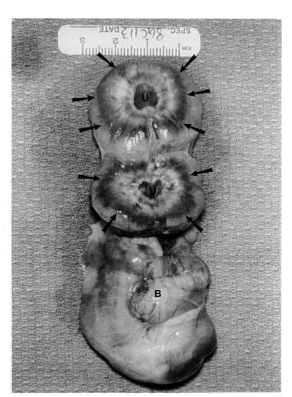

Figure 19–2. Block specimen of bladder (B) and prostate resected immediately after heat treatment. Prostate has been sectioned transversely in half, and the halves are pulled apart. Arrows show acute demarcation of coagulative necrotic extension, which in some areas extends to the capsule region of the gland. The urethral (U) channel also has widened significantly.

involved, and accomplished in a single treatment on an outpatient basis. Therefore, our research has changed completely the previously established clinical and experimental protocols.

Our goal is to produce central prostatic tissue ablation (Fig. 19–2), with subsequent debulking (Fig. 19–3) of the

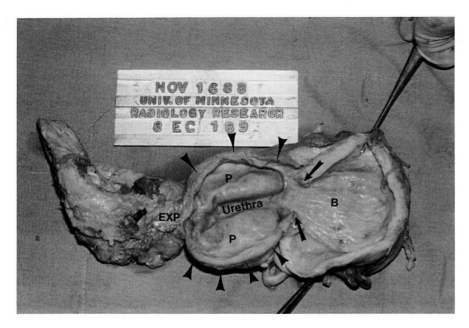

Figure 19–3. Block specimen of bladder (B), prostate (P), and external sphincter and perineal tissues (EXP) sectioned longitudinally in half 2 months after heat treatment exposure. This shows that only a very small amount of prostatic tissue remains in contiguity to the prostatic capsule (arrowheads), but for the most part the prostatic fossa (P) is empty and covered by normal urothelium. Black arrows point to the bladder neck.

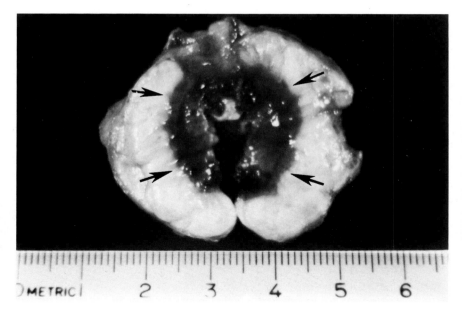

Figure 19–4. Gross prostatic specimen transversely sectioned, showing precise demarcation of coagulative necrosis of central adenoma after hyperthermia tissue ablation using the 7 F computer-controlled catheter, limited to the central periurethral tissue.

periurethral adenomatous tissue by a retrograde transurethral approach using much higher temperatures in the range of 80–90°C for a single exposure period ranging from 15 to 60 min. The heat is delivered through two different mechanisms, by a balloon catheter that is filled with a heated medium and by a 7 F specially designed computer-controlled, heat-emitting catheter. Both are centered in the prostatic urethra using fluoroscopic guidance. Both designs depend entirely on tissue thermal conduction rather than on microwave, which is the mode of heat delivery used by other methods.

The first prototype (balloon catheter) was very effective in accomplishing this purpose. However, the depth of tissue coagulative necrosis and ablation was hard to predict and control because balloons of the same size would compress the tissues differently, producing different degrees of ischemia and heat diffusion coefficients. This prototype was abandoned for the now more reliable and predictive 7 F system. With this prototype, the depth and amount of tissue to be ablated (Fig. 19–4) and subsequently debulked (Fig. 19–5) from the central periurethral adenoma can be controlled adequately.

Histopathologic findings have shown coagulative necrosis that extended to different depths depending on the treatment and length of exposures used (Fig. 19–6). After treatment and complete resolution of the initial inflammatory response, reepithelialization, widening of the prostatic urethra, atrophy of the periurethral prostatic tissue glands, maintenance of the normal architecture of the periurethral prostatic tissue glands, and maintenance of the normal architecture of the periurethral connective tissue were seen on subsequent follow-ups (Fig. 19–7).

Our technique is novel in the sense that it uses much higher temperatures, and, therefore, the principle of selective ab-

normal cell destruction is not applicable with this method. Rather, the high-dose hyperthermia is used to ablate adjacent tissue completely and to debulk and produce a larger central lumen to resolve the bladder outlet obstruction caused by the central adenomatous tissue (Figs. 19–8, 19–9, 19–10). This limited resection of a central channel has been proposed by some urologists[35] in high-risk patients in an effort to limit the intervention.

This technique accomplishes our goal in a single treat-

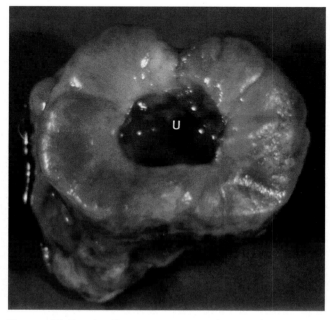

Figure 19–5. Another gross prostatic specimen transversely sectioned obtained 1 month posttreatment. This shows the new, much larger prostatic fossa and urethra (U).

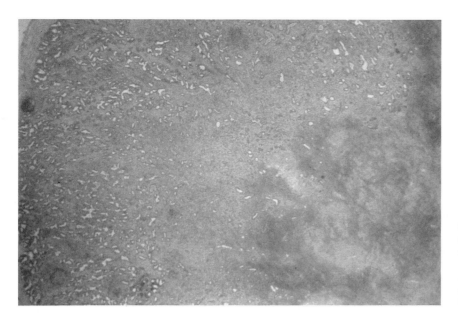

Figure 19–6. Photomicrograph showing central coagulative necrosis changes (left lower corner) immediately after treatment, extending into the more normal peripheral adenomatous changes, bordered by the capsule periphery (right upper corner).

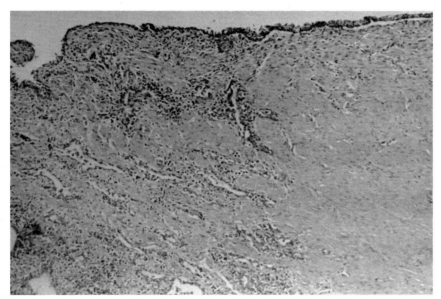

Figure 19–7. Photomicrograph of specimen resected 2 months after treatment showing reconstitution of the urothelium (top margin) with residual atrophy and fibrosis with persistent inflammatory changes of the remaining prostatic tissue.

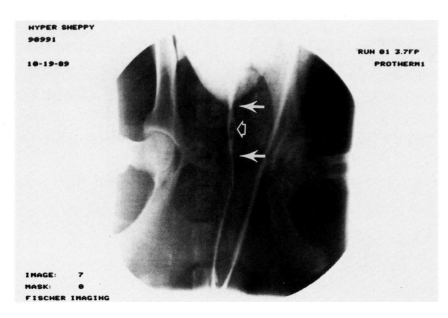

Figure 19–8. Baseline retrograde urethrogram of one of the canines with BPH used for the study shows the length of prostatic urethra (white arrows) and the central filling defect representative of the verumontanum (open arrow).

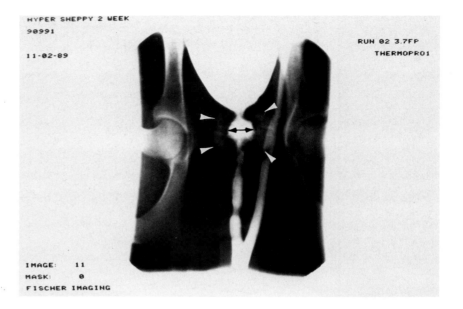

Figure 19–9. Retrograde urethrogram obtained 2 weeks after prostatic thermal ablation showing central adenomatous prostatic tissue debulking, as evidenced by an increase of prostatic urethral caliber (black arrows). Arrowheads show demarcation of more peripheral adenoma, as evidenced by reflux and opacification of intraprostatic glands, which denote persistent edema at 2 weeks.

ment, and since it is easy to control and selectively ablate the desired amount of periurethral tissue, the chances of complications are diminished. We doubt that other complications, such as strictures, would develop because of the normal appearance of the regenerated tissues. Impotence, another condition that might be of concern, probably will not occur if we limit the ablation to shallow depths, only deep enough to open a reasonable channel, since the major nerve networks are more toward the periphery. This procedure may be performed on an outpatient basis, since there is no bleeding or need for external drainage. The necrosed tissue sloughs off gradually, without sequelae. This procedure requires regional anesthesia because of the higher temperatures used.

This can be obtained easily and effectively by a perineal block, which uses local anesthetics injected in the perineum. This type of block is used widely in obstetrics and urology with excellent results. This blockade would not preclude the performance of this procedure on an outpatient basis.

Some of these clinical issues will be resolved only when the clinical trial begins. However, experimental animal studies suggest that this technique may be a nonsurgical, minimally invasive way of debulking the central prostatic adenoma. The ongoing clinical series using low temperatures have not produced results comparable with those of transurethral resection of the prostate, the standard mode of BPH treatment. Although the proposed high-temperature debulk-

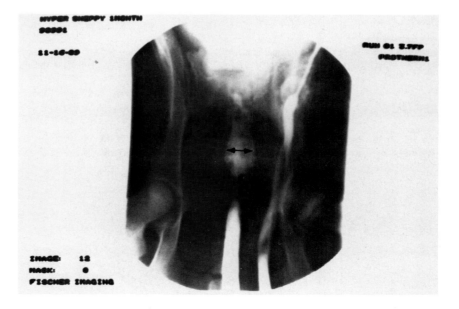

Figure 19–10. Retrograde urethrogram obtained at 1 month postprocedure, showing that further increase of prostatic lumen has occurred (black arrows). This demonstrates further tissue debulking. Note that at this time, no reflux of contrast is noted into the prostatic glands due to resolution of glandular edema.

ing of the periurethral central adenoma has not reached the clinical stage, it has many theoretical advantages over previous methods.

REFERENCES

1. Busch W. Ober den Einfluss welchen Heftigere Erysipeln Zuweilen auf Organisierte Neubildungen Ausuben. *Verhandl Naturh Preuss Rhein Westphal* 1866;23:28–30
2. Bruns P. Die Heilwirkung des Erysipels auf Geschwulste. *Beitr Klin Chir* 1877;3:443–466
3. Coley WB. The treatment of malignant tumors by repeated inoculations of erysipelas—with a report of ten original cases. *Am J Med Sci* 1893;105:487–511
4. Rohdenburg GL. Fluctuations in the growth of malignant tumors in man, with special reference to spontaneous recession. *J Cancer Res* 1918;3:193–225
5. Nauts HC, Fowler GA, Bogatko FH. A review of the influence of bacterial infections and bacterial products (Coley's toxin) on malignant tumors in men. *Acta Med Scand* (Suppl) 1953; 267:1–103
6. Westermark F. Ober die Behandlung des Ulcerirended Cervix-carcinomas. Mittel Konstanter Warme. *Zentralbl Gynakol* 1898;1335–1339
7. Gottschalk S. Zur Behandlung des Ulcerirenden inoperablen Cervixcarcinoms. *Zentralbl Gynakol* 1899;79–80
8. Vidal E. Travaux de la Deuxieme Conference Internationale pour l'Etude du Cancer. Paris, 1911:160
9. Percy JF. Heat in the treatment of carcinomas of the uterus. *Surg Gynecol Obstet* 1916;22:77–79
10. Goetze O. Ortliche Homogene Oberwarmung Gesunder und Kranker Gliedmassen. *Deutsch Z Chir* 1932;234:577–589
11. Warren SL. Preliminary study of the effect of artificial fever upon hopeless tumor cases. *AJR* 1935;33:75–87
12. Woodhall B, Pickrill KL, Georgiade NG, Mahaley MS, Dukes HT. Effect of hyperthermia upon cancer chemotherapy—application to external cancer of head and face structures. *Ann Surg* 1960;151:750–759
13. Crile G Jr. Selective destruction of cancers after exposure to heat. *Ann Surg* 1962;156:404–407
14. Shingleton WW, Bryan FA, O'Quinn WL, Krueger LC. Selective heating and cooling of tissue in cancer chemotherapy. *Ann Surg* 1962;156:408–416
15. Kirsch R, Schmidt D. Erste Experimentelle und Klinische Erfahrungen mit der Gaszkorper-Extrem-Hyperthermie. In: Doerr W, Linder F, Wagner G (eds). *Aktuelle Probleme aus dem Gebiet der Cancerologie.* Heidelberg: Springer-Verlag. 1966:53–70
16. Cavaliere R, Ciocztto EC, Giovanella BC, et al. Selective heat sensitivity of cancer cells. *Cancer* 1967;20:1351–1381
17. Bicher HI, Hetzel FW, Sandhu T, et al. Effects of hyperthermia on normal and tumor microenvironment. *Radiology* 1980;137:523–530
18. Song CS, Kang MS, Rhee JG, Levitt SH. The effect of hyperthermia on vascular function, pH, and cell survival. *Radiology* 1980;137:795–803
19. Emami B, Song CW. Physiological mechanisms in hyperthermia: a review. *Int J Radiat Oncol Biol Phys* 1984;10:289–295
20. Astrahan MA, Norman A. A localized current field hyperthermia system for use with 192-iridium interstitial implants. *Med Phys* 1982;9:419–424
21. Samaras GM. Intracranial microwave hyperthermia: heat induction and temperature control. *IEEE Trans Biomed Eng (BME)* 1984;31:63–69
22. Strohbehn JW, Trembly BS, Douple EB. Blood flow effects on temperature distributions from an invasive microwave antenna array used in cancer therapy. *IEEE Trans Biomed Eng (BME)* 1982;29:649–661
23. Lyons BE, Britt RH, Strohbehn JW. Localized hyperthermia in the treatment of malignant brain tumors using an interstitial microwave antenna array. *IEEE Trans Biomed Eng (BME)* 1984;31:53–62
24. Stauffer PR, Cetas TC, Jones RC. Magnetic induction heating of ferromagnetic implants for inducing localized hyperthermia in deep seated tumors. *IEEE Trans Biomed Eng (BME)* 1984;31:235–251
25. Brezovich IA, Atkinson WJ, Lilly MB. Local hyperthermia with interstitial techniques. *Cancer Res* 1984;44 (Suppl): 4752s–4756s
26. Yerushalmi A. Localized, non-invasive deep microwave hyperthermia for the treatment of prostatic tumors: the first 5 years. *Recent Results Cancer Res* 1988;107:140–146
27. Mendecki J, Firedenthal E, Botstein C. Microwave applicators for localized hyperthermia treatment of cancer of the prostate. *Int J Radiat Oncol Biol Phys* 1980;6:1583–1588
28. Kaver I, Ware J, Koontz W. The effect of hyperthermia on human prostatic carcinoma cell lines: evaluation in vitro. *J Urol* 1989;141:1025–1027
29. Lindner A, Golomb J, Siegel Y, Lev A. Local hyperthermia of the prostate gland for the treatment of benign prostatic hypertrophy and urinary retention. A preliminary report. *Br J Urol* 1987;60:567–571
30. Servadio C, Lieb Z, Lev A. Diseases of the prostate treated by local microwave hyperthermia. *Urology* 1987;30:97–99
31. Yerushalmi A, Fishelovitz Y, Singer D, et al. Localized deep microwave hyperthermia in the treatment of poor operative risk patients with benign prostatic hyperplasia. *J Urol* 1985; 133:873–886
32. Servadio C, Lieb Z, Lev A. Further observations on the use of local hyperthermia for the treatment of diseases of the prostate in man. *Eur Urol* 1986;12:38–40
33. Astrahan MA, Sapozink MD, Cohen D, et al. Microwave applicator for transurethral hyperthermia of benign prostatic hyperplasia. *Int J Hyperthermia* 1989;5:283–296
34. Leib Z, Rothem A, Lev A, Servadio C. Histopathological observations in the canine prostate treated by local microwave hyperthermia. *Prostate* 1986;8:93–102
35. Blandy JP. The history and current problems of prostatic obstruction. In: Blandy JP, Lytton BJ (eds). *The Prostate.* Chicago: Butterworths, 1986:17–18

20

Canine Transurethral Laser-Induced Prostatectomy

Dean G. Assimos, David L. McCullough,
Ralph D. Woodruff, Lloyd H. Harrison,
Lois J. Hart, Wei-Jia Li

During the last decade, a number of treatment alternatives for patients with benign prostatic hyperplasia (BPH) have been developed. Urologists have used laser technology for the treatment of patients with a variety of disorders.[1] Other investigators have reported using an Nd:YAG laser to ablate human and canine prostatic tissue.[2-4] Tissue removal was based on vaporization in these studies. We report our experience with transurethral laser incision of the prostate (TULIP) using an Nd:YAG laser in a canine model. In contrast to previous studies, tissue is ablated through coagulation necrosis in this technique. This technology was developed by the Intra-Sonix Company, Burlington, MA.

MATERIALS AND METHODS

Instrumentation

The main components of the TULIP system are a probe and an ultrasound imager. The probe consists of a rigid, 22 F stainless steel sheath that contains a laser fiber, a 90-degree microprism laser port, and paired 7.5 MHz ultrasound transducers. The laser port, which is located at the distal end of the sheath, has ultrasonic transducers on each side that are driven simultaneously to provide a 90-degree sector cross-sectional image with 2 mm spatial resolution. This probe is coupled to a Surgilase YAG 100 Nd:YAG laser system and a modified Hewlett-Packard Sonos 200 ultrasound unit (Fig. 20–1A). A sterile plastic sheath having an optically clear low-pressure 36 F balloon at its distal end is placed over the probe to cover the ultrasound transducers and laser port.

The balloon is inflated with sterile water to 1–2 atm of pressure during treatment to stabilize the probe in the prostatic urethra, provide a fluid environment for ultrasound transmission, and uniformly compress the surrounding prostatic tissue (Fig. 20–1B). A plastic probe handle with a spring-loaded hand grip is placed over the base of the probe. When the hand grip is moved proximally by the operator, the laser-emitting portion of the probe is brought through the prostatic urethra in a slow continuous manner. Pull distances are assessed by monitoring a linear measurement device located on top of the probe handle. A dial on the handle is manipulated to change the direction of the laser port.

Animals

Five- to seven-year-old male fox hounds weighing 25–35 kg were used. The animals were housed in separate cages in the medical school vivarium. They received standard dog chow feedings, and water was provided ad libidum.

Surgery

All animals were anesthetized initially with IV sodium thiamylal and subsequently underwent oral endotracheal intubation. Halothane, 1.5%–2%, was used for maintenance inhalational anesthesia. The animals were given 1 g of cefazolin IV. A perineal urethrostomy was performed using aseptic technique. The urethral mucosa was sutured to the adjacent skin with interrupted 3-0 chromic sutures. The proximal urethra was dilated to 26 F with a coaxial dilation

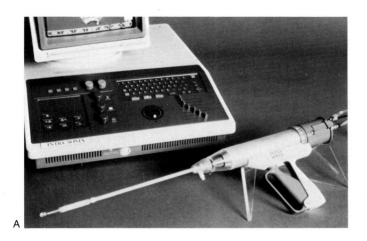

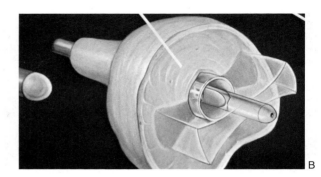

Figure 20–1. The TULIP system. **A.** Probe with spring-loaded hand grip and ultrasound unit. **B.** Balloon surrounding laser probe inflated in the prostatic urethra.

system. Urethroscopy and cystoscopy were performed using a 19 F sheath and a 30 degree lens. These examinations were video recorded. The bladder was filled with sterile irrigant, the laser probe was passed through the perineal urethrostomy, and the balloon was inflated. An ultrasonic examination of the bladder and prostatic urethra was conducted.

Twelve dogs received laser treatment of the prostatic urethra, usually performed in four quadrants: 2, 4, 8, and 10 o'clock positions. These areas were treated with either 25 W or 35 W of laser energy at a pullout speed of 1 cm/5 sec. In two of these animals, only three quadrants were treated because of technical difficulties. The length of the prostatic urethra measured endoscopically ranged from 2.5 to 3 cm. Laser energy was directed using ultrasonic guidance starting just distal to the bladder neck and terminating at the prostatic apex. The pullout speed was regulated through stopwatch monitoring. Two animals were subjected to control procedures in which the same mechanical procedures were performed but without laser activation. Another videorecorded endoscopic examination was performed after the laser and sham procedures. Because of problems with postoperative hematoma formation at the perineal urethrostomy site in one of the first three laser-treated animals, the bladders of all the subsequent dogs were drained with an 18 F urethral catheter for 72 h after laser or sham treatments. All animals received 1 g of cephalexin orally daily during the first 5 postoperative days.

Necropsy

Four laser-treated dogs were humanely killed at 3, 7, and 12 weeks postoperatively, and one control animal was euthanized at 7 and another at 12 weeks postoperatively. A thorough laparotomy was performed. Urine was aspirated from the bladder using aseptic technique and cultured. The bladder, prostate, and urethra were removed en bloc and fixed in formalin. The rectum underlying the bladder and prostate was removed and fixed similarly. The tissue was cross-sectioned at 2–3-mm intervals, photographed, and processed for light microscopy with hematoxylin and eosin staining. The kidneys and ureters underwent careful macroscopic inspection.

RESULTS

There were no perioperative deaths. Posttreatment videoendoscopy demonstrated linear yellow-white areas 2–3 mm wide just inside the bladder neck and extending to the prostatic apex in the various quadrants of the laser-treated animals. Bleeding was not encountered. No similar lesions were present in the controls. One of the animals treated early in the series developed a hematoma at the perineal urethrostomy site causing urinary retention, which resolved after 72 h of catheter drainage. All subsequent animals, who underwent planned postoperative bladder catheterization, had no voiding difficulties or gross hematuria.

The laser-treated animal who developed the perineal hematoma had a positive urine culture, *Streptococcus faecalis*, at necropsy. However, there was no histologic evidence of cystitis in this animal. Urine cultures were all negative in the other respective animals.

At necropsy, there was no hydronephrosis or gross evidence of bowel or other visceral abnormalities in the laser-treated and control animals. Histologic examination of the rectum adjacent to the bladder and prostate demonstrated no abnormalities in the treated and control animals. The bladders of all the dogs were uniformly normal on light microscopic examination. The urethra distal to the prostatic apex was patent in all animals. Macroscopic examination of the sectioned prostatic urethras of all laser-treated animals demonstrated well-defined reurethelialized cavitation channels similar to defects observed after TURP (Fig. 20–2). Such defects were not observed in the control animals (Fig. 20–3). Although the defects appeared somewhat larger in the quadrants treated with 35 W, this could not be assessed objectively. Histologic analysis demonstrated areas of glandular

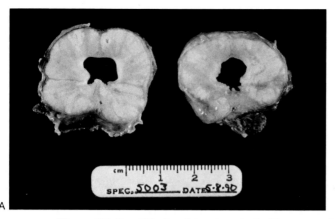

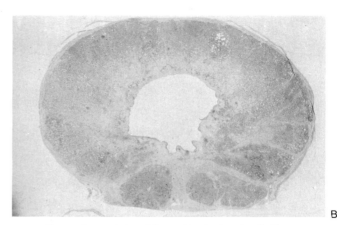

Figure 20–2.   Effects of treatment. **A.** Macroscopic cross-sections of prostate of laser-treated animal. **B.** Microscopic cross-section of prostate of same animal.

hyperplasia compatible with canine BPH in all of the animals (Fig. 20–4). There were no laser effects outside the prostatic capsule in the treated animals. At 3 weeks after laser treatment, there were areas of mild coagulation necrosis, almost complete reepithelialization, and atrophy of the prostatic glands. At 7 and 12 weeks after laser treatment, there was complete reepithelialization, mild chronic inflammation, atrophy of the prostatic glands, and a few scattered areas of squamous metaplasia (Fig. 20–5). Histologic analysis of the prostatic tissue of the control animals demonstrated mild chronic inflammation but none of the other features present in the laser-treated specimens.

DISCUSSION

The results of this feasibility study indicate that the TULIP procedure creates defects in the canine prostatic urethra that are similar to those produced in humans undergoing TURP. The intraluminal cavitation defects occurring after TULIP appear to result from coagulation necrosis, a process characterized by cell necrosis in tissue retaining its original configuration because of heat (60–100°C) protein denaturation. The glands peripheral to the areas of coagulation necrosis atrophied, as evidenced by the presence of flattened epithelial cells in dilated acini and ducts. We have designated this process *cystic atrophy,* which we believe results from central ductal mechanical obstruction or direct laser effects.

The TULIP device combines two technologies familiar to most urologists: therapeutic laser energy and ultrasound imaging. The Nd:YAG laser energy, which is minimally absorbed by water and can be transmitted through semiflexible fibers easily adaptable to endoscopic equipment, has been used by urologists for the treatment of a variety of genitourinary lesions.[1] The action of this laser is based on the conversion of light into thermal energy. Other investigators have used this laser to ablate prostatic tissue by vaporization.[2–4] Vaporization occurs when the tissue temperature is rapidly increased above 100°C. Although there was some reported enthusiasm for this technique, it was abandoned for a variety of reasons. Tissue vaporization often was awkward

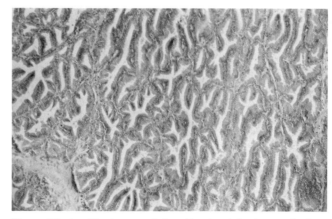

Figure 20–3.   Macroscopic cross-section of prostate of control animal.

Figure 20–4.   Canine prostate with glandular hyperplasia.

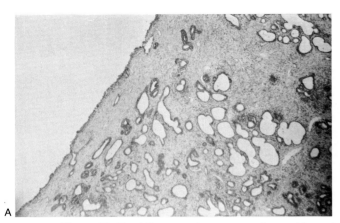
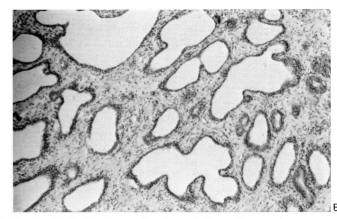

Figure 20–5. Microscopic cross sections of laser-treated animals. **A.** Reepithelialized prostatic urethra and atrophic glands in a laser-treated animal. **B.** Higher-power view of atrophic glands.

and inefficient for removal of bulky tissue, and Nd:YAG energy was less effective than electrocautery for controlling hemorrhage encountered during endoscopic removal of prostatic tissue. In addition, the depth of tissue penetration was difficult to assess.

There are a number of unresolved issues regarding the TULIP procedure. Canine BPH is characterized primarily by diffuse glandular hyperplasia, whereas in human BPH, there are both stromal and glandular components. Therefore, it cannot be predicted whether human prostatic tissue will react similarly. It also is not known whether these tissue effects will be longlasting or whether there will be delayed deleterious sequelae. Because our study demonstrated no discernible laser effects exterior to the prostatic capsule, we do not anticipate any untoward long-term extraprostatic side effects. The urodynamic and functional consequences of TULIP are likewise unknown. The appropriate amount of laser energy and the rate of delivery have not been established. Others who have investigated TULIP in a canine model found that lower power levels delivered per unit length of the urethra were associated with a lower depth of tissue penetration and less coagulation necrosis. However, with power levels greater than 40–50 W, those investigators demonstrated no increased depth of tissue penetration. The maximum tissue penetration in these studies was 8.5 mm.[5]

The true use of TULIP for treatment of BPH as contrasted to TURP in humans will be established only by carefully performed clinical trials. Advantages envisioned for TULIP are that it will be a shorter procedure, possibly conducted in an outpatient setting, associated with minimal bleeding and no dilutional electrolyte complications. A significant disadvantage is that tissue is not obtained, which would limit the diagnosis of stage A prostate cancer. Therefore, measures to help detect occult prostate cancer, such as transrectal ultrasonography, serum prostatic-specific antigen assessments, and fine-needle aspiration of the prostate, may need to be undertaken before TULIP.[6,7]

REFERENCES

1. Smith JA Jr, Dixon JA. Laser photoradiation in urologic surgery. *J Urol* 1984;131:631–635
2. Bloiso G, Warner R, Cohen M. Treatment of urethral diseases with neodymium:YAG laser. *Urology* 1988;32:106–110
3. Kandel LB, Harrison LH, McCullough DL, Boyce WH, Woodruff RP, Dyer RB. Transurethral laser prostatectomy: creation of a technique for using the neodymium:yttrium aluminum garnet (YAG) laser in the canine model. *J Urol* 1986;135:Abstract 110
4. Sander S, Beisland HO. Laser in the treatment of localized prostatic carcinoma. *J Urol* 1984;132:280–281
5. Roth RA, Aretz TH, Lage AL. "TULIP": transurethral laser induced prostatotomy under ultrasound guidance. *J Urol* 1990;143:Abstract 285
6. Cooner WH, Mosley BR, Rutherford CL Jr, Beard JH, Pond HS, Bass RB Jr, Terry WJ. Clinical application of transrectal ultrasonography and prostate-specific antigen in the search for prostate cancer. *J Urol* 1988;139:758–761
7. Agatstein EH, Hernandez FJ, Layfield LJ, Smith RB, deKernion JB. Use of fine needle aspiration for detection of stage A prostatic carcinoma before transurethral resection of the prostate: a clinical trial. *J Urol* 1987;138:551–553

Reprinted from *Journal of Endourology* 1991;5:145–149.

21

Single-Session Transurethral Microwave Thermotherapy for the Treatment of Benign Prostatic Obstruction

S. St. C. Carter, A. Patel, P. Reddy, P. Royer, J.W.A. Ramsay

For the last 60 years, the transurethral surgical approach (TURP) has dominated prostatic surgery because of the high success rates and low morbidity obtained in the hands of experienced urologists.[1] The success of the operation and the ever-aging population impose a high demand on health care systems throughout the western world.[2] In addition to the established population already treated by TURP, many men suffering with symptoms of early bladder outflow are not considered candidates for operative treatment but might benefit from a minimally invasive treatment.[3] Although TURP is widely perceived by urologists as a successful operation, there is some morbidity and a small failure rate.[4–6] The necessity for spinal or general anesthesia, postoperative catheterization, and hospitalization has led to a search for safer but equally effective treatment.[3,7] A satisfactory alternative to TURP should neither require admission to the hospital nor need anesthesia. Neither transurethral incision of the prostate nor balloon dilation meets these criteria, as at least spinal anesthesia and sometimes hospital admission are required.[8,9] Stenting of the prostatic urethra may be performed with topical anesthesia alone in ambulatory patients, but concern remains about the long-term risks of prosthetic materials within the urinary tract.[10,11] The great hope of finding a medication to replace the TURP still seems to be some way off. In selected patients, alpha-blockade may produce symptomatic and objective improvement.[7,12] The place of antiandrogen therapy has yet to be established, but it

is known that a lifetime commitment to treatment is required because of the rapid regrowth of the prostate once normal testosterone stimulation resumes.[13]

The application of heat has been held to have therapeutic benefits since the earliest origins of medicine. Many ingenious methods of heating the prostate have been described since the mid-19th century and were advocated for the relief of obstruction or the symptoms of prostatitis.[14] There was limited success because of the superficial nature of prostatic heating obtained by conduction from the urethral or rectal surface. The development of radiative heating by microwaves allowed the application of thermal energy deep within the lateral lobes of the prostate.[15] The first clinical devices employed a shielded antenna within the rectum with simultaneous cooling of the rectal wall.[16,17] Because the microwave field has to encompass the nontarget tissues behind the prostate, only limited power application is possible, and multiple sessions are required to obtain any clinical success. Furthermore, microwaves from a rectal antenna predominantly affect the peripheral zone of the prostate rather than the obstructive adenoma growing from the more anterior transition zone.

Recent technologic advances in microwave engineering have allowed the development of flexible antennas that can be introduced into the urethra and used to apply heat directly to the obstructive prostatic tissue. Sapozink et al. described a system for transurethral heating of the prostate using three

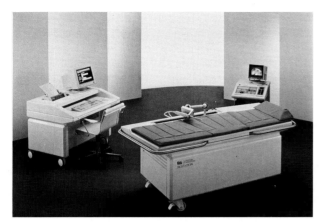

Figure 21–1. The Prostatron showing the separate treatment module and control console. The device is designed to be operated with a freestanding transrectal ultrasound scanning unit. (Courtesy of Technomed International.)

separate antennas and subsequently a single spiral antenna mounted on the surface of a urethral catheter.[18,19] Multiple treatments of 1-h duration were used to avoid painful and damaging heating of the urethral surface. Significant clinical benefit was found in patients with benign prostatic obstruction using eight treatments of 1 h each.[18,19]

We have described a new system (Prostatron, Technomed International) for heating of the prostate by a transurethral microwave applicator incorporating simultaneous conductive cooling of the urethra (Fig. 21–1).[20] Urethral surface cooling permits greater power application, limits urethral pain, and preserves the integrity of the urethral mucosa. Temperatures in excess of 45°C can be generated within the lateral lobes, producing focused tissue destruction. The complete treatment can be performed in a single session without sedation or analgesia. The combination of irradiative heating and conductive cooling has been termed transurethral microwave thermotherapy (TUMT). An investigation into the clinical effects of the treatment is reported here.

PATIENTS AND METHODS

Patients

Fifty men aged 46–91 with symptomatic benign prostatic obstruction that otherwise would have been treated by TURP or a long-term indwelling catheterization underwent TUMT during the period April–September 1990. The criteria for entry into the study are given in Table 21–1. Certain patients were excluded from the study on the theoretical grounds of

Table 21–1. Inclusion and Exclusion Criteria for TUMT

INCLUSION CRITERIA	EXCLUSION CRITERIA
Benign prostatic hyperplasia as determined by clinical examination and transrectal ultrasonography with *Either* Symptoms of bladder outflow obstruction for more than 3 months and peak urine flow rates of less than 15 mL/sec on two occasions with voided volumes of >100 mL *Or* Acute retention of urine requiring an indwelling catheter; failure of at least one trial withdrawal	*Local factors* Clinical or sonographic findings suspect for prostatic cancer Prostate <30 mL as judged by transrectal ultrasound Upper tract dilation or biochemical evidence of renal failure Urethral stricture Clinical and bacteriologic evidence of bacterial prostatitis Urinary tract infection at the time of treatment Bladder calculus Previous TURP or other prostatic surgery other than biopsy *Factors likely to interfere with response to microwave irradiation* Significant arterial disease leading to clinical evidence of Leriche's syndrome Previous pelvic surgery or radiotherapy Previous rectal surgery other than hemorrhoidectomy The presence of metallic pelvic or femoral joint replacement *General medical factors* Mental incapacity or inability to give informed consent to the procedure Medical or physical deformity that would prevent conventional TURP Neurologic disorders, such as multiple sclerosis or cord injury Evidence of disorders of hemostasis Uncontrolled cardiac dysrhythmias or presence of cardiac pacemaker

Table 21–2.   Preliminary Investigations Before TUMT

Madsen symptom score
Creatinine, urea, and electrolytes[a]
MSU for culture[a]
Upper tract imaging[a] (IVU or ultrasound)
Transrectal ultrasound to determine prostatic dimensions
    and exclude cancer
Flow rates × 2
Residual urine (ultrasound; catheter)
Flexible cystoscopy[a]
Pressure flow urodynamic studies[a]

[a]Follow-up studies not reported.

impaired blood supply to the prostate leading to an increase in tissue heating. No patients with metallic implants in the pelvis or hip were treated for fear of distortion of the microwave field and consequent eccentric or excessive heating. Patients with recurrent outflow obstruction after a previous TURP were excluded to avoid the possibility of misplacement of the treatment applicator by distal migration of the positioning balloon into the resection fossa.

Methods

Patients were seen in a specialized prostate unit and underwent preliminary investigation, both to establish their suitability for treatment and to quantify the degree of obstruction (Table 21–2). All patients had symptoms for more than 3 months, and particular importance was attached to a close analysis of the symptom status using the Madsen scoring system.[21] Patients without indwelling catheters had the diagnosis of outflow tract obstruction confirmed by voiding urodynamic studies. Urinary performance was assessed throughout the study period by the objective criteria of peak urinary flow rates (measured on several occasions) and residual volume measured either by catheterization or by

postmicturition ultrasound examination. Careful evaluation excluded other causes of bladder outflow obstruction. Transrectal sonographic images (Proscan, Teknar) were obtained to ascertain the benign nature of the prostate and to assess the size of the gland. Measurements of the length of the prostate were used to define the treatment parameters and as an objective means of follow-up. All patients were free of infection at the time of treatment.

A leaflet explaining the treatment and research protocol was given to each patient. Informed consent was obtained at the outset of the clinical investigation. Transurethral thermotherapy was undertaken at least 2 days after the preliminary investigations in order to avoid excessive urethral irritation. Urodynamic flow measures, urethral length, and residual volume were measured at 6, 12, and 24 weeks after treatment.

Description of the Prostatron

The Prostatron is an integrated unit consisting of a microwave generator, a urethral cooling system, a fiberoptic temperature monitoring system, and a treatment couch (Fig. 21–1). The Prostatron is controlled by a dedicated computer software system operated from a separate control module. The device is used in conjunction with a disposable transurethral applicator and rectal thermometry probe (Fig. 21–2).

The microwave antenna is mounted within a flexible 20 F urethral applicator with a Foley balloon self-retaining device. The treatment applicator contains two channels for the circulation of coolant. The tip of one thermosensor is positioned on the surface of the catheter to measure the applicator surface temperature at the hottest point of the microwave field. Two applicators with different antenna positions were available for treatment of prostates from 30 to 40 mm and 41 to 65 mm in length. The antenna is positioned in a precise relation to the Foley balloon so that the predictable micro-

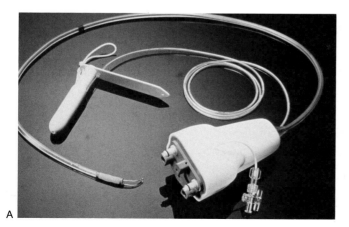
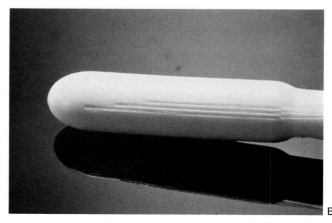

A   B

Figure 21–2.   Parts of Prostatron. **A.** Disposable treatment applicator and rectal thermometry probe. **B.** Close-up view of rectal thermometry probe showing the fiberoptic thermosensors, which are positioned 80, 90, and 100 mm from anal verge. (Courtesy of Technomed International.)

wave field can treat the greatest volume of the prostate without compromising the external sphincter.

The integral thermometry system is of the optical fiber type, designed to measure temperature accurately within a microwave field, and is consistently accurate to 0.1°C. In addition to the urethral thermosensor, three fibers are mounted on a rectal probe to monitor the temperature of the anterior rectal wall. The rectal thermosensors are placed at 80, 90, and 100 mm from the anal verge, positions that have been shown to indicate the maximum rectal wall temperature most reliably during treatment (Fig. 21–2B).

The cooling system is comprised of both a refrigeration and a heating unit, providing precise control of applicator temperature during treatment. The coolant is circulated at a constant rate, although the temperature can be varied from 20°C to 40°C. The microprocessor controls the power output of the Prostatron in response to preset parameters of achieved temperature within the rectal and urethral thermosensors. Multiple safety devices are incorporated to prevent the excessive or misplaced delivery of energy, and the treatment remains under the physician's control at all times. The details of the treatment are displayed on a video monitor and recorded by the computer for subsequent analysis. Printouts of the treatment details and temperature tracings are available for inclusion in the individual patient records.

Technique

The relevant transurethral treatment catheter was selected. The proximal antenna position was used for patients with a prostate length of less than 40 mm. The catheter assembly was sterilized by immersion in 2% glutaraldehyde. Gentamicin 80 mg was administered IV at the commencement of the treatment, and trimethoprim 200 mg twice daily was prescribed for the 5 following days. The rectal temperature monitoring probe was covered by a standard condom to prevent contamination or damage to the thermosensors.

The patient was placed supine on the couch, the penis was cleaned, and 1% lignocaine jelly was applied transurethrally. The bladder was first emptied by catheterization with a 14 F Lofric catheter (Astra Meditech, Sweden) and then refilled with 50 mL of saline. Additional lignocaine gel was applied through the catheter to ensure adequate lubrication and analgesia of the prostatic and posterior urethra. The treatment applicator was passed, the self-retaining balloon was inflated with 15 mL of saline, and the catheter was withdrawn until it rested gently at the bladder neck.

The patient was repositioned in the left lateral position, and a clinical mercury thermometer was used to measure the rectal temperature for calibration of the fiberoptic thermosensors. A multiplane transrectal ultrasound probe (Proscan, Teknar USA) was used to check the correct placement of the applicator by identifying the balloon at the bladder neck.

The rectal temperature probe was inserted so that the flange lay at the anal margin. A string attached to the posterior part of the flange was laid along the crease between the buttocks and strapped to the patient's back under tension so as to tilt the anal probe onto the anterior rectal wall.

With the patient once more in the supine position, the machine was switched on, and the treatment catheter assembly was connected. The patient details, including the prostatic dimensions, as determined by transrectal ultrasound, and rectal temperature were entered into the computer.

The treatment sequence was commenced. The coolant temperature was circulated at 20°C for at least 5 min until the urethral temperature reached a stable state (approximately 25°C). The microwave power application was started at levels between 15 and 35 W, depending on the length of the prostate. Throughout the treatment, increasing power levels were applied in 5-W increments every 3 min until either a rectal thermosensor registered 42.5°C or a maximum of 60 W was reached. If the temperature measured by a rectal sensor exceeded 42.5°C, the power was switched off until the thermosensor reached 42.0°C, when the power was recommenced at a level 5 W lower.

Two distinct parts of the treatment were defined. During the phase of increasing power buildup, the coolant temperature was maintained at 20°C. Once either the maximum rectal temperature was reached, the maximum power output was obtained, or after 20 min of treatment, the urethral coolant temperature was allowed to increase in 3°C increments to raise the applicator surface temperature to a maximum of 45.5°C. If the temperature in the applicator sensor exceeded 45.5°C, the power was stopped until it cooled to 45.0°C.

If the patient complained of discomfort, the positioning of all catheter and probes was checked carefully. The power level or coolant temperature was reduced by the operator if the patient was unable to tolerate the sensation of urethral heating.

The treatment was continued for 55 min from the start of microwave application. At the conclusion of the treatment, the applicator and rectal probe were removed. If the patient was catheter free before the treatment, he was asked to wait in the department until he passed urine. Patients with catheters before treatment were recatheterized with a 16 F Silastic catheter and either returned to the ward or discharged home while awaiting a trial of voiding 3–6 weeks later.

RESULTS

Patients have been allocated to four groups for analysis, as shown in Table 21–3. Overall, TUMT was easy to perform and was well tolerated by the patients. No anesthesia or sedation was required during any of the treatments. No complications occurred during the treatment, and no treatment was discontinued as a result of patients experiencing pain. Most patients felt minor urethral discomfort and a sensation of local heating within the pelvis. Some felt

Table 21–3. Results of TUMT According to Pretreatment Condition

	TOTAL
Indwelling catheter (n = 19)	
Treated (n = 15)	
Trial of catheter removal	
Success	6
TURP	7
Long-term catheter	2
Patient died (disseminated kidney cancer)	1
Awaiting catheter removal	3
Bladder outflow obstruction	
(symptom score > 8, peak flow rate < 15 mL/sec, residual urine < 350 ml)	
Treated (n = 23)	
Follow-up	
24 weeks	5
12 weeks	9
6 weeks	19
Obstruction with abnormal bladder	
(flow rates < 15 mL/sec, history of infection)	
Treated (n = 6)	
High residual volume	3
Low symptom score	2
Parkinson's disease	1
Unsuccessful treatment (n = 2)	
Retention of urine	2
Total	50

systemically hot toward the end of the treatment. Bladder spasm with bypassing of the treatment catheter (which contains no drainage lumen) was experienced by a few patients. A rapid decrease in urethral temperature was seen as soon as the power was turned off or reduced, providing easy control for the patient's safety and comfort. The rectal temperature took longer to fall when the power application was stopped, and consequently, the treatment in some patients was of an intermittent pattern. It was not possible to reach the rectal temperature maximum of 42.5°C or the urethral maximum of 45.5°C in all patients.

Group 1 (Acute Retention)

Nineteen patients with urethral catheters placed for episodes of acute retention have been treated. A Silastic catheter was replaced after treatment in all patients for periods of up to 6 weeks. Three patients are awaiting a trial of voiding, and one patient with disseminated renal cancer died from metastatic disease before the catheter was withdrawn. Eight of fifteen men voided normally on withdrawal of the catheter. One 90-year-old man required recatheterization for social reasons despite voiding normally. A second man voided well for 10 weeks and went back into retention after a further surgical procedure and subsequently required TURP. Six men (40%) are voiding satisfactorily 6 weeks to 5 months later. Four are known to have flow rates between 4.4 and 22.5 mL/sec

(average 7.7 mL/sec) with minimal postmicturition residual urine in the bladder.

Nine patients either have had the catheter replaced (2) or have undergone TURP (7). Of the 7 patients who have undergone TURP, 5 were noted during the resection to have areas of black or dark brown tissue to the depth of approximately 15 mm. The tissue response in these patients who had failed with TUMT often was seen to be eccentric, affecting one lateral lobe more than the other. Histologic examination of the prostatic chips showed marked changes of inflammation and necrosis affecting a variable proportion of the resected gland. Cystoscopy in the patient who underwent TURP 3 months after treatment showed evidence of lateral lobe retraction distally but continuing proximal obstruction. Histology showed minor inflammation only. No complications have been noted in the patients who underwent surgery after TUMT.

Group 2 (Outflow Obstruction)

All patients have had an improvement in their symptom score status at 6 weeks and 12 weeks after treatment (Table 21–4). This supports the general statement from most patients that they find micturition easier 2–3 weeks after treatment. Follow-up data at 24 weeks after treatment are available in 5 patients. One man has had a deterioration in symptoms and poor flow rate, which is disappointing, but he does not want any further treatment. The other 4 have maintained the improvement in symptoms.

The average of all flow rates for patients in group 2 before treatment was 8.2 mL/sec (range 4.4–13.0). After treatment, the increase in peak flow rate at 6 weeks was 4.7 mL/sec and at 12 weeks 6.1 mL/sec. A normal flow rate of more than 15.0 mL/sec was seen in 37% and 33% of men at 6 and 12 weeks, respectively. The peak flow rate had increased by more than 5 mL/sec in the same percentage of men.

The apparent increase in postvoiding residual volume at 6 weeks is attributable mainly to one patient whose volume increased from 200 mL to 470 mL. He has been shown subsequently to again have a residual volume of 200 mL at 24 weeks. Of the six patients with an accurate assessment of residual volume by catheterization before treatment and at 24 weeks, the mean volume left in the bladder has fallen to 41 mL.

Before treatment, no patient had a prostatic urethral length greater than 60 mm and the average was 44 mm, representing a prostatic volume of approximately 50 mL and a resectable weight of 30 g. A decrease of greater than 15% of the mean (6 mm) was seen in 31% of patients at 6 weeks and in 57% at 12 weeks. Patients with an increase in peak flow rate of greater than 5 mL/sec at both 6 weeks and 12 weeks were seen to have a greater decrease in the urethral length (Table 21–5).

Although it was difficult to assess in a small group of patients, sexual function generally has been preserved, together with prograde ejaculation.

Table 21–4. Results of TUMT in Patients with Outflow Obstruction Before Treatment

| | | WEEKS AFTER TREATMENT | | |
	BEFORE	6	12	24
Number	19	19	9	5
Symptom score	12.0	3.0	2.8[a]	1.4
No. >8	100%	0	11	0
No. <3	0	14 (73%)	6 (75%)	4 (80%)
Peak flow (mL/sec)				
Mean	8.2	12.9	14.3	14.3
Range	4.4–13.0	7.6–22.7	8.2–26.0	5.9–23.1
No. >15	0	7 (37%)	3 (33%)	2 (40%)
No. increase >5	—	7 (37%)	3 (33%)	2 (40%)
Residual (mL)				
Mean	64	137	41[a]	58
Range	0–200	0–470	0–200	0–140
% > 50 ml	61%	40%	71%	60%
Prostatic length (mm)	44	36	39[a]	45[a]
Range	35–60	28–63	31–45	37–52
Fall > 15%	—	6 (31%)	4 (57%)	0

[a]Incomplete data.

Group 3 (Obstruction with Abnormal Bladder)

All patients in group 3 had a history of recurrent urinary tract infection as a result of outflow obstruction. Three patients with large postvoiding residual volumes (800, 550, 450 mL) were treated, of whom only one had a significant reduction at 12 weeks (150 mL). One of the two men with a low symptom score but low flow rates has had an increase in flow rate of 6 mL/sec, whereas the other has had no significant change in objective measures. The single patient with Parkinson's disease had marked obstructive and irritative symptoms before treatment and has had a dramatic symptomatic improvement associated with an increase in voided volume. All men from this group remain well and have had no further urinary tract infections to date.

Group 4 (Unsuccessful Treatment)

One patient was unable to have a treatment because the urethral applicator could not be passed through a narrow urethra, and one patient was not treated because of a technical failure with the applicator. No ill effects have been noted from the instrumentation in either patient.

Table 21–5. Flow Rate Related to Decrease in Prostatic Urethral Length

FOLLOW-UP	INCREASE IN FLOW RATE (mL/SEC)	CHANGE IN PROSTATE LENGTH (mm)
6 weeks	>5	−8.5
	<5	+0.3
12 weeks	>5	−9.6
	<5	−3.0

Complications

Side effects have not been a prominent feature in this series. Immediately after treatment, most patients had some urethral bleeding, which was generally short lived and innocuous. During the first few days after treatment, the outflow symptoms often became slightly worse, presumably because of urethral edema. The increase in urethral resistance has been sufficiently severe to cause a short-lived retention necessitating catheterization in five patients from groups 2 and 3. In four men, this occurred at the end of treatment, and in two, it may be attributed to the bladder becoming overfull. The fifth patient developed retention 3 days after treatment. The retention was relieved by urethral catheterization. All five passed urine spontaneously once the catheter was removed between 3 and 6 days later. No evidence of rectal injury was detected by clinical examination at 1 week. No systemic complications have been encountered.

DISCUSSION

The term *thermotherapy* has been coined because we believe there is a difference between generalized heating associated with hyperthermia and the deliberate tissue destruction by a targeted heat field. The rationale of thermotherapy assumes that temperatures above 45°C can kill a significant proportion of benign prostatic cells. Such temperatures also will cause thermal destruction of nontarget tissues, and consequently, the technique requires sonographic control of applicator positioning and adequate safety mechanisms to prevent extraprostatic heating. We see the precise targeting and accurate temperature monitoring required with high-power treatments as being a primary difference between TUMT using the Prostatron and other microwave devices produced for prostatic therapy.

It has become apparent that benign prostatic hyperplastic tissue contains cell types of differing thermosensitivity and that at all temperatures in the range of 45°C to 50°C achieved by TUMT with the Prostatron, not all cells perish. As a result, a full necrotic process does not ensue, and no sloughing of the prostate has been identified in this series. In addition, temperatures of 45°C and above will cause pain in areas where there are sensory nerve endings. In the prostate, the majority of the pain fibers are found on the surface of the urethra, whereas the adenomatous tissue is sparsely innervated. The addition of simultaneous applicator cooling in the Prostatron not only limits the thermal injury to the urethra, further preventing prostatic sloughing, but also increases patient tolerance during treatment. The two effects of microwave radiative heating and conductive cooling do not cancel each other out, and it is this physical phenomenon that allows deep heating within the prostate during TUMT.

Single-session transurethral microwave thermotherapy has been well tolerated by the patients. The symptom response has been excellent. In particular, the nocturia that most often troubles patients has been greatly decreased, and patients feel that they can pass urine more freely than before even when there is little evidence of objective improvement. Thus far, all but one patient with outflow symptoms have been pleased with the results of treatment. The reduction in Madsen symptom score to below 3 in 75% with a general increase in flow rates suggests that the great majority would not be recommended for further treatment if presenting anew at this stage.

Our study does not provide controls, and any conclusions drawn must take into account the widely recognized placebo effect. However, approximately one third of individual patients have had sufficient increases in flow rate to be in the normal range as defined for this study (>15 mL/sec with a voided volume of greater than 100 mL). The sustained increase of peak flow rate of 74% of the baseline at 12 and 24 weeks is greater than that seen in most trials of alpha-blocker drug therapy.[12] Studies of the flow rate before and after TURP suggest that there is likely to be a 100% increase at 3 months.[4,22] In a study comparing TURP and terazosin therapy, Lepor reported the increase in flow rates as 108% and 42%, respectively, suggesting that the efficacy of TUMT lies between these two treatments.[23]

Treatment of benign prostatic obstruction by transrectal microwave therapy in multiple sessions has been reported as having a success rate of 50% in rendering patients catheter free, with 40% still voiding at 1 year, which is similar to the result reported in this series at 3 months using a single session.[17] Large increases in flow rate in patients treated by transrectal microwave hyperthermia were initially reported by Lindner et al. in 1987.[16] Subsequently, the average increase in patients with symptomatic outflow obstruction has been observed to be as low as 23% at 3 months.[24] A 45%

increase in flow rate was achieved by eight sessions of transurethral heating without cooling by Sapozink et al.[18] Recently, Baert et al. demonstrated a doubling of the flow rate in patients treated with between 5 and 10 sessions of transurethral microwave hyperthermia (without cooling).[19] Transurethral microwave application gives better results than transrectal techniques, and the addition of applicator cooling allows effective treatment in a single session.

The change in residual urine volume after TUMT is less impressive than the changes in flow rate and may represent a degree of detrusor failure in some of our patients.[25] The effect of TUMT is not the same as a TURP, where the prostatic component of the urethral resistance is almost abolished, and patients with a poorly contracting detrusor may succeed in completely emptying the bladder by a combination of gravity and staining. Caine et al. have suggested that an absence of observed change in the residual volume may be attributable to a short period of observation, and data from further follow-up of our patients will be important in this respect.[26]

The results suggest that TUMT reduces the bladder outflow resistance. The place of TUMT in the urologist's armamentarium remains to be defined. The reduction in urethral resistance is not as great as that achieved by TURP but is sufficient to decrease symptoms and improve peak urinary flow rates. The role for TUMT will be at either end of the natural history of benign prostatic obstruction. A simple nonoperative ambulatory treatment is attractive for younger patients with early obstruction and well-preserved detrusor function because it requires little disruption of a man's life. At the other extreme, TUMT offers the possibility of improving urinary performance or rendering a patient catheter free at the risk of little or no morbidity for those unable to undergo TURP because of medical or social reasons. Further groups of patients who are suitable for this treatment are those in whom preservation of prograde ejaculation and sexual function is important and those with an unstable bladder or other neurologic problem, such as Parkinson's disease, where the outcome of TURP is less satisfactory.

REFERENCES

1. Blandy J. The history and current problems of benign prostatic obstruction. In: *The Prostate*. London: Butterworths, 1986:12–22
2. Barry MJ. Epidemiology and natural history of benign prostatic hyperplasia. *Urol Clin North Am* 1990;17:495
3. McCloughlin J, Williams G. Alternatives to prostatectomy. *Br J Urol* 1990;65:313
4. Neal DE, Ramsden PD, Sharples L, et al. Outcome of elective prostatectomy. *Br Med J* 1989;299:762
5. Mebust WK, Holtgrewe HL, Cockett ATK, et al. Transurethral prostatectomy: immediate and postoperative complications: a cooperative study of 13 participating institutions evaluating 3,885 patients. *J Urol* 1989;141:243
6. Fowler FJ, Wennberg JE, Timothy RP, et al. Symptom status and quality of life following prostatectomy. *JAMA* 1988;259:3018

7. Lepor H. Nonoperative management of benign prostatic hyperplasia. *J Urol* 1989;141:1283

8. Orandi A. Transurethral resection versus transurethral incision of the prostate. *Urol Clin North Am* 1990;17:601

9. Dowd JB, Smith JJ. Balloon dilation of the prostate. *Urol Clin North Am* 1990;17:671

10. Chapple CR, Milroy EJ, Rickards D. Permanently implanted urethral stent for prostatic obstruction in the unfit patient: preliminary report. *Br J Urol* 1990;66:58

11. McLoughlin J, Jager R, Abel PD, El Din A, Adam A, Williams G. The use of prostatic stents in patients with urinary retention who are unfit for surgery. *Br J Urol* 1990;66:66

12. Caine M. Alpha-adrenergic blockers for the treatment of benign prostatic hyperplasia. *Urol Clin North Am* 1990;17:641

13. McConnell JD. Androgen blockade in the treatment of benign prostatic hyperplasia. *Urol Clin North Am* 1990;17:661

14. Edwards LE. History of nonsurgical treatment. In: Hinman F Jr (ed). *Benign Prostatic Hypertrophy*. New York: Springer-Verlag, 1983:30

15. Yerulshami A, Servadio C, Leib Z, et al. Local hyperthermia for treatment of carcinoma of the prostate: a preliminary report. *Prostate* 1982;6:623

16. Lindner A, Golomb J, Siegal Y, Lev A. Local hyperthermia of the prostate gland for the treatment of benign prostatic hypertrophy and urinary retention: a preliminary report. *Br J Urol* 1987;60:567

17. Lindner A, Braf Z, Lev A, et al. Local hyperthermia of the prostate gland for the treatment of benign prostatic hypertrophy and urinary retention. *Br J Urol* 1990;65:201

18. Sapozink MD, Boyd S, Astrahan MA, Gabor J, Petrovich Z. Transurethral hyperthermia for benign prostatic hyperplasia: preliminary clinical results. *J Urol* 1990;143:944

19. Baert L, Ameye F, Willemen P, Vandenhove J, Lauweryns J, Astrahan M, Petrovitch Z. Transurethral microwave hyperthermia for benign prostatic hyperplasia: preliminary clinical and pathological results. *J Urol* 1990;144:1383

20. Devonec M, Cathaud M, Carter S, Dutrieux-Berger N, Perrin P. Transurethral microwave application: temperature sensation and thermokinetics of the human prostate. *J Urol* 1990;143: Abstract 414

21. Madsen OM, Iverson P. A point system for selecting operative candidates. In: Hinman F Jr (ed). *Benign Prostatic Hypertrophy*. New York: Springer-Verlag, 1983:763

22. Christensen M, Aagaard J, Madsen P. Transurethral resection versus transurethral incision: a prospective randomized study. *Urol Clin North Am* 1990;17:621

23. Lepor H. Role of long-acting selective alpha$_1$-blockers in the treatment of benign prostatic hyperplasia. *Urol Clin North Am* 1990;17:651

24. Saranga R, Matzkin H, Braf Z. Local microwave hyperthermia of the prostate gland in the treatment of benign prostatic hypertrophy. *Br J Urol* 1990;65:349

25. Hinman F Jr. Residual urine: measurements and influence in obstruction. In: *Benign Prostatic Hypertrophy*. New York, Springer-Verlag, 1983:589

26. Caine M, Perlberg S, Meretyk S. A placebo-controlled double-blind study of the effect of phenoxybenzamine in prostatic obstruction. *Br J Urol* 1981;50:542

Reprinted from *Journal of Endourology* 1991;5:137–144.

22

Self-Expandable Metallic Prostatic Urethral Stents

Euan Milroy

Anxiety about the risks of carrying out prostate surgery on elderly and unfit patients has generated considerable interest in a variety of recently developed urethral devices for mechanically holding open the prostatic urethra, thereby avoiding the need for prostate surgery.

Problems caused by leaving foreign material in the urinary tract are well recognized. Catheters, indwelling stents of any type, and sutures inevitably will become infected and encrust with phosphatic deposits when left in contact with urine. Newer materials will reduce these problems but have failed to prevent them completely. Once infection or encrustation has occurred, it is always necessary to remove the implanted material in order to deal with the problem satisfactorily. These difficulties have meant that implanted material in the lower urinary tract can be used only as a temporary measure to drain urine or to relieve obstruction while awaiting more definitive treatment.

A major development was the finding that woven mesh stents manufactured of fine superalloy wire would cover with normal urothelium if the wire was held against the wall of the urinary tract by the radial spring force of the device. Rapid covering with urothelium prevents contact of the wire with urine and thus avoids the complications of infection and encrustation.[1,2]

SELF-EXPANDABLE METALLIC STENTS

We first used the Urolume Wallstent 4 years ago for the treatment of recurrent bulbar urethral strictures.[3] It proved so successful that we then started using it in patients with prostatic obstruction.[4]

The Urolume Wallstent is a woven tubular mesh of corrosion-resistant superalloy wire manufactured in various lengths and diameters (Fig. 22–1). When expanded from its

delivery system, the stent is stable but flexible. This device was invented by Hans Wallsten of Medinvent, Lausanne, Switzerland, and was first designed for endovascular use, where it has been employed successfully for 6 years in the prevention of restenosis after transluminal angioplasty.[5] It is now manufactured and marketed by American Medical Systems, Minnesota.

We first used a modification of the device developed for endovascular use. This consisted of a small-diameter (9 F) delivery catheter on which a doubled-over plastic membrane held the stent in a compressed and elongated form. The

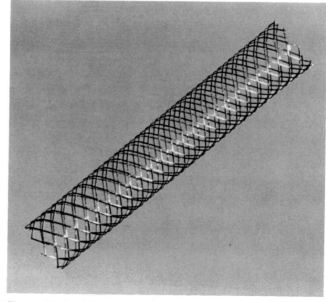

Figure 22–1.   Urolume urethral Wallstent, American Medical Systems.

double-membrane system could be pressurized to 3 atm, after which the outer layer of the membrane was progressively withdrawn to allow the stent to expand once it had been positioned within the prostate cavity or previously dilated urethral stricture. The expansile force of the mesh held it in position, preventing any possibility of displacement and allowing urothelium to grow over the implanted material while holding open the urethra. Because of difficulties with the considerable shortening of the stent as it expanded from its small-diameter delivery catheter, resulting in inaccurate positioning of the stent, we developed, with Hans Wallsten, a new delivery system for the stent. This consists of an endoscopic delivery tool developed specifically for the urologist (Fig. 22–2). With this device, the stent emerges as the outer retaining sheath is pulled back. Because the endoscopic system is much larger than the original small-diameter delivery catheter, far less shortening of the stent takes place as it expands into its final position. A standard 0° telescope fits down the center of the device and may be moved longitudinally, allowing the full length of the stent to be observed as it opens (Fig. 22–3). This ensures that both ends of the stent are positioned correctly. The device includes a locking mechanism to prevent final deployment of the stent until it has been positioned correctly. Until the lock is released, the stent can be recovered into the delivery system by advancing the outer sheath back over the stent. The device can then be repositioned before the stent is opened once more and deployed finally. The outer sheath of the new delivery system measures 21 F.

The internal diameter of the Urolume stent is large enough to permit endoscopic surgery or catheterization if necessary, although these are not advisable until the stent has epithelialized. The stents used for prostate obstruction have all been 14 mm diameter (43 F) in lengths of 20 mm or 30 mm. These

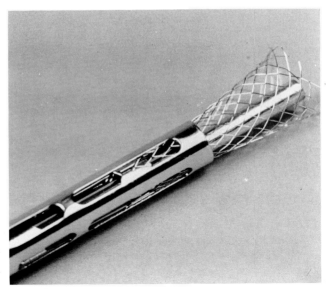

Figure 22–3. Close-up view of stent within sheath of introducer. Note telescope within lumen of stent.

dimensions are measured with the stent unconstrained and exerting no radial force. When used in the prostatic urethra, the diameter will be somewhat smaller, since the stent will then exert a radial force against the prostatic urethra. In this situation, the length of the stent is, of course, correspondingly greater.

EXPERIMENTAL WORK

The first experimental work on the Urolume Wallstent in the blood vessels of experimental animals was carried out by Sarramon in Toulouse, France. He demonstrated rapid covering of the stent with normal endothelium. In collaboration with Sarramon, we carried out studies using the same stent in the normal posterior urethra of a number of male dogs. Stents 4.5 mm in diameter and 10 mm in length were placed in the dogs' urethras using the original small-diameter delivery catheter. The stents were introduced to lie in the bulbar part of the urethra proximal to the os penis. Urethras were examined at between 2 and 12 months after implantation, and scanning electron microscopy showed excellent covering of the stent. Very little surrounding inflammation or fibrosis was found on routine histologic examination.[1,2]

CLINICAL EXPERIENCE

Prostate Obstruction

We have developed two techniques for inserting the Urolume Wallstent into the prostatic urethra. These stents have all been inserted using local urethral lignocaine with additional IV short-acting benzodiazepine as necessary because of the

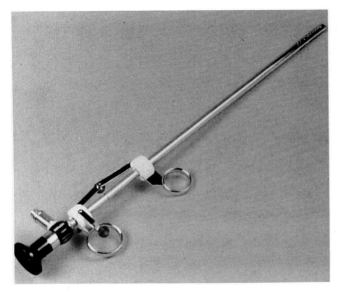

Figure 22–2. New introducer for Wallstent.

mainly elderly and unfit population being treated. With a few patients, we have used a spinal or epidural anesthetic.

Ultrasound Guided Technique

The first technique uses transrectal ultrasound guidance with the stent loaded on the original small-diameter catheter delivery system. The patient lies in the left lateral position, and after local urethral anesthesia, a careful cystourethroscopy is carried out using a flexible cystoscope. Following this, a transrectal ultrasound probe is inserted, and the length of the prostate is measured. The Urolume stent on the catheter system is threaded over a guidewire into the bladder. The compressing double-membrane system is pressurized to 3 atm with normal saline, and the outer layer of the membrane is peeled back to open approximately one third of the stent. The whole device is then gently withdrawn using ultrasound guidance until the inner margin of the stent lies exactly at the bladder neck. The membrane can then be withdrawn fully, allowing the stent to be released into the prostatic urethra. In a few cases where the prostatic urethra is longer than the largest 3 cm stent, a second overlapping stent can be inserted. The position of the stent can be checked with the flexible cystoscope if necessary. Occasionally, the stent fails to expand completely from the catheter delivery system (Fig. 22–4), and in these patients, a 12 mm diameter dilating balloon catheter can be passed over the guidewire and inflated within the lumen of the stent.

The main difficulty with this stent delivery system is that we have found that the considerable shortening that takes place from the small diameter delivery catheter up to the final expanded size of the stent results in such shortening of the stent that exact positioning within the prostatic urethra is difficult. It is vitally important that no wires are left remain-ing within the bladder, since this will prevent the stent covering with urothelium and will allow encrustation to take place. At the distal end of the urethra, any encroachment of the stent on the distal sphincter mechanism will, of course, cause urinary incontinence.

The ultrasound guidance system of stent delivery remains a useful technique for patients whose immobility or other medical condition prevents them being put in the lithotomy position, which is necessary for the more accurate endoscopic delivery technique that we now use for all Urolume stent insertions using the new stent delivery system (Fig. 22–2).

Endoscopic Technique

Because of the difficulties with the ultrasound guided technique, we now use the new endoscopic delivery system for all prostate stent insertions. With this device, more accurate positioning of the stent can be ensured (Figs. 22–2, 22–3).

Urethral lignocaine anesthesia and IV sedation are given, and the patient is placed in the extended lithotomy position. A careful cystoscopy is carried out to check for any bladder abnormality and also to check on the length of the prostatic urethra that has been measured previously using transrectal ultrasound. This preoperative ultrasound scan is used also to confirm the digital diagnosis of a benign prostate. If any suspicious areas are found, ultrasound guided biopsies are taken before proceeding to stent insertion. Prostatic length is measured endoscopically either with a calibrated cystoscope sheath or a calibrated ureteric catheter. This is easier if a balloon occlusion calibrated ureteric catheter is used with the balloon inflated just inside the bladder neck to prevent movement during the measurement.

Having selected an appropriate length stent in its endo-

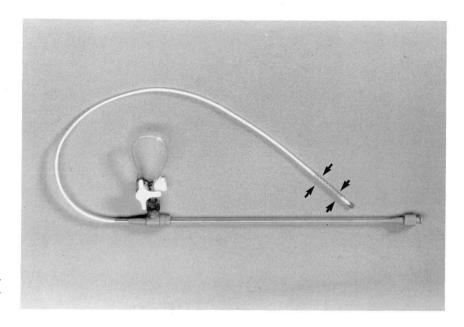

Figure 22–4. Original catheter delivery system. Arrows mark compressed stent.

scopic delivery system—the stents are supplied preloaded and sterile packed by the manufacturer—this is introduced into the prostatic urethra under direct vision using a standard 0° telescope. The first safety lock, which prevents premature opening of the stent as the device is passed down the urethra, is removed, and the stent is deployed within the prostatic urethra under direct vision by pulling back the outer sheath from the stent, allowing it to expand. Once the sheath has been pulled back as far as the second safety lock, the position of the stent is checked by moving the telescope along the full length of the stent within the prostatic urethra. The verumontanum and the position of the distal sphincter mechanism can be observed through the slots cut in the outer covering sheath for this purpose. If the position of the stent is not correct, the outer sheath can be pushed back over the device, which then will close inside the sheath, allowing repositioning if necessary. The inner end of the stent should lie exactly at the bladder neck, and the outer distal margin of the stent should cover fully the lateral lobes of the prostate. Once this final position is confirmed, the final safety lock is removed, and the outer sheath is fully retracted to allow the stent to spring open into its final position. Before removing the delivery system, it is very important to check that the three stent-retaining clasps have been fully released from the wires of the stent. This can be determined by direct observation of the outer end of the stent while gently rotating the delivery system. If it is found that one or other of the clamps is still attached to the wires, gentle manipulation of the delivery sheath will free it without difficulty. Before withdrawal of the delivery system, the three clamping jaws should be withdrawn into the covering sheath for at least the length of the safety clip to prevent any damage to the distal urethra as the device is removed from the urethra. If necessary, once these grasping jaws have been withdrawn into the sheath and the safety clip is reapplied, the delivery system can be introduced down the length of the stent to check its position. If it is necessary to carry out a cystoscopy at this stage, great care must be taken not to damage the wires of the outer end of the stent with the beak of the cystoscope as it passes through the sphincter mechanism.

RESULTS

We have treated 45 patients with prostate obstruction using the Urolume Wallstent. Thirty-two patients had acute retention (Table 22–1). Forty-two patients are fully satisfied with the stent and are passing urine normally, with significantly reduced residual urines. Where possible, full urodynamic videocystograms have been carried out before stent insertion and at 3–6 months postoperatively. Postoperative studies have not been possible in a number of these patients because of the severe medical problems that prevented prostate surgery when they first were seen. Some idea of the general condition of these patients can be gained from Table 22–2.

Table 22–1.   Features of Prostate Patients Treated with Urolume Stent

45 patients	32 acute retention
	7 chronic retention
	3 severe symptoms
	3 symptoms prostate/Parkinson's disease symptoms (therapeutic trial)
39 benign	
6 malignant	
Mean age 74.8 (range 49–95 years)	

As with all other types of urethral stents, we have found that most patients suffer frequency, urgency, and occasional urge incontinence following stent insertion, presumably because of the mechanical irritation of the prostatic urethra caused by these devices. We have found that using the Urolume Wallstent, these symptoms settle as the stent covers with epithelium over a period of 1–2 months. Only 2 patients, both of whom have severe detrusor instability, still have persistent symptoms of frequency and urgency. Six patients failed to pass urine immediately after stent insertion and required suprapubic catheterization. It is important that no urethral catheter is passed in these patients for the first month to avoid the risk of damaging the stent. Providing care is taken, no damage should result from catheterization or cystoscopy once epithelial covering is under way. Voiding commenced in all these patients without difficulty during the next 2 or 3 days, and all suprapubic catheters (except one inserted preoperatively for chronic retention and advanced prostate cancer) were removed by 6 weeks. These stents seemed to cause remarkably few other symptoms, and no patient experienced pain other than the dysuria associated with a urinary infection in 3 patients after insertion of the stent. All of these settled with a standard course of antibiotics and did not affect healing of the stent. Any preexisting urinary infection was treated vigorously before stent insertion, and all procedures were covered with broad-spectrum antibiotics for the perioperative period.

Whenever possible, we carried our regular cystoscopies on these patients under local anesthetic to check on healing of the stent. A number of our patients were unfit or unwilling to undergo these procedures because of failing health. The stent covers with urothelium in a similar fashion to what we have

Table 22–2.   American Society of Anesthesiology Patient Fitness Status

ASA GRADE	STATUS	NO. OF PATIENTS
1	Health	2
2	Mild systemic disease	5
3	Severe disease	15
4	Threat to life	23
5	Moribund	0

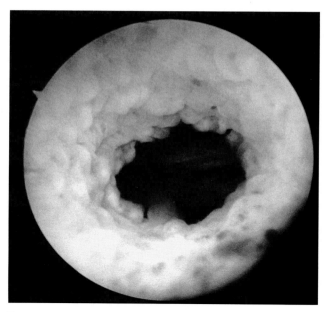

Figure 22–5. Endoscopic appearance of prostate stent covered with hyperplastic urothelium 5 months after insertion. Patient has no symptoms.

observed in urethral strictures. There is a considerable hyperplastic reaction (Fig. 22–5) that seems to last longer in prostate stents than in those used for urethral strictures but settles between 12 and 18 months after stent insertion (Fig. 22–6). We have seen no encrustation of stents within the prostatic urethra, although a number of our earlier patients, in whom some of the wire mesh was left within the bladder

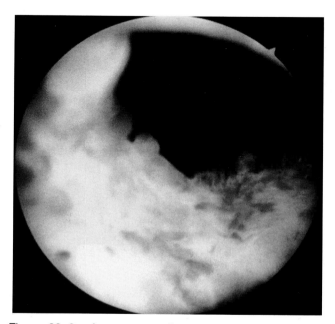

Figure 22–6. Appearance of prostate stent 1 year after insertion. The stent is covered, and little hyperplasia remains.

proximal to the bladder neck, have developed fine encrustation on the wire after a period of 6–12 months. None of these have yet caused symptoms or needed removing.

Stent Removal

Five stents had to be removed subsequent to deployment. Two of these were removed at the time of surgery because of poor position, one was removed after 1 week, and one was removed after 1 month because the stent was encroaching on the distal sphincter mechanism, causing a degree of urinary incontinence. All these stents were removed easily by grasping the stent at the bladder neck and pushing it into the bladder using standard grasping forceps. The stent can be pulled into a large resectoscope sheath or simply pulled out through the urethra. As the stent is pulled, it lengthens and narrows, causing remarkably little damage to the distal urethra as it is pulled out. One stent was removed 11 months after implantation at the request of the patient because of persistent severe detrusor instability. The hyperplastic lining epithelium was resected endoscopically without difficulty, and the stent was pushed into the bladder and removed as described. This patient did not improve but has declined further treatment.

Several patients have noticed a minor degree of intermittent hematuria for the first 3–6 months, and one experienced clot retention 3 months after implantation. This was treated with suprapubic catheterization, and spontaneous voiding recommended 48 h later, with no further bleeding or other symptoms.

No patient has reported any change in potency as a result of stent insertion, although the majority of these patients were elderly and suffering from severe chest and heart disease, which prevented normal sexual intercourse. Most of those patients having regular sexual intercourse report retrograde ejaculation, although it is interesting that two state that normal ejaculation has been maintained. The mean age of these patients was 74.8 years (49–95 years), with a mean follow-up of 10.6 months (range 4–18 months).

INDICATIONS FOR PROSTATE STENT

Recent anxieties about the risks of prostate surgery have stimulated great interest in the medical profession and among a well-informed public in alternative treatments for prostate obstruction.

In the elderly and unfit patient for whom prostate surgery would be a major risk and in whom pharmacologic treatment might cause unacceptable side effects, some form of prostate stenting to relieve acute retention or severe prostate symptoms offers an excellent alternative providing that treatment can be carried out rapidly and local anesthesia is used.[4,6] Included in this group may be patients who for some reason or other refuse prostate surgery or other forms of treatment. Until other new treatments are assessed and evaluated fully, there will remain in many parts of the word long waiting lists for prostate surgery. These patients are particularly suited to the various temporary prostate stents, which are, in general, less expensive than the permanent stents.

We also have used the Urolume Wallstent as a therapeutic trial in 3 patients with Parkinson's disease, whose urinary symptoms are difficult to distinguish symptomatically and urodynamically between those caused by prostate obstruction and those caused by Parkinson's disease. Insertion of a prostate stent relieved prostate obstruction in our 3 patients, and since both the symptoms and urodynamic results improved, the stents were left in place. If there is no improvement, the stent can be removed easily.

Other Indications for Urethral Stents

We have now used the Urolume Wallstent in over 60 patients with recurrent bulbar urethral strictures. Although further follow-up is needed, at 3 years the results remain very good for the vast majority of these patients, and there is no doubt that this device will continue to make a major contribution to the treatment of difficult strictures.[3,7]

We also have used the Urolume Wallstent for the treatment of patients with traumatic high cervical spinal injuries causing tetraplegia and dyssynergic sphincters. All these patients had high pressure voiding and were unsuitable for intermittent catheterization. Stents were inserted using the same device as that used for urethral strictures and prostate obstruction, and the procedure was notable for its simplicity and lack of complications. Although some difficulties have been experienced in these patients after stent insertion, it seems that this is an excellent alternative to endoscopic sphincterotomy.[8]

The stent also is being used successfully for the treatment of biliary strictures[9] and in a number of cases of tracheal and esophageal obstruction. The hyperplastic reaction seen when the stent is first inserted, particularly in experimental models, has prevented widespread use of the Urolume Wallstent in ureteric obstruction. Clinical trials are continuing, however, in carefully selected patients with ureteric obstruction, and early results are promising.

FUTURE DEVELOPMENTS

There is no doubt that the concept of a mechanical device to hold open the obstructed prostate will continue to play an important role in the elderly unfit patient. Permanently implanted devices that cover with epithelium may well find an important role in a far larger group of patients.

There are still problems with the delivery systems. A greater range of sizes of stents is necessary, and ensuring accurate positioning remains a vital requirement. Changes in the design and structure of the stent may improve the ease of delivery and also may help to reduce the early symptoms of irritation when the stents are first implanted. Similar changes may help to improve the speed of epithelial covering and reduce the hyperplastic reaction. Careful positioning and rapid epithelial covering remain vitally important to prevent the inevitable encrustation and infection that otherwise will occur with any foreign material left in contact with urine.

CONCLUSION

Temporary prostate stents inserted under local anesthesia offer a useful alternative for the short-term relief of urinary retention and prostate symptoms in patients with limited life expectancy or awaiting prostate surgery. Because of problems with encrustation and infection, the stents cannot be left in place for a long period of time without changing the stent. Permanent prostate stents, such as the Urolume Wallstent, which is known to cover with epithelium while holding open the prostatic urethra, will, if long-term results confirm the early successes with these devices, offer a simple and effective alternative to prostate surgery for many patients.

REFERENCES

1. Milroy EJG, Chapple CR, Cooper JE, et al. A new treatment for urethral strictures. *Lancet* 1988;1:1424–1427
2. Sarramon JP, Joffre F, Rischmann P, et al. Prosthese endourethrale wallstent dans les stenoses recidivantes de l'urethre. *Ann Urol* 1989;23:383–387
3. Milroy EJG, Chapple CR, Eldin A, Wallsten H. A new treatment for urethral strictures: a permanently implanted urethral stent. *J Urol* 1989;141:1120–1122
4. Chapple CR, Milroy EJG, Rickards D. Permanently implanted urethral stent for prostate obstruction in the unfit patient—preliminary report. *Br J Urol* 1990;66:58–65
5. Sigwart U, Puel J, Mirkovitch V, et al. Intravascular stents to prevent occlusion and restenosis after transluminal angioplasty. *N Engl J Med* 1987;316:701–706
6. Williams G, Jager R, McLoughlin L, et al. Use of stents for treating obstruction of urinary outflow in patients unfit for surgery. *Br Med J* 1989;298:1429
7. Milroy EJG, Chapple CR, Eldin A, Wallsten H. A new stent for the treatment of urethral strictures. *Br J Urol* 1989;63:392–396
8. Shaw PJR, Milroy EJG, Eldin A. Permanent external sphincter stents in spinal injured patients. *Br J Urol* 1990;66:297
9. Dick R, Gillams A, Dooley JS, Hobbs KEF. Stainless steel mesh stents for biliary strictures. *J Intervent Radiol* 1989;4:95–98

23

Preshaped Metallic Prostatic Urethral Stent

J. Vicente, J. Salvador, F. Izquierdo

In recent years, the technique of transurethral resection of the prostate (TURP) for benign prostatic hyperplasia (BPH) has undergone close scrutiny in terms of opportunity,[1] exact indications,[2,3] and efficacy,[4] comparing its results and morbidity and mortality with those obtained with open surgery.[5]

The controversy about this topic has brought about the appearance of different alternatives to surgery for BPH: medical treatment (e.g., LH-RH agonists, alpha-blockers), prostatic hyperthermia, balloon urethroplasty or divulsion, and transurethral prostatic incision.

Newer techniques, such as ultrasonic prostatic aspiration, robot prostatectomy, and transurethral lasertherapy, are alternatives that need larger numbers of cases and longer follow-up to be assessable. Another alternative to surgery for BPH is placement of an endourethral prosthesis as a temporary deobstructive maneuver.

There are different models of endourethral prostheses on the market: prostakath,[6] double malecot,[7,8] and the expandable tube.[9,10] The most used to date has been the preshaped metallic spiral stent (PMS), described initially as the *urologische Spirale* by Fabian in 1980.[11] A literature search has uncovered a total of 172 PMS inserted up to the present time,[12–21] and we have 49 cases in our experience.

This chapter deals with an intraurethral prosthesis, the preshaped metallic spiral stent.

PATIENT SELECTION

Indications

The PMS can be used as an alternative to surgery for BPH in patients who have the following characteristics.

1. Older patients, mean age 81.5 years in our experience, whose age and medical conditions make them an in-creased anesthetic risk and who have a short life expectancy.[13,19,22]
2. Patients with long-term indwelling bladder catheters, a mean of 10.5 months in our series, who experience problems with infection, hematuria, or intolerance to the catheter.
3. Patients with severe concomitant systemic illnesses that contraindicate any type of prostatic surgical maneuver;[17,23] approximately 85% of our patients were ASA IV.
4. As a temporary alternative to surgery for BPH—awaiting an intercurrent illness to stabilize enough to allow definitive surgery or for sociologic or sanitary conditions to permit the admittance of the patient into a medical center.[20]

Apart from placement of the PMS as an alternative to surgery for BPH (40 cases in our experience), it also is indicated in prostatic cancer with bladder outlet obstruction (7 cases)[24] and in cases of cervicoprostatic sclerosis.[16]

Contraindications

General. Important bleeding disorders, arthritis that makes endoscopic positioning impossible (usually hip problems), and cortical (cerebral) incompetence that precludes normal control of voiding.[4,9]

Local. Urethral stricture disease, urethral length that does not correspond to the available prosthetic lengths, bacterial prostatitis, and preferential growth of the prostatic middle lobe.[14,22,23]

INSTRUMENTS

The instruments necessary for placement of the intraurethral PMS are simple and available in any urologic endoscopy suite: local anesthesia with lidocaine gel, 6 F–7 F ureteral catheters, and a 21 F panendoscope with a foreign body forceps. The spiral metallic prosthesis must be purchased separately and it is available commercially in four different lengths, 45, 55, 65, and 75 mm.

The PMS consists of three metallic parts joined together. The prostatic portion, or body, which is formed by a series of spirals with a tapered proximal (endovesical) tip and a width of 21 F (7 mm), continues with a straight portion 2 cm in length that is placed in the membranous urethra. The distal portion of the prosthesis consists of two spirals that anchor the prosthesis in the bulbar urethra (Fig. 23–1).

TECHNIQUE

The length of the prostatic urethra should be measured prior to the placement of the prosthesis. This can be done directly with a numbered ureteral catheter under endoscopy[15] but we prefer to use linear transrectal ultrasound to measure the length of the prostatic urethra[13,18,21,22,23] (Fig. 23–2). To the length of the prostatic urethra, we add 1 cm, which gives the correct prosthetic length. The prosthesis is placed endoscopically, and its correct position is confirmed radiologically.

Once the patient has been placed on the table in a lithotomy position, the external urethral meatus is prepared with clorhexidine solution, and the urethra is filled with 2% lidocaine gel. A 6 F–7 F ureteral catheter is introduced into the bladder transurethrally, and the prosthesis is threaded onto this

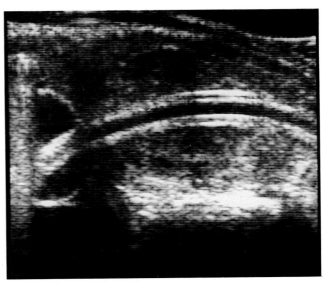

Figure 23–2. Linear transrectal ultrasound as a way to measure prostatic urethral length.

catheter and manually introduced into the penile urethra until it disappears from view. A 21 F panendoscope is then introduced, and using the foreign body forceps, the base of the body of the prosthesis is grasped. The prosthesis slides easily into the urethra following the ureteral catheter in a well-lubricated environment, with excellent patient tolerance.

Under direct endoscopic view, the prosthesis is pushed toward the bladder cavity, situating the body of the prosthesis at the level of the verumontanum, an easily identifiable landmark. In this situation, the straight portion is positioned in the membranous urethra with the two distal spirals in the bulbar urethra (Fig. 23–3).

A retrograde voiding urethrogram is then performed using a hydrosoluble iodinated contrast solution to verify correct

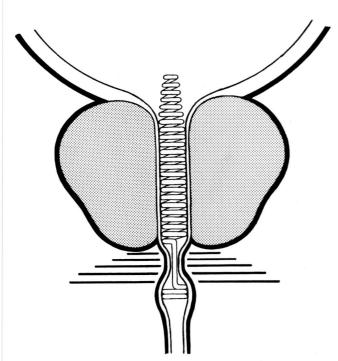

Figure 23–1. Schematic view of the prosthesis.

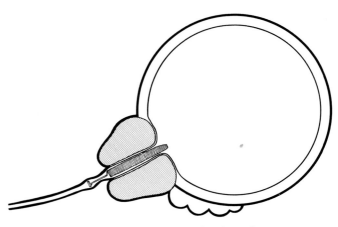

Figure 23–3. Transverse schematic view of correct prosthetic placement.

placement, adequate micturition, and absence of significant postvoid residual urine.[22,23] If position or voiding is not satisfactory, the prosthesis is repositioned immediately.

The prosthesis is removed endoscopically, usually with poor patient tolerance.[22] Another possibility for removal that appears to be better tolerated consists of the introduction of a Fogarty catheter through the prosthesis, filling the balloon with 1.5 mL of water, and removing the prosthesis by pulling on the catheter (atraumatically) under radiologic control.[17]

DISCUSSION

The PMS prosthesis is a good alternative to surgery for BPH in a selected group of patients who because of their age (mean 81.5 years), intolerance to the catheter over the long term (mean 10.5 months), or poor general health (ASA IV in 85% of patients) have an anesthetic contraindication to surgery.[13,17,19,22,23] We consider interesting the use of the prosthesis in patients who must wait a determined period of time before their definitive prostatic surgery can take place.[20]

In our experience, 6 patients (30%) carried the prosthesis for a mean of 11.8 months, allowing the patient's general status to improve enough for a definitive prostatic surgical procedure to take place—1 prostatic incision, 1 open prostatectomy, and 4 transurethral resections. Other advantages are that the prosthesis adapts well to the normal curvature of the prostatic urethra (Fig. 23–4) and that its metallic composition offers minimal adherence to calcium salts, with only 2 cases reported of partial prosthetic calcification.[17,22] Its capacity to adapt well to the curvature of the prostatic urethra and its excellent biotolerance account for the absence of histologic lesions in 5 operative specimens (1 open surgery and 4 TURs) in patients who used the prosthesis for a mean of 11.8 months. Routine endoscopic equipment is used for placement, the procedure is performed under local anesthesia, and the technique is both simple and precise.

The PMS prosthesis also has some disadvantages. Only four lengths are commercially available, and they sometimes do not coincide with the proper prostatic urethral length. A number of patients do not tolerate the prosthesis because of the consistency of its material and local factors. In our experience with 40 prostheses, 5 (15.5%) required removal because of extreme intolerance less than 30 days after placement.

The prosthesis is not effective in patients whose prostate has a prominent middle lobe.[22,23]

Inadequate fixation of the prosthesis is responsible for spontaneous mobilization and other complications and side effects. Exceptionally, the prosthesis can be displaced accidentally, as occurred in one of our patients after introduction of a bladder catheter without knowing that a urethral prosthesis was in place (Fig. 23–5).

The usual scenario is spontaneous mobilization, which occurred in 7 cases in our experience. When the proximal

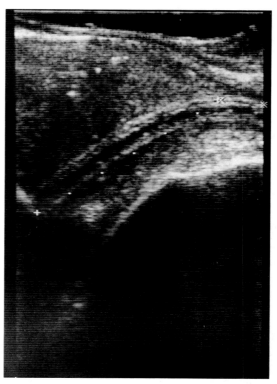

Figure 23–4.   Linear transrectal ultrasound: adaptation of the prosthesis to the normal prostatic urethral curvature.

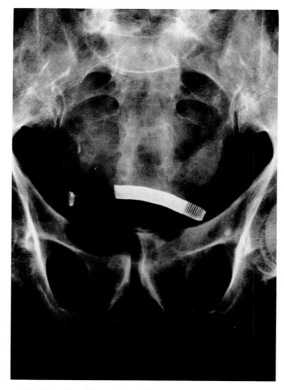

Figure 23–5.   Accidental mobilization of the prosthesis after bladder catheterization when it was not known that a prosthesis was in place.

(cranial) tip of the prosthesis does not reach the bladder cavity (2 cases), the patient experiences urinary retention (Fig. 23–6). If the body of the prosthesis on mobilization locates itself at the level of the membranous urethra (2 cases), the patient experiences incontinence, necessitating repositioning of the prosthesis. Mobilization of the prosthesis can cause the urethra to become transfixed and perforated by the distal tip (1 case) (Fig. 23–7) or bulbar urethral stricture by prosthetic decubitus (1 case) (Fig. 23–8). In both cases, cystotomy was required for removal of the prosthesis.

Results vary according to whether the prosthesis was placed in patients with chronic or acute urinary retention[15] and, most importantly, according to the length of time the prosthesis is left in place.[19] Good results are, therefore, determined by the length of follow-up and the number of patients who die during the time of follow-up (elderly patients with severe systemic illnesses). This explains the diversity of good results published in the literature: 80%,[13] 77%,[20] 76%,[18] 75%,[14] 52%,[19] and 47%.[15]

In our experience of 18 cases with a mean follow-up of 21.6 months (range 12–28 months), we have achieved good results, globally, in 51.4% of cases. All patients were evaluated with history (subjective): normal voiding in 72%; radiology/ultrasound: correct positioning in 86% and less than 50 mL postvoid residual in 87%; uroflowmetry: < 6 mL $\dot{Q}$max in 38% with $\dot{Q}$max 6–14 mL/sec in 62%; normal urine

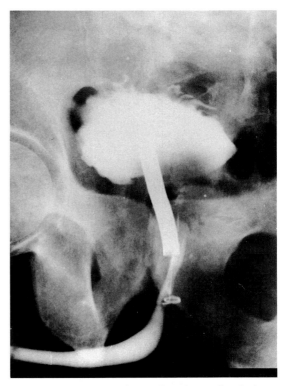

Figure 23–7. Urethra perforated and transfixed after mobilization of the distal end of the prosthesis.

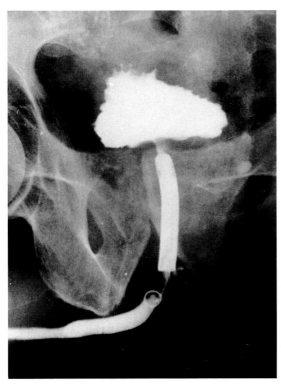

Figure 23–6. Radiologic view. The proximal end of the prosthesis does not reach the bladder cavity. This patient had acute urinary retention.

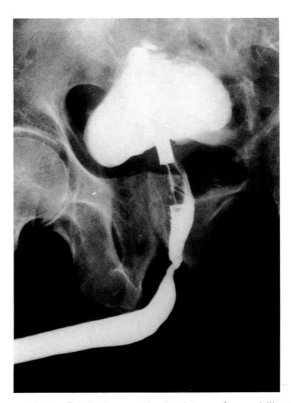

Figure 23–8. Postbulbar urethral stricture after mobilization and decubitus in a prosthesis used for 36 months.

sediments: 58% of patients. Good results were obtained with the PMS prosthesis in 65%–70% of patients within 12 months of follow-up, falling to 50%–55% when the prosthesis was indwelling for more than 1 year.

Perhaps the future of the prosthesis as an alternative to surgery for BPH will evolve with the creation of a prosthesis that conserves the advantages of the PMS but avoids its inconveniences: better tolerated material of a modifiable length with a good fixation system and easily removable.

REFERENCES

1. Barry MJ, Mulley AG, Flower FJ, Wennenberg JW. Watchful waiting vs immediate transurethral resection for symptomatic prostatism. *JAMA* 1988;259: 3010
2. Graversen PH, Gasser TC, Wasson JH, Hinman F, Burskewitz RC. Controversies about indications for transurethral resection of the prostate. *J Urol* 1989;141:475
3. Vela Navarrete R. Controversia sobre la resección transuretral de próstata. *Arch Esp Urol* 1989;42:487
4. Lepor H, Riagud G. The efficacy of transurethral resection of the prostate in men with moderate symptoms of prostatism. *J Urol* 1990;143:533
5. Roos NP, Wennberg JE, Malenka DJ, Fisher ES, McPherson K, Anderson TF. Mortality and reoperation after open and transurethral resection of the prostate for benign prostatic hyperplasia. *N Engl J Med* 1989;320:1120
6. Norling J, Nielsen KK, Kromann MJ, Absalon MJ, Fowler CG. The Prostakath intraprostatic stent: a simplified technique for insertion. *Eur Urol* 1990;18 (suppl 1):Abstract 37
7. Nissenkorn I. Experience with a new self-retaining intraurethral catheter in patients with urinary retention: a preliminary report. *J Urol* 1990;142:92
8. Nissenkorn I, Richter S. A new self-retaining intraurethral device. *Br J Urol* 1990;65:197
9. Chapple CR, Milroy EJG, Rickards D. Permanently implanted urethral stent for prostatic obstruction in the unfit patient. *Br J Urol* 1990;66:58
10. Mcloughlin J, Jager R, Abel PD, Eldin A, Adam A, Williams G. The use of prostatic stents in patients with urinary retention who are unfit for surgery. *Br J Urol* 1990;66:66
11. Fabian KM. Der intraprostatische partiale Katheter (urologische Espirale). *Urologe A* 1980;19:236
12. Garbit JL, Blitz M, Bonell J, Pin P, Paillot J. La prothese endoprostatique Spirale de Fabian. *J Urol* 1988;94:265
13. Nordling J, Holm HH, Klarskon P, Nielsen KK, Andersen JT. The intraprostatic spiral: a new device for insertion with the patients under local anesthesia and with ultrasonic guidance with 3 months of follow-up. *J Urol* 1989;142:756
14. Nielsen KK, Kroman-Andersen B, Nordling J. Relation between detrusor pressure and urinary flow rate in males with an intraurethral prostatic spiral. *Br J Urol* 1989;64:275
15. Birch BRP, Parker CJ, Chave H, Miller A. Endoprostatic helicoplasty: the Porges urospiral. *Eur Urol* 1990;18 (suppl 1):Abstract 37
16. Parra RO. Titanium urethral stent in the management of prostatomembranous urethral strictures. *Eur Urol* 1990;18 (suppl 1):Abstract 38
17. Garofalo F. Emprego de spiral endouretral em pacientes con hiperplasia benigna da prostata e risco operatorio elevado. *J Bras Urol* 1990;16:106
18. Billiet J, Mattelaer J, Van Brien P. Use of transurethral longitudinal sonography in the placement of a prostatic coil. *Eur Urol* 1990;17:76
19. Harrison NW, De Souza JV. Prostatic stenting for outflow obstruction. *Br J Urol* 1990;65:192
20. Yadia D, Lask D, Robinson S. Self-retaining intraurethral stent. *AJR* 1990;154:111
21. Braf Z, Chen J, Matzkin H. Experience with the insertion of two different intraurethral metal spiral catheters in BPH. *J Urol* 1990;143:Abstract 874
22. Vicente J, Salvador J, Chechile G. Spiral urethral prosthesis as an alternative to surgery in high-risk patients with benign prostatic hyperplasia. Prospective study. *J Urol* 1989;142: 1504
23. Vicente J, Chechile G, Salvador J, Izquierdo F. Long-term follow-up of patients with intraurethral prostheses. *Semin Int Radiol* 1989;6:82
24. Vicente J, Chechile G. Chirugie endoscopique palliative dans le traitement des cancers de prostate. In: Khoury S, Chatelain C (eds). *Urologie: Cancer de la Prostate*. Paris, FIIS, 1988:432

24

Balloon Expandable Titanium Prostatic Urethral Stents

Ramon Perez-Marrero, Laurel E. Emerson

The concept of using metallic stents to treat prostatic obstruction is fairly recent. In the 1980s, Fabian and others[1-4] used an intraprostatic metal coil as a stent. This spiral was inserted endoscopically after measuring the prostatic urethral length, but this was found to be somewhat complicated and did not achieve wide acceptance. In 1988, Nordling reported on a Danish gold-plated spiral (ProstaKath) that was inserted under ultrasound guidance. Although good results were reported in 41 patients, these stents may migrate and require repositioning or removal.[5-7] Most recently, Williams et al. used a stainless steel self-expandable stent in prostatic obstruction.[8] These stents were designed originally for intravascular use[9] but have been modified for use in the treatment of urethral strictures.[10] Excellent results have been reported by several authors,[11,12] and Milroy has updated his series in Chapter 22 of this book. One disadvantage of this system is that it may require secondary balloon dilation of the stent itself to attain a lumen of 12 mm in diameter.[12] All of these stent systems can be inserted under endourethral anesthesia and are used most often as a permanent implant in patients with prostatic obstruction unfit for other forms of intervention. Vicente et al., however, have used stents successfully on a temporary basis while patients' medical condition improved or to allow for hormone treatment of an obstructive prostatic tumor.[6]

We have experience with a titanium mesh stent produced by the Advanced Surgical Intervention Incorporated of California (ASI) (Fig. 24–1). This stent is supplied collapsed and mounted over a high-pressure balloon (Fig. 24–2) that deploys it to its full diameter, obviating secondary dilations (Fig. 24–3). It is available in several lengths from 22 mm to 58 mm in 7-mm increments, and it is supplied with its own introducing sheath, graduated catheter, and high-pressure insufflator device.

TECHNIQUE

The insertion procedure is simple and uses techniques already familiar to those with experience in prostatic balloon dilation (Chapter 12). Endourethral anesthesia with 2% lidocaine jelly is sufficient for this short procedure, and IV sedation rarely is necessary. Cystoscopy is performed, and the prostatic urethra is measured using the graduated catheter in a similar manner as is done for transcystoscopic urethroplasty. The stent will shorten as it expands by as much as 6 mm, so, in selecting the appropriate length, the expanded

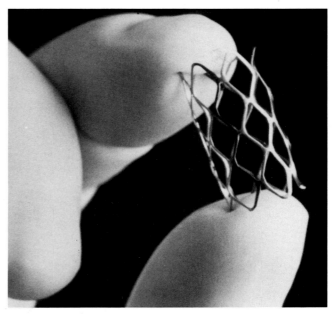

Figure 24–1. Expanded titanium stent.

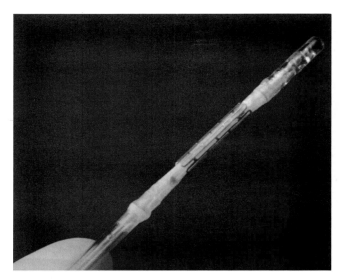

Figure 24–2. Stent collapsed over high-pressure balloon delivery catheter.

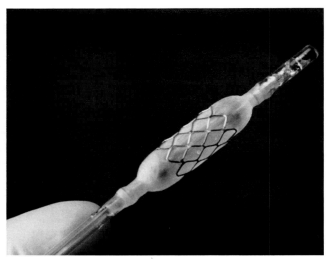

Figure 24–3. Stent expanded to its full diameter (11 mm) by high-pressure balloon.

length of the stent should be used. This is indicated clearly on the packaging label.

The disposable sheath is introduced into a partially full bladder, and the balloon catheter with the appropriate stent is inserted through it with a 0 or 30° cystoscope lens alongside it. Although the balloon catheter has a blue band that helps us in the initial placement, the stent should be positioned using its most distal edge as a marker. I like to position this edge 1 mm or 2 mm distal to the verumontanum so that, when the stent expands and foreshortens, it will cover the verumontanum (Fig. 24–4). Under visual control, the high-pressure balloon is inflated using the pressure insufflator with gauge provided by the company. A pressure of 130 psi is main-

tained for 30 sec (Fig. 24–5). Once the stent is deployed to its full diameter (11 mm, 33 F), the balloon is deflated and withdrawn into the sheath, leaving the stent firmly anchored in place (Fig. 24–6). Its position is then checked using a 15 F rigid cystoscope or a flexible cystoscope. It should be located over the verumontanum proximally and should keep the bladder neck open, protruding only 1–2 mm into the bladder. If it protrudes more than this, it may cause severe frequency and urgency postoperatively. The company provides a removal tool that can be used to remove and replace the stent if necessary. Repositioning may be done using simple grasping forceps. We have had to reposition the stent in 2 of our early cases, and this proved to be quite straightforward and well tolerated by the patient.

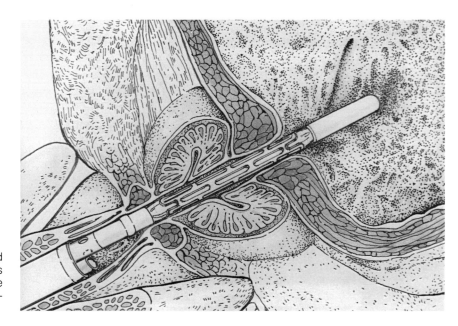

Figure 24–4. Delivery balloon and stent in place. The cystoscope lens is in place, and the distal edge of the stent is placed between verumontanum and sphincter.

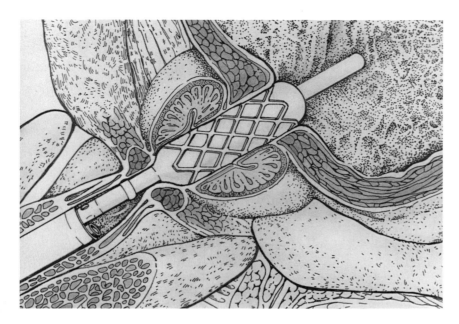

Figure 24–5. The stent is deployed by inflating the delivery balloon to 130 psi. The blue band in the catheter allows detection of any migration of the delivery system into the bladder.

Most patients tolerate the procedure well. There is minimal bleeding and postinsertion discomfort, but most patients complain of frequency and terminal dysuria. This resolves over the first 1 or 2 weeks. If catheterization becomes necessary, it should be done with a 14 F or 16 F Foley catheter. Smaller catheters may get caught in the holes of a freshly inserted stent, and larger ones may dislodge it. Patients are given a wallet card stating that they have a urethral implant and advising physicians how to catheterize the bladder.

CLINICAL RESULTS

There have been over 140 insertions of the ASI stent worldwide, 56 of which are in the company's database. Of these, 27 patients were in retention before the procedure. Table 24–1 details the follow-up peak flow rates after insertion. Of the rest, 17 patients had evaluable symptom scores and underwent a significant reduction in their scores after insertion persistent in follow-up (Table 24–2). Four of these patients have had their stents removed and undergone a

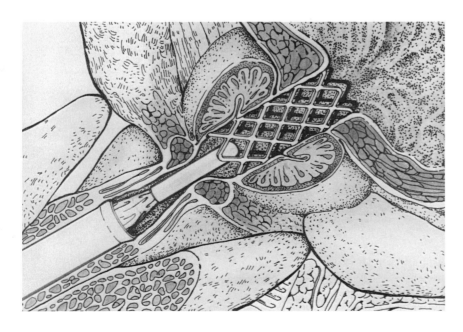

Figure 24–6. The delivery balloon is deflated and withdrawn into the sheath, leaving the stent in optimal position, keeping the bladder neck open, with minimal intrusion into the bladder, and extending well into the apical urethra.

Table 24–1. Balloon Expandable Prostatic Stent Average Peak Uroflow (Patients in Retention prior to Treatment)

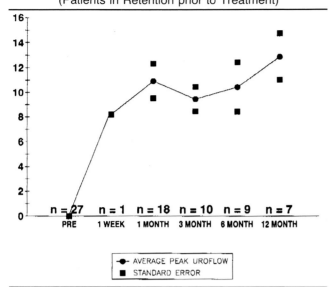

Table 24–2. Balloon Expandable Prostatic Stent Average Symptom Score

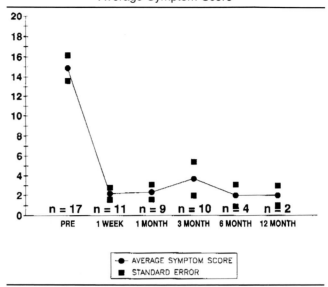

TURP. Two of these patients failed to void after resection, suggesting the presence of a decompensated detrusor. Three others have died with their stents in place and functioning.

Our series is comprised of 8 patients in chronic urinary retention who, for various reasons, were not candidates for regional or general anesthetics. Their mean age was 74 years, and they had been catheterized for 2–14 months. They have all been followed for a minimum of 6 months, with a mean follow-up of 10 months (range 6–14 months). All but 2 patients voided spontaneously after stent insertion, 1 required catheterization for 4 days, and another was never able to void and underwent removal of the stent. He is still on intermittent catheterization 6 months after removal.

To date, 5 patients' stents remain in place and are functioning well, with flow rates at or above 10 mL/sec and residual urines less than 20% of total bladder capacity as measured by ultrasound (Table 24–3). These 5 patients underwent flexible cystoscopy at several intervals postinsertion, and this confirms Chapple's findings of a hyperplastic reaction to the stent that culminates on complete epithelialization around 6–9 months (Fig. 24–7). There has been no migration of these stents.

Two of our patients underwent stent removal around 3 months postinsertion. One of the patients had an adequately working stent that was dislodged by an emergency catheterization. His medical condition precluded removal of the stent, which is still in his bladder, and he is being managed by

Table 24–3. Patient Details and Outcome

PATIENT	AGE (YEARS)	DURATION OF CATHETERIZATION (MONTHS)	OTHER MEDICAL PROBLEMS	FLOW RATE		POST-OPERATIVE RESIDUAL (%)[a]	FOLLOW-UP[b] (MONTHS)	OUTCOME
				Pre-operative	Post-operative			
MP	85	3	ASHD[c]	—	12.5	8	12	Stent in place, voiding
WB	76	4	COPD	—	10.0	11	6	Stent dislodged Indwelling catheter
DS	71	2	ASHD	—	11.0	7	8	Stent removed TURP
AH	55	14	COPD	—	1.0	80	9	Detrusor decompensation Stent removed on CIC
HW	78	9	ASHD COPD	—	10	2	14	4 days urine retention Stent in place, voiding
PD	75	3	COPD	—	14	10	10	Stent in place, voiding
OM	71	6	MI	—	11.5	4	11	Stent in place, voiding
AW	79	8	COPD	—	13	8	9	Stent in place, voiding

[a]Residual is expressed as a percentage of total bladder capacity.
[b]The flow rate is the last recorded one in follow-up (mL/sec).
[c]ASHD, arteriosclerotic heart disease; COPD, chronic obstructive pulmonary disease; MI, myocardial infarct; CIC, clean intermittent catheterization.

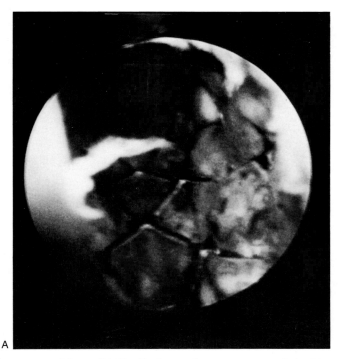
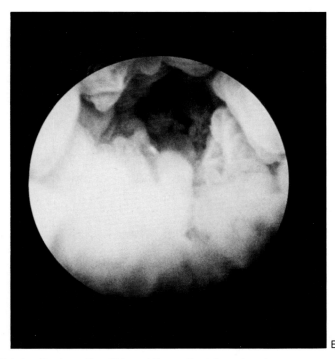

A   B

Figure 24–7. Endoscopic appearance of stent immediately after insertion (**A**) and 7 months later, showing complete epithelialization (**B**). (Photographs courtesy of Advanced Surgical Intervention, Inc.)

indwelling catheterization. This episode has made us require all our patients to wear a Medic-Alert bracelet stating the presence of a urethral stent and recommending safe catheter sizes. The other patient developed persistent and severe frequency and urgency unresponsive to anticholinergic agents. His stent was removed suprapubically by another urologist whose operative note suggests that the stent was protruding too much into the bladder.

In summary, 5 of our 8 patients have had good response to stenting, with normal flow rates and acceptable residuals (63%). There has been no spontaneous migration, secondary retention, or incontinence. There has been no encrustation or stone formation in our 5 long-term patients, but 1 of our failures did form some stones in the intravesical portion of the stent. Complete epithelialization of the stent occurs around 6–9 months postinsertion but does not seem to progress further.

BIOCOMPATIBILITY OF MATERIALS

One of the most important differences between these prostatic urethral stents is their metallic characteristics. Metals implanted into the body are subject to corrosion, particularly in a strong chloride environment, such as urine. This produces a release of metal ions into the surrounding tissue, and these ions induce an inflammatory or foreign body reaction. Stainless steel is highly susceptible to corrosion in the body[13]

and may be subject to excessive long-term inflammatory response and implant failure.[14]

Titanium was first used for biologic implants in the 1940s and, in recent years, has become the most commonly used implant metal, mainly due to its resistance to corrosion, particularly in environments high in chloride ions, such as urine.[15] It also produces minimal inflammatory response and necrosis.[16] Although titanium and stainless steel are equally well tolerated initially, titanium may be a superior choice when the implantation is intended to be long term.

DISCUSSION

Metallic prostatic stenting is still a developing technology. It offers a therapeutic alternative to indwelling catheterization for those patients who are medically unfit for other procedures. This may be of particular use in those patients postmyocardial infarction.

We believe that the ASI titanium stent offers several advantages over the other metallic stents. Titanium is a more biocompatible material and may be a safer long-term implant. The techniques used in inserting this stent are familiar to most urologists, particularly if they have experience with cystoscopic balloon urethroplasty. Endoscopic balloon delivery is simpler, more accurate, and safer than other methods of delivery. It avoids secondary dilations of the stent, since it is always deployed to its maximum diameter. No delayed failures have occurred in our series.

As we gain more experience with stent placement, we probably will decrease the incidence of postinsertion urgency and frequency and the need for stent replacement or removal.

In short, prostatic stenting promises to be a viable therapeutic alternative for selected patients with prostatic obstruction, reducing the need for long-term indwelling catheterization. It is still a fairly new technology, and its place in our therapeutic armamentarium needs to be clarified by further clinical trials.

REFERENCES

1. Fabian KM. Der intraprostatische "Partielle katheter" (urologische Spirale) I. *Urolge (A)* 1980;19:236–238
2. Fabian KM. Der intraprostatische "Partielle katheter" (urologische Spirale) II. *Urologe (A)* 1984;23:229–233
3. Fabricus PG, Matz M, Sepnick H. Die Endourethral spiral—eine Alternative zum Dauer Katheter? *Z Arzt Forbild* 1983;77:482–483
4. Eller G, Seppelt U. Erfahrungen mit der Urologischen Spirale. *Urologe (B)* 1987;27:304–307
5. Nordling J, Klarskov P, Nielsen KK, et al. Voiding patterns after relief of retention with the Danish intraprostatic spiral (Prostakath). *Neurourol Urodyn* 1988;No. 41
6. Vicente J, Salvador J, Chechile G. A spiral urethral prosthesis as an alternative to surgery in high-risk patients with benign prostatic hyperplasia: prospective study. *J Urol* 1989;142:1504–1506
7. Nordling J, Holm HH, Klarskov P, Nielsen KK, Andersen JT. The intraprostatic spiral: a new device for insertion with the patient under local anesthesia and with ultrasonic guidance with three month follow-up. *J Urol* 1989;142:756–758
8. Williams G, Jager R, McLoughlin J, et al. Use of stents for treating obstruction of urinary outflow in patients unfit for surgery. *Br Med J* 1989;298:1429
9. Palmaz JC, Windler SA, Garcia F, Tio FO, Sibbit RR, Reuter SR. Atherosclerotic rabbit aortas: expandable intraluminal grafting. *Radiology* 1986;160:723–726
10. Milroy EJG, Chapple CR, El-Din A, Wallsten H. A new stent for the treatment of urethral strictures. Preliminary report. *Br J Urol* 1989;63:392–396
11. Chapple CR, Milroy EJG, Rickaards D. Permanently implanted urethral stent for prostatic obstruction in unfit patient. Preliminary report. *Br J Urol* 1990;66:58–65
12. McLoughlin J, Jager R, Abel PD, El Din A, Adam A, Williams G. The use of prostatic stents in patients with urinary retention who are unfit for surgery. An interim report. *Br J Urol* 1990;66:66–70
13. Harris B. Corrosion of stainless steel surgical implants. *J Med Eng Technol* 1979;3:117
14. Bundy M, Hockman RF. In vivo and in vitro studies of stress corrosion cracking behavior of surgical implant alloys. *J Biomed Mater Res* 1983;17:467–487
15. Williams DF (ed). *Titanium and Titanium Alloys in Biocompatibility of Clinic Implant Materials.* Boca Raton, FL: CRC Press, 1981, vol 1
16. Rae T. The biological response to titanium and titanium-aluminum-vanadium alloy particles. *Biomaterials* 1986;7:37–39

25

Pathophysiology and Medical Management of Benign Prostatic Hyperplasia

Jorn Aagaard, Reginald C. Bruskewitz

Transurethral resection of the prostate (TURP) is the standard treatment of symptomatic benign hyperplasia of the prostate (BPH). Approximately 425,000 prostatectomies for benign disease were performed in the United States in 1989, according to the draft reports of the National Kidney and Urologic Disease Board. Prostatectomy has gained this widespread acceptance because the procedure is relatively free of serious complications and because the majority of the patients experience satisfactory resolution of their micturation symptoms. Dørflinger et al.[1] reported that 86% of men experienced marked symptomatic improvement after transurethral prostatectomy. Studies by Lepor et al.[2] agree with these findings, reporting that 84% of patients received marked symptomatic improvement.

Although the quality of life is improved dramatically after prostatectomy for most patients, it is a concern that 15% of patients experience no benefit. Furthermore, Roos et al.[3] reported that transurethral prostatectomy possibly is associated with a greater long-term mortality rate than is open prostatectomy.

These concerns about prostatectomy and the patient's objection to surgery provide the impetus for the development of effective nonsurgical alternatives.

A variety of medical alternatives are under investigation. Among these are the alpha-blockers, which reduce contraction of the prostatic smooth muscle, and manipulation of prostatic epithelium to reduce overall prostatic size by blocking the action of the androgenic hormones. To understand the rationale underlying these treatments, it is necessary first to review briefly (1) the basic anatomy of the prostate and the pathophysiologic changes in BPH, (2) the autonomic innervation, and (3) the hormonal milieu that acts on the prostate.

ANATOMY AND PATHOPHYSIOLOGY

The prostate is the largest male sexual accessory gland. It lies under the urinary bladder and rests on the urogenital diaphragm. The blood supply of the prostate is from the inferior vesical artery branch of the internal iliac artery. Innervation is primarily from the autonomic nervous system via the hypogastric, aortic, or pelvic plexus. McNeal[4] describes the prostate as a fibromuscular and glandular portion divided by the urethra. The glandular portion is divided into a peripheral zone, a central zone, a transitional zone, and a periurethral glandular region (Fig. 25–1). The ventral fibromuscular portion, which is approximately one third of the tissue within the prostate capsule, appears distinct from the glandular tissue and its surrounding stroma. Smooth muscle exists in the stroma as well as in the prostate capsule. The initial lesion of BPH occurs in the periurethral area proximal to the verumontanum. BPH develops at the intersection of prostate ducts and glands that reside in or are adjacent to the urethral wall.

AUTONOMIC INNERVATION OF THE PROSTATE

The autonomic nervous system is divided into sympathetic and parasympathetic components. The sympathetic system produces its effect by liberation of the neurotransmitter

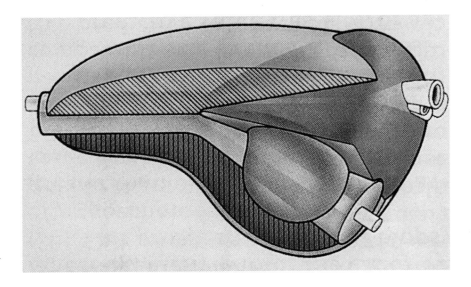

Figure 25–1. Prostatic zonal anatomy as described by McNeal.

norepinephrine from the postganglionic nerve endings, which act on adrenergic receptors in the target cells. Acetylcholine is liberated from the postganglionic fibers of the parasympathetic nerves and acts on muscarinic receptors in the target cells. The adrenergic receptors are divided into two main groups, alpha and beta, according to effects produced in the target cell. In the lower urinary tract, smooth muscle stimulation by the alpha-receptors produces contraction, whereas stimulation of the beta-receptors causes relaxation.

The alpha-receptors are further classified into two subgroups. Alpha$_1$-receptors are found on the target cell and mediate the effect produced on it. Alpha$_2$-receptors are found on the postganglion nerve terminals, where they control the reabsorption of excessive norepinephrine into the neuron. In recent years, receptors having the same characteristics as alpha$_2$-receptors have been identified on the target cells, where they mediate a contractile response.

In a normal prostate, alpha$_1$-receptors predominate, but in BPH, there are equal amounts of alpha$_1$- and alpha$_2$-receptors. The alpha$_1$-receptor is more sensitive to various alpha-agonists than is the alpha$_2$-receptor.[5,6]

Autonomic nerves enter smooth muscle in the wall of the prostatic urethra, prostatic capsule, and prostatic stroma. In the capsule, there are both muscarinic and alpha-adrenergic receptors. In the stroma, there are only alpha-adrenergic receptors. When the tone of the smooth muscle increases, the pressure exerted on the urethra will increase above the relatively fixed degree of obstruction caused by the mechanical effect of the bulky prostate. The pressure produced by the smooth muscle is referred to as the dynamic aspect, and the pressure produced by the enlarged prostate itself is the mechanical aspect of the obstruction. Furuya et al. have shown that 40% of the total urethral pressure in patients with BPH is due to alpha-adrenergic tone.[7] Administration of alpha-antagonists prevents contraction of the smooth muscle and results in reduced resistance to urinary flow in the prostatic urethra. This is accomplished without altering the contractile components of the bladder body, which contains few alpha-receptors.

HORMONAL INFLUENCE ON THE PROSTATE

For many years, it has been known that the gonadal hormones are related to the pathogenesis of BPH. In 1944, Moore[8] showed that the absence of testicular function from either castration or pituitarectomy up to the age of 40 prevents the occurrence of BPH or prostate cancer.

As previously mentioned, the initial lesion of BPH occurs in the periurethral area proximal to the verumontanum and develops at the intersection of the prostatic ducts and the glands that are adjacent to the urethral wall. Prostatic epithelial growth is under the control of testosterone (and perhaps estrogen or other factors as well) and, therefore, is subject to hormonal influence. The testes secrete both estrogen and testosterone. Testosterone is a prehormone for dihydrotestosterone, which is the prime mediator of androgen action within prostate cells. Testosterone is also the major substrate for peripheral transformation to estradiol in men (Fig. 25–2).

SYMPTOMS OF BPH

BPH is manifested by bladder outlet obstruction resulting from narrowing of the prostatic urethra and is associated with a spectrum of obstructive and irritating symptoms. These include urinary straining, hesitancy in initiating urinary flow, diminished stream caliber, interruption of stream, postvoid dripping, nocturia, urinary frequency, dysuria, urgency, and urge incontinence. In most patients with BPH, symptoms of obstruction vary from day to day. This variability of symptoms can in some part be explained by the dynamic neuromuscular component.

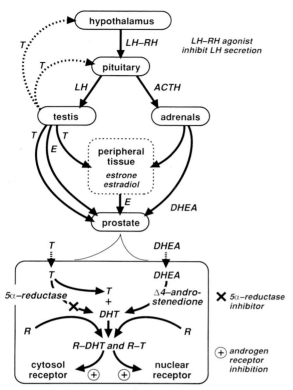

Figure 25–2. Hormonal milieu involved in development and maintenance of BPH.

CLINICAL TRIALS WITH ALPHA-BLOCKERS

The first clinical trial using an alpha-blocker was published by Caine et al.[9] This study was conducted on 49 patients who received phenoxybenzamine 10 mg twice a day. Administration of the drug resulted in improvement in daytime and nighttime frequency and overall symptomatic improvement. Two other studies by Abrams et al.[10] and Brooks et al.[11] were not able to identify urodynamic or symptomatic improve-

ment in patients receiving medication. Because blockers using phenoxybenzamine caused side effects, such as hypertension (orthostatic), nasal congestion, or absent ejaculation, and because it has been associated with intestinal malignancy in rats, trials of several other blockers, mostly selective alpha$_1$-blockers have been undertaken (Table 25–1).

Results

As seen from Table 25–1, clinical trials of alpha-blockers are of short duration, and some are not placebo controlled or blinded. The number of patients often is small, and the criteria for including patients are seldom well defined. Therefore, definite conclusions are difficult to draw.

HORMONAL TREATMENT WITH ANTIANDROGENS

A number of different approaches have been used in the hormonal treatment of BPH. One group of antiandrogen drugs works centrally and prevents production of testosterone. Another group acts peripherally on the prostatic cell. This peripherally acting group prevents transformation of testosterone to dihydrotestosterone (5-alpha-reductase inhibitor) or competes for binding to the androgen receptor. Peters and Walsh[18] demonstrated a positive effect of medical castration using a centrally acting antiandrogen, a luteinizing hormone/releasing hormone (LH-RH) analog. The prostate size regressed by approximately 25% based on ultrasound measurement. Biopsy from the prostate confirmed that regression was in the glandular tissue. There was no change in stromal tissue. Gabrilove et al.[19] describe the use of the analog leuprolide.

These centrally working drugs have many side effects, including impotence, and drugs that do not substantially alter sexual function would be more desirable.

In a study by Stone[20] investigating flutamide, which blocks the uptake of dihydrotestosterone by the cytoplasmic androgen receptor, 84 patients were randomized into equal groups of drug or placebo. Twelve patients were studied for

Table 25–1. Clinical Studies

DRUG	NO. OF PATIENTS	TYPE OF STUDY	DURATION	OVERALL	FLOW	REFERENCE
Phenoxybenzamine	49	Double-blind, placebo-controlled	2 weeks	Improved	Improved	9
Phenoxybenzamine	28	Double-blind, placebo-controlled	4 weeks	No effect	No effect	10
Phenoxybenzamine	41	Double-blind, placebo-controlled	4 weeks	No effect	No effect	11
Prazosin	55	Double-blind, crossover	3 weeks	Improved	Improved	12
Prazosin	20	Double-blind, crossover	4 weeks	No effect/improved	Improved	13
Prazosin	127	Double-blind, placebo-controlled	4 weeks	No effect	Improved	14
Terazosin	15	Uncontrolled	6 months	Improved	Improved	15
Doxazosin	91	Double-blind, placebo-controlled	9 weeks	Improved	No effect	16
YM-617	270	Double-blind, placebo-controlled	4 weeks	No effect	No effect	17

6 months, and 58 had been in the study for 12 or more weeks. At 6 weeks, peak urinary values had increased by 12% in the placebo group and 30% in the placebo group. However, symptom reduction was identical in both groups. The study is not completed, but at this time, it can be concluded that antiandrogens should be taken for a prolonged time to achieve maximum efficacy.

Geller et al.[21] described the effect of megestrol acetate in the treatment of BPH. Sixty-one patients were randomized to placebo or megestrol acetate and studied over a 5-month period. Improvement in symptoms of prostatism was similar in both groups. Seventy percent of the drug-treated patients reported a reduction of libido. Sexual side effects have kept the steroidal antiandrogens, such as megestrol, from being used widely for BPH.

A large clinical prospective randomized trial comparing a 5-alpha-reductase inhibitor to placebo is being conducted in the United States and abroad. Results of this investigation are not available, but preliminary reports suggest that administration of synthetic alpha$_1$-reductase inhibitor causes regression of prostate size on a magnitude similar to that with LH-RH analog administration. Very few side effects, including impotence, have been reported.

Results

Prevention of contraction of the smooth muscle should, from a theoretical point of view, provide the patient relief from obstruction. However, there is an important factor that has not been considered. Stereometric studies by Bartsch et al.[22-24] demonstrated that although the prostate is usually considered to be a glandular organ, it contains a large quantity of fibromuscular stroma. In normal prostates, the ratio of stroma to epithelium is 2:1, whereas the stroma to epithelial tissue in BPH is approximately 5:1. The stroma consists of smooth muscle and intermuscular components, such as collagen. The extractability of collagen is the limiting factor in the contraction/release of the smooth muscle. The effect of the alpha-blockers will, therefore, depend on nonmuscular components. At this moment, very little is known about age-related changes in these components.

Hormonal treatment of BPH has resulted largely in regression of the epithelial component. There is no apparent effect on the stroma. It is important to keep in mind that prostate involution because of regression of the epithelial part may not necessarily decrease urethral resistance and, therefore, may not reduce the symptoms of prostatism. Again, BPH is characterized by more stromal than epithelial enlargement.

SUMMARY

Research and medical treatment of BPH have intensified through the last two decades. The new approaches, however, have not yet established efficacy and safety to the degree that they represent an alternative to well-established treatments, such as urethral resection or incision of the prostate, for patients suffering from symptoms of BPH.

REFERENCES

1. Dørflinger G, England DM, Madsen PO, et al. Urodynamic and histological correlations of benign prostatic hyperplasia. *J Urol* 1988;140:1487
2. Lepor H, Gup DI, Baumann M, et al. Laboratory assessment of terazosin and alpha-blockade in prostatic hyperplasia. *Urology* 1988;32(Suppl):21
3. Roos NP, Wennberg JC, Malenka DJ, et al. Mortality and reoperation after open and transurethral resection of the prostate for benign prostatic hyperplasia. *N Engl J Med* 1989;320:1120
4. McNeal JE. The zonal anatomy of the prostate. *Prostate* 1981;2:35–49
5. Hedlund H, Anderson KE, Larsson B. Alpha-adrenoceptors and muscarinic receptors in the isolated human prostate. *J Urol* 1985;134:1291–1298
6. Shapiro E, Tsitlik JE, Lepor H. Alpha$_2$-adrenergic receptors in canine prostate: biochemical and functional correlations. *J Urol* 1987;137:565–570
7. Furuya S, Kumamoto Y, Yokoyama E, et al. Alpha-adrenergic activity and urethral pressure in prostate and in benign prostatic hyperplasia. *J Urol* 1982;128:836
8. Moore RA. Benign hypertrophy and carcinoma of the prostate. Occurrence and experimental production in animals. *Surgery* 1944;16:152–167
9. Caine M, Perlberg S, Meretyk S. A placebo-controlled double-blind study of the effect of phenoxybenzamine in benign prostatic obstruction. *Br J Urol* 1978;50:551
10. Abrams PH, Shah PJR, Stone R, Chou RJ. Bladder outflow obstruction treated with phenoxybenzamine. *Br J Urol* 1982;54:527
11. Brooks ME, Sidi AA, Hanani Y, Braf ZF. Ineffectiveness of phenoxybenzamine in treatment of benign prostatic hypertrophy: a controlled study. *Urology* 1983;21:474–478
12. Kirby RS, Coppinger SWC, Corcoran MO, Chappel CR, Flannigan M, Milroy EJG. Prazosin in the treatment of prostatic obstruction: a placebo-controlled study. *Br J Urol* 1987;60:136
13. Hedlund H, Anderson KE, Ek A. Effects of prazosin in patients with benign prostatic obstruction. *J Urol* 1983;130:275
14. Yamaguchi O, Shiraiwa Y, Kobayashi M, et al. Clinical evaluation of effects of prazosin in patients with benign prostatic obstruction. *Urol Int* 1990;45:40–46
15. Dunzendorfer U. Clinical experience: symptomatic management of BPH with terazosin. *Urology* 1988;32:27–31
16. Holme JB, Husted SE, Jacobsen F, et al. Doxazosin: a new efficient and safe drug in the treatment of benign prostatic obstruction. *J Urol* 1990;143:Abstract 257
17. Kawabe K, Veno A, Takimoto Y, Aso Y, Kato H. Use of an α-blocker YM 617, in the treatment of benign prostatic hypertrophy. *J Urol* 1990;144:908–911
18. Peters CA, Walsh PC. The effect of nafarelin acetate, luteinizing hormone/releasing hormone agonist on benign prostatic hyperplasia. A placebo-controlled study. *N Engl J Med* 1987;317:599
19. Gabrilove JL, Levine AC, Kireschenbaum A, Droller M. Effect of long-acting gonadotropin-releasing hormone analog (leuprolide) therapy on prostatic size and symptoms in 15 men

with benign prostatic hypertrophy. *J Clin Endocrinol Metab* 1989;68:461

20. Stone N. Flutamide in the treatment of benign prostatic hypertrophy. *Urology* 1989;34 (Suppl):64

21. Geller J, Nelson CG, Albert JD, Pratt C. Effects of megestrol acetate on uroflow rates in patients with benign prostatic hypertrophy. *Urology* 1979;14:467

22. Bartsch D, et al. Electron microscopic stereological analysis of the normal human prostate and of benign prostatic hyperplasia. *J Urol* 1979;122:481

23. Bartsch D, et al. Light microscopic stereological analysis of the normal human prostate and of benign prostatic hyperplasia. *J Urol* 1979;122:487

24. Ohrh P, Bartsch D. Human benign prostatic hyperplasia: stroma disease. New prospective by quantitative morphology. *Urology* 1980;16:625

26

Transurethral Incision of the Prostate: An Alternative Therapeutic Modality for Obstructive Prostatic Hypertrophy

Judy Fried Siegel, Joseph Banno, Arthur D. Smith

Transurethral resection of the prostate (TURP) is the treatment of choice for bladder outlet obstruction caused by a moderately hypertrophied gland. However, the combination of outlet obstruction and a small gland has been a diagnostic and therapeutic dilemma. Until recently, obstruction by a small gland was not a recognized disease entity. To resect such a gland seemed unnecessary and posed unacceptable risk, and application of nonsurgical therapies often was ineffective. With the advent of cystourethrography, various configurations of an obstructed bladder outlet, regardless of absolute prostate volume, have been identified. Incising such glands has been therapeutically effective, making transurethral incision of the prostate (TUIP) an elegant procedure for treatment of symptomatic bladder obstruction caused by a small prostate. TUIP is a timely procedure with few postoperative complications. As such, its application has been extended to include patients who are poor operative risks and patients for whom likely complications of prostate resection are unacceptable. More than 150 years after its first description, TUIP has become an accepted procedure in the armamentarium of a urologist.

This chapter reviews the history of TUIP, its indications, preoperative and postoperative care, technique, and results.

HISTORY

The history of TUIP parallels that of transurethral surgery. As early as 1834, Guthrie described blind transurethral incision of the bladder neck.[1]

"When, however, in spite of the continued use of the . . . (catheter), the disease (of the bladder neck) increases, and renders life miserable, . . . (I) would suggest that an operation be performed. The object is to divide the bar, dam, or stricture, with as little injury as possible to any of the neighboring parts. . . . The knife being projected just as the instrument is felt to be passing over the bar, will cut it; and if, after it has just passed into the bladder, it be withdrawn, the little knife, in coming back, will enlarge the original cut. . . . I have no doubt of the possibility of dividing . . . (the bar) without doing mischief; and in two cases in which I have tried it, I have reason to believe the object was effected, from the greater facility with which the catheter passed into the bladder. . . ."

At the same time in France, Mercier, Civiale, and LeRoy D'Etoilles modified the lithotrite with a sharpened blade that was passed transurethrally to incise the bladder neck. Further modification occurred in 1877, when Bottini developed the galvanocautery incisor using electrical energy to obliterate the bladder neck. Transurethral surgery was still performed without vision.

By the early twentieth century, the cystoscope evolved to permit use of the electrocautery under direct vision. In 1924, Keye and Collings employed a vacuum tube current to incise median bar contractures using oil distention of the bladder. In 1933, Beer described "incision of the internal sphincter at 5 and 7 o'clock with the point electrode."[2] Thirty years later, Aboulker et al. described forceful rupture of the prostatic urethra with expandable sounds to create anterior and posterior commissures.[3] Finally, in the 1970s, Orandi and Turner-Warwick separately wrote descriptions of transurethral incision of the bladder neck, which is still performed today.

156

INDICATIONS

The indications for TUIP are still being defined. At this time, prostate incision is indicated for symptomatic outlet obstruction caused by a gland less than 20–35 g on digital rectal examination without suspicion of malignancy. Additional indications include radiographically proven dyssynergic bladder neck with intolerable symptoms of obstruction,[4] the prostate trapped in an unforgiving capsule, or the young, symptomatic patient who wishes to preserve fertility.[5] TUIP has been used successfully under local anesthesia for symptomatic patients with small glands who are poor anesthetic risks.[6] Exclusion has been described for patients who have obscured anatomy from previous TURP, urethral stricture disease, or previous major intrapelvic surgery.[7] Detrusor instability has been described as a relative contraindication to TUIP.[8]

In general, the indications for TUIP are fourfold.

Symptomatic Obstruction

Symptoms of outlet obstruction have been divided arbitrarily into obstructive (weak stream, abdominal straining, hesitancy, intermittency, incomplete bladder emptying, and terminal dribble) and irritative (frequency, nocturia, and urgency). These symptoms are subjective variables reflecting patients' perceptions and attitudes. Symptoms of obstruction are often a strong impetus for surgical intervention and should be included in the preoperative evaluation.

A Small Gland

Initial evaluation of TUIP focused on incising glands 15–20 g in size as estimated by digital rectal examination and verified by cystoscopy. The procedure met with such success that surgeons incised glands up to 40 g in size. Incising glands larger than 20 g proved to be technically difficult, requiring deep incisions that enter venous sinuses, causing excessive venous bleeding. Extensive fulguration within the deep incisional clefts increases the risk of retrograde ejaculation. For these reasons, prostate incision currently is best indicated for glands less than 20 g in size. Furthermore, resection of prostate glands less than 20 g in size is associated with postoperative bladder neck contracture. This observation has led some urologists to perform prophylactic bladder neck incisions at the time of prostate resection.[9,10] Incising rather than resecting small glands circumvents this problem.

No Clinical Suspicion of Malignancy

Prostate tissue is not harvested during prostate incision. Thus, incidental prostate cancer will not be identified. Studies of random biopsies of apparently benign glands have yielded a 0–20% rate of cancer.[11] If 10% of all prostatectomies will reveal occult malignancy, performing TUIP will inherently miss identification of these cancers. In response to this dilemma, some urologists perform random prostate biopsies at time of TUIP. Still other urologists treat stage A disease expectantly and question the significance of the discovery of occult malignancy. Consequently, digital rectal examination and serum markers are advised prior to performing TUIP to decrease the suspicion of malignancy. Prostate malignancy, suspected or biopsy proven, is a contraindication to performing TUIP.

Relative Contraindication to TURP

When preservation of antegrade ejaculation is paramount, prostate resection is an unacceptable treatment of bladder outlet obstruction because of the high incidence of postoperative retrograde ejaculation. Indeed, retrograde ejaculation is a complication of both prostate resection and prostate incision. Edwards et al. report retrograde ejaculation in 100% of TURP patients as compared to 18% of TUIP patients.[8] Turner-Warwick reports an even lower rate of retrograde ejaculation (5%) in patients undergoing unilateral TUIP as compared to TURP, which is further diminished with unilateral modifications of TUIP.[12] When the desire to preserve fertility is paramount, prostate incision provides an alternative to resection, albeit an imperfect one.

Management of BPH in the frail elderly is a dilemma. These patients often pose a poor surgical risk, and prostate resection may prove to upset the balance that preserves their independence and stability.[13] In this population, prostate incision may prove to be an attractive therapeutic option, since it is a timely procedure associated with limited fluid resorption and minimal blood loss. Moreover, TUIP can be performed under local anesthesia, which eliminates common problems associated with general anesthesia, such as nausea, vomiting, painful throat, drowsiness, and disorientation. It also prevents the precipitous blood pressure fluctuation associated with spinal anesthesia.[10] Indeed, prostate incision has been used successfully as a therapeutic option in the older patient with significant medical disease.[14]

PREOPERATIVE EVALUATION

Preoperative evaluation for TUIP is designed to select that patient population for which it is best indicated, namely, patients with symptoms of obstruction caused by a small, benign gland.

Objective scoring schemes have been developed in an attempt to quantify subjective symptoms of obstruction. The Madsen-Iversen score is an example of one scoring scheme. In a prospective study of 84 patients with BPH, Bruskewitz et al. found that the symptom score system alone did not reliably predict which patients will benefit from surgery.[15] Rather, such scores provide a quantitative gauge of deterioration or improvement of symptoms over time.

The use of uroflowmetry is another attempt to gain objective evidence of obstruction. The goal of this technique is to analyze a representative recording of micturition, and more than one recording may be necessary. The peak flow rate is the value most closely correlated with the extent of outflow obstruction. The obstructed patient has a peak flow rate more than 2 standard deviations below the mean after correction for intravesical volume.[16] The peak flow rate in asymptomatic elderly males has been found to decrease to 6.5 mL/sec at age 80, suggesting that the mean peak flow rate also must be corrected for advancing age.[17] Appropriately interpreted, uroflowmetry is another attempt to objectify obstruction over time.

Urine culture is part of the routine preoperative evaluation of outlet obstruction. This ensures that infection is not mimicking outlet obstruction.

At this time, digital rectal examination is the most important part of the physical examination for detecting prostate cancer. Prostate ultrasound, serum prostatic acid phosphatase, and prostate-specific antigen (PSA) are helpful adjuvants in evaluating the prostate for malignancy. Specifically, PSA appears helpful in following prostate malignancy over time. The role of transrectal ultrasound of the prostate is currently under investigation. Ultrasound may prove helpful in estimating prostatic volume when considering TUIP, but it is not essential at this time.

Orandi has studied the worth of evaluating the configuration of the bladder neck using cystourethrography and endoscopy in TUIP candidates. After analyzing 5000 endoscopic photographs of bladder outlets in cervical, midprostatic, and apical positions, empty and full, he identified two configurations appropriate for TUIP, circular with a deep bas fond and bulging lateral lobes with a distant median lobe. In addition to obstruction of the prostatic urethra, Orandi observed postvoid residual, sacculation of the bas fond on lateral projection, trabeculation, cellule formation, diverticulum, occasional vesicoureteral reflux, and frequent bladder calculi in his patient population.[18,19] After this study, Orandi bases his patient selection on the estimated size of the prostate and the endoscopic configuration of the bladder neck—small prostates and short urethras. Other findings are considerations rather than indications for intervention.

Cystometrography often is used in the preoperative evaluation of outlet obstruction. Micturition is a delicate balance between detrusor mechanical energy and bladder outlet resistance.[20] Increased bladder outlet resistance is manifested as symptomatic prostatic obstruction, a clinical assessment rather than a urodynamic assessment. Urodynamics are useful to assess detrusor activity, especially when a neurologic deficit is suspected, but urodynamics do not indicate surgery.

The irritative symptoms of outlet obstruction can be caused by bladder cancer. Thus, a patient with hematuria and irritative symptoms must be evaluated for possible urothelial carcinoma. Urine cytology, excretory urography, and cys-

toscopy are, therefore, indicated in the evaluation of the TUIP candidate with hematuria.

TECHNIQUE

Anesthesia

TUIP is performed efficiently under conventional general or spinal anesthesia but also may be performed under local anesthesia with sedation. Lidocaine jelly is instilled transurethrally, and a soft penile clamp is applied for at least 10 minutes. Lidocaine anesthetic (1%) is injected directly into the four quadrants of the bladder neck and the lateral lobes of the prostate at the 3 o'clock and 9 o'clock positions, starting at the bladder neck and advancing toward the apex using a resectoscope needle, such as the Orandi needle[21] (Fig. 26–1).

An alternative form of anesthesia is transperineal instillation of local anesthetic. This is performed with the patient in the lithotomy position. The physician's finger is placed in the rectum. Using a 20-gauge 5-inch spinal needle, 5–10 mL of 1% lidocaine is delivered along the lateral borders of the prostate to the junction of the prostate and seminal vesical through previously anesthetized skin. Patients report minor discomfort, and adequate anesthesia is readily obtained[22] (Figs. 26–2, 26–3).

Bladder Neck Incision

Various procedures have been described to incise the prostate. These range in location, depth, and number of incisions. The patient is placed in the lithotomy position and examined bimanually and endoscopically to confirm a small, benign

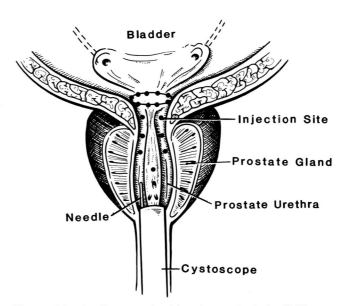

Figure 26—1. Transurethral local anesthetic for TUIP.

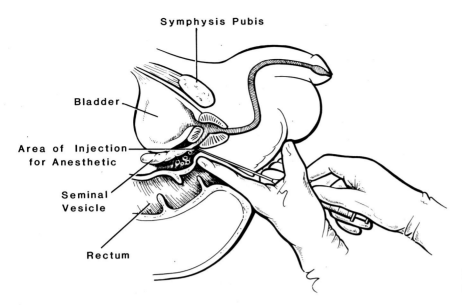

Figure 26–2. Transperineal local anesthetic for TUIP.

gland. Landmarks are identified, the ureteral orifices for proximal margins and the verumontanum for distal margin (Fig. 26–4). A cut is extended from the level of the ureteric orifice until just lateral to the verumontanum. The cut is deepened as desired, usually until capsular fibers and fat globules are seen. Deeper incisions are believed to provide more lasting, definitive therapy. However, they also increase the risk of retrograde ejaculation via pooling of seminal fluid and increase the risk of bleeding from venous sinuses. Consequently, for younger patients, shallower incisions may be indicated, realizing that additional therapy may be required in the near future.

The significance of which prostate incision is used to incise the gland is not known. Turner-Warwick utilizes a single full-thickness incision of the bladder neck ring from the bladder base to the verumontanum in the 7 o'clock to 8 o'clock position. He avoids the posterior midline and thus the underlying rectum. He believes that this technique minimizes postoperative bleeding, maintains antegrade ejaculation, and avoids subsequent stricture formation.[12]

Orandi favors the use of a continuous resectoscope via a transperineal urethrotomy, maintaining a bladder pressure of 40–50 cm of water. He utilizes two incisions at the 5 o'clock and 7 o'clock positions of the bladder neck, extending distally to the sides of the verumontanum. The incisions are deepened until the prostatic capsule is reached. Concomitant prostate biopsies are taken to identify occult malignancy.[23]

We favor the use of two incisions in the 5 o'clock and 7 o'clock positions, extending from the ureteric orifices to the verumontanum. The incision usually is extended through the prostatic capsule. Use of the electrocautery in the incisional cleft is minimized. Biopsy is performed selectively. The procedure is modified for younger patients with less electrocautery, shallower incisions, and consideration of unilater-

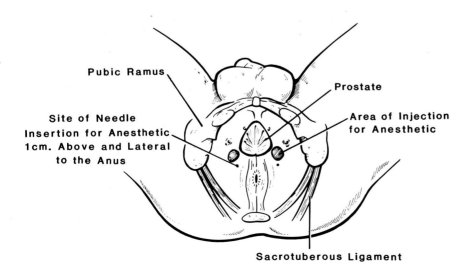

Figure 26–3. Perineal view for transperineal local anesthetic.

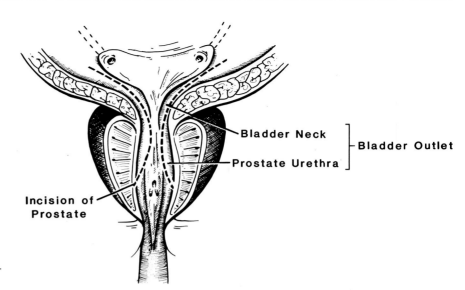

Figure 26–4. Anatomy of the incision for TUIP.

ally. The patient undergoing modified prostate incision must understand that shallower and unilateral incisions may necessitate additional therapy in the near future and deeper incisions may have better long-term results. For this reason, we advise against shallow incisions.

Various knives are available commercially for performing TUIP (Fig. 26–5). These vary in configuration and angulation of the working instrument tip. All knives utilized electric current, providing cutting and cautery capability. Instrument selection is based primarily on availability and personal experience.

RESULTS

Preliminary data comparing prostate incision with resection suggest comparable efficacy with regard to system score, subjective improvement, and uroflow evaluation (Table 26–1). Hospital stay, catheter time, urine infection, and complication rates appear variable from study to study. TUIP appears superior for treatment of small glands because of the decreased operative time, lesser incidence of retrograde ejaculation, and diminished transfusion requirement. Reoperation rates appear greater for unilateral prostate incision,

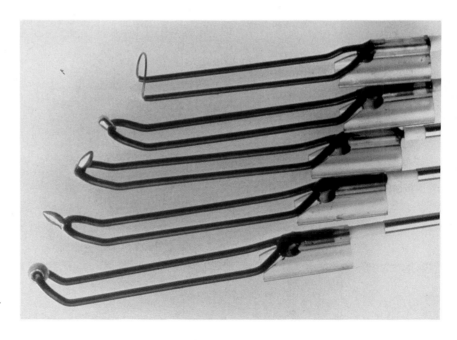

Figure 26–5. Various instrumentation for TUIP.

Table 26–1. Authors Reporting on TUIP

AUTHOR (INCISION)	SYMPTOM SCORE Pre-operative	SYMPTOM SCORE 3 months	SYMPTOM SCORE 12 months	PEAK FLOW Pre-operative	PEAK FLOW 3 months	PEAK FLOW 12 months	OR TIME (MIN)	BLOOD LOSS	CATHETER TIME (DAYS)	HOSPITAL DAYS	ADDITIONAL SURGERY (%)	RETROGRADE EJACULATION (%)
Larsen (6:00)												
TUIP	17	2	2	7.4	14.4	18.5	NR[a]	NR	1	2.5	NR	28
TURP	17	2	2	8.6	16.3	20.6	NR	NR	2	4.5	NR	100
Li et al.[27] (4:00 + 8:00)												
TUIP		NR		NR	23		19	7%[b]	2.5	5.6	NR	NR
TURP		NR		NR	19		36	43%[b]	2.5	8	NR	NR
Nielson[28] (5:00 + 7:00)					2 months							
TUIP		NR		5	10	9	18	4%[b]	1	3	NR	NR
TURP		NR		5	17	12	45	80%[b]	1	3	NR	NR
Orandi[29] (5:00 + 7:00)												
TUIP		Improved		8.2	13.7		NR	NR	NR	NR	1	31
TURP		Improved		7.6	12.7		NR	NR	NR	NR	3	42
Christensen et al.[24] (6:00)												
TUIP		NR		7.8	12.7	13.5	50	150 mL	2	4	10	13
TURP		NR		9.7	16.6	18.5	20	25 mL	1	3	NR	37
Edwards et al.[25] (7:00)												
TUIP		NR			Improved		NR	1.6%[b]	2.01	6.9	16	NR
TURP		NR			Improved		NR	19.6%[b]	3.23	6.7	18	NR
Bruskewitz et al.[15] (6:00)												
TUIP	17	3		7.1	12.7		NR	NR	NR	NR	NR	NR
TURP	17	3		9	17.2		NR	NR	NR	NR	NR	NR
Laguna et al.[26] (5:00 + 7:00)												
TUIP	13	3		8.1	13.7		NR	NR	NR	NR	13	10.5

[a]NR, not reported.
[b]% patients requiring transfusion.

which is concordant with the progressive disease course of prostatic hypertrophy. Randomized, long-term studies are required to verify these results.

CONCLUSION

Transurethral incision of the prostate has become an acceptable alternative therapy for outlet obstruction caused by a small, benign prostate gland. The indications for incision currently are being defined further. Evaluation is aimed at identifying symptomatic obstruction caused by a benign gland. Incision does not identify stage A prostate carcinoma. It does lessen the operative time, decrease the transfusion requirement, and decrease the risk of retrograde ejaculation. This is especially true with procedure modification, namely, unilaterally with shallower incisions. Thus far, results appear comparable to those of TURP. In short, TUIP is a viable alternative therapy for outlet obstruction.

REFERENCES

1. Nesbit RM. A history of transurethral prostate resection. In: Silber SJ, Nesbit RM (eds). *Transurethral Resection*. New York: Appleton-Century-Crofts, 1977:1
2. Beer E. Discussion on surgery of the neck of the bladder. *Br J Urol* 1933;5:362
3. Aboulker P, et al. La divulsion de la prostate d'apres 218 observations personelles. *J Urol Nephrol* 1964;70:337
4. Turner-Warwick R, et al. A urodynamic view of the clinical problems associated with bladder neck dysfunction and its treatment by endoscopic incision and transtrigonal posterior prostatectomy. *Br J Urol* 1973;45:44
5. Mebust WK. Transurethral prostatectomy. *Urol Clin North Am* 1990;17:575–585
6. Loughlin KR, et al. Transurethral incisions and resections under local anesthesia. *Br J Urol* 1987;60:185
7. Larsen EH, et al. Transurethral incision versus transurethral resection of the prostate for the treatment of benign prostatic hypertrophy. A preliminary report. *Scand J Urol Nephrol* 1987;104 (suppl):83
8. Edwards LE, et al. An objective comparison of transurethral resection and bladder neck incision in the treatment of prostatic hypertrophy. *J Urol* 1982;128:325
9. Kulb TP, et al. Prevention of postprostatectomy vesical neck contracture by prophylactic vesical neck incision. *J Urol* 1987;137:230
10. Lo JN. Anesthetic block. In: Kaye KW (ed). *Outpatient Urologic Surgery*. Philadelphia: Lea & Febiger, 1985:63
11. Morse RM, et al. Detection of clinically occult prostate cancer. *Urol Clin North Am.* 1990;17:575
12. Turner-Warwick R. The sphincter mechanism. The relation to prostatic enlargement and its treatment. In: Hinman F, Boyorsky S (eds). *Benign Prostatic Hypertrophy*. New York: Springer-Verlag, 1983:821
13. Fried Siegel J. The prostatic urethral stent as an alternative treatment for obstructive prostatic hypertrophy in the frail elderly. Unpublished

14. Graversen PH, et al. Transurethral incisions of the prostate under local anesthesia in high-risk patients: a pilot study. *Scand J Urol Nephrol* 1987;194(suppl):87

15. Bruskewitz RC, et al. Critical evaluation of transurethral resection and incision of the prostate. *Prostate* 1990; 3(suppl):27

16. Siroky MB. Interpretation of urinary flow rates. *Urol Clin North Am* 1990;17:537

17. Balslev JJ, et al. Uroflowmetry in asymptomatic elderly males. *Br J Urol* 1986;58:390

18. Orandi A. Transurethral incision of the prostate (TUIP): 646 cases in 15 years—a chronological appraisal. *Br J Urol* 1985;57:703

19. Orandi A. Transurethral incision of the prostate (TUIP). *J Endourol* 1990;4:S43

20. Shafer W. Principles and clinical application of advanced urodynamic assessment of voiding function. *Urol Clin North Am* 1990;17:553

21. Kaye KW. Surgery using local anesthesia in the elderly. *Clin Geriatr Med* 1990;6:85

22. Reddy PK. New technique to anesthetize the prostate for transurethral balloon dilatation. *Urol Clin North Am* 1990; 17:55

23. Orandi A. Transurethral incision of the prostate. *J Urol* 1973;110:229

24. Christensen MM, et al. Transurethral resection versus transurethral incision of the prostate. A prospective randomized study. *Urol Clin North Am* 1990;17:621

25. Edwards LE, et al. An objective comparison of transurethral resection and bladder neck incision in the treatment of prostatic hypertrophy. *J Urol* 1982;128:325

26. Laguna MP, et al. Bladder neck incision (BNI) as an alternative to transurethral prostatectomy (TURP). Unpublished

27. Li K, et al. Bladder neck resection and transurethral resection of the prostate: a randomized prospective trial. *J Urol* 1987; 87:807

28. Nielson HO. Transurethral prostatotomy versus transurethral prostatectomy in benign prostatic hypertrophy. *Br J Urol* 1988;61:435

29. Orandi A. Transurethral incision of prostate compared with transurethral resection of prostate in 132 matched cases. *J Urol* 1987;138:810

27

Use of Robots in Surgery: Development of a Frame for Prostatectomy

A.G. Timoney, W.S. Ng, B.L. Davies, R.D. Hibberd, J.E.A. Wickham

The immediate morbidity rate of a transurethral prostatectomy is 18% and has remained stationary in three large series over a 27-year period.[1-3] Transurethral prostatectomy has been regarded as a safe procedure, and the immediate mortality rate has declined over the same time period. Both immediate morbidity and mortality rates are related to the time of operation, the size of the gland, and the age of the patient. There is concern that the long-term mortality rate is higher than after open prostatectomy and that this may be attributable to irrigant absorption.[4-5] Transurethral prostatectomy is associated with a significant decrease in cardiac output and an increase in vascular resistance,[6] and this effect increases with operation time and occurs even during apparently uneventful procedures. Our aim in automating prostatectomy is to reduce the operation time and fluid absorption and thus reduce morbidity and mortality rates.

One of the main reasons that robotics have not been applied previously to surgical practice relates to safety requirements. A safety frame was designed to hold a resectoscope during transurethral prostatectomy in such a way that the resectoscope can be moved through controlled incremental motions to sweep out a predetermined resection cavity while the maximum range of movement is physically limited by the hardware.[7,8] Motorization of this frame with the addition of control software would result in a special-purpose robotic prostatectomy device. Thus, this frame can be viewed as the first stage in the development of a surgeon-assistant robot.

The aim of this study was to determine if a resection carried out with the frame would relieve prostatic outflow obstruction in patients awaiting a transurethral prostatectomy.

METHODS

The frame has been described in detail previously.[7,8] Briefly, it consists of an outer metal frame, which is fixed to the end of the table after the patient is placed in the lithotomy position. A wheel is mounted on this fixed frame and carries a pin that locates in 24 peripheral indents positioned around the fixed frame. An arc-shaped crossbeam is mounted on the wheel and carries eight similar indents. These indents allow the resectoscope to rest in various defined positions during the procedure. A sliding carriage is mounted on the arc, and the resectoscope can be mounted rigidly on this carriage.

After preliminary cystoscopy, the resectoscope is positioned at the level of the verumontanum by the operator and then mounted on a central locking mechanism. The resectoscope is locked rigidly to this mechanism and can be rotated through 360 degrees and traverse the crossbeam. The frame pivots the resectoscope at a point 37 mm proximal to the distal tip of the resectoscope loop. Movement of the resectoscope across the arch and rotation of the ring resects a symmetrical truncated cone of tissue.

The original design of the frame permitted resection of a cavity of 23–25 mm in length. The radius of the base, toward the bladder neck, could be varied from 5.25 mm to a maximum of 24 mm by increasing the distance the resectoscope travelled across the crossbeam (Table 27–1). The

Table 27–1. Resected Radius at Bladder Base (R_b') and Verumontanum (R_a') for Various Indent Values

ARC INDENT NO.	R_b (mm)	R_a (mm)	RESECTION VOLUME (mL)
1	5.25	4.0	1.4
2	8.25	5.0	3.3
3	11.75	7.0	5.8
4	16.0	8.75	10.3
5	19.25	9.5	13.7
6	21.25	10.25	15.5
7	24	10.5	18.2

resection volume could be increased to a maximum of 18.2 mL. A longitudinal travel of 25 mm was subsequently introduced, increasing the length of the cavity that can be resected to as much as 48 mm and the maximum volume to 60 mL (Fig. 27–1). During this stage, the resectoscope is moved manually by the surgeon, and hemostasis is obtained after the resection is complete.

A trial in patients awaiting elective prostatectomy was undertaken. Before entry into the trial, the patient provided three flow rates with at least 150 mL voided. Any patient with a flow rate in excess of 15 mL/sec was excluded. Conventional pressure–flow studies, using an Ormed Urodynamic Investigation System 5000, were carried out after drainage of the residual urine. Fluid-filled lines (4 F) were used to measure bladder and rectal pressures, with zero reference being at the level of the symphysis pubis. A 10 F catheter was used to fill the bladder at a medium rate, as defined by the International Continence Society.[9] Transrectal ultrasound estimation of prostatic dimensions and volume and transabdominal estimation of bladder urine volume were carried out using the Proscan ultrasound imaging system with a 7.5-MHz biplanar transrectal probe and a 5-MHz general purpose probe, respectively.

The "resection time" refers to the time taken to resect the

Longitudinal Section

Pivot Point

← 14 → mm   ← 48 mm →

Maximum Resection Volume = 60 ccs

Verumontanum

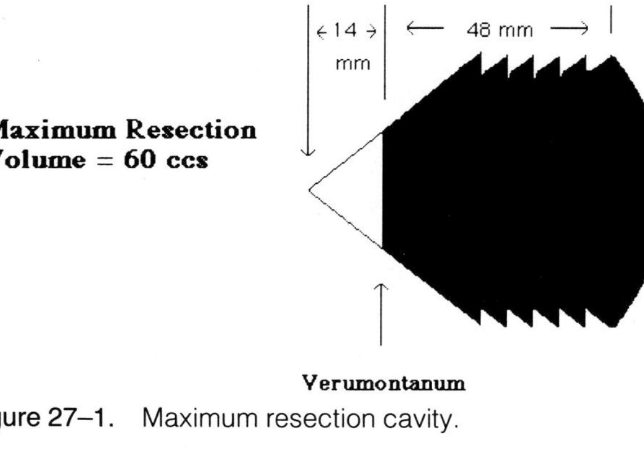

Figure 27–1. Maximum resection cavity.

prostatic tissue and carry out diathermy during the resection but excludes the setting-up time and the time required to achieve hemostasis at the end of the resection. Postoperative bladder drainage was via a three-way continuous drainage system.

Postoperatively, a free flow rate and transabdominal ultrasound estimation of residual urine volume were planned on discharge, at 6 weeks, at 3 and 6 months, and at 1 year and repeat transrectal ultrasonography at 3 months. Relief of obstruction was considered achieved if, after the operation, the flow rate was greater than 15 mL/sec. Repeat pressure–flow studies were planned at 6 months if flow rates fell below this figure.

RESULTS

To date, 30 patients have been entered in the trial. Their mean age was 67 years (range 55–81). The mean preoperative peak flow rate of 26 patients was 9.8 mL/sec (range 4.2–13.6). Preoperative flow rates for 4 patients are not available because of inadequate voided volume, but on urodynamic testing, all 4 had peak detrusor pressures at maximum flow of 90 cm H_2O or greater. The mean catheter-determined residual urine volume was 230 mL (range 15–1100). On urodynamic assessment, 7 patients had a detrusor pressure at peak flow of less than 70 cm H_2O. The transrectal ultrasound assessment of prostatic weight was 48 g (range 20–86) and length 41 mm (range 29–59). The average setting up time was 11 min (2–35), and the resection time was 28 min (20–45).

At the end of the frame resection, 2 patients had residual median lobe tissue, and a manual resection was carried out. Therefore, 28 patients had a frame resection alone. Postoperative flow rates are available on 26 of these patients. The mean peak flow rate was 22.2 mL/sec (9–40.5); the mean ultrasound-determined residual urine volume was 121 mL (0–589). Postoperatively, 1 patient failed to void and had a conventional transurethral prostatectomy. One patient voided less than 150 mL on discharge. Five patients have flow rates less than 15 mL/sec: 1 at discharge, 1 at 6 weeks, and 3 at 6 months (Fig. 27–2). Repeat pressure–flow studies on these 3 patients confirm outflow obstruction. Two patients have had further surgery: 1 a bladder neck incision for stenosis and 1 removal of residual prostatic tissue. One patient has declined further surgery because of subjective improvement. Five patients had a coincidental carcinoma on histologic examination.

DISCUSSION

As a robot is equipped with position sensors, it always knows where it is with reference to its working space. Thus, a robot can insert a surgical instrument to a desired position and orientation, deep within the body, with an accuracy impos-

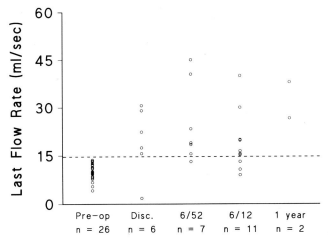

Figure 27–2. Peak flow rates in patients before and after frame prostatectomy.

sible for a surgeon. The potential use of an industrial robot to complete an experimental resection using a potato as a model was first demonstrated in 1989.[10] In this experiment, a precise and predictable cavity was resected in approximately 5 min. This pilot study was thought to demonstrate the feasibility of a robotized procedure.

The main reason for the limited application of robots in surgery has been considerations of safety. Two centers have used robots to guide the surgeon during a brain biopsy.[11,12] The robot positions the cannula adjacent to the skull with a predefined orientation and position. The surgeon then inserts the biopsy needle through the cannula to a predefined depth. Regulations on industrial robot safety require that when a robot is working, humans remain outside the operating environment. The application of robotics in surgery, however, requires that the robot may be within reach of the patient, surgeon, anesthetist, or theater staff. To satisfy safety requirements of both patients and surgeons, a device to limit the movement of any roboticized system to within a predetermined envelope of tissue was required. The frame is such a safety device, as it is intended to confine a motorized resectoscope to a given volume of space as determined by a preoperative transrectal or perioperative transurethral ultrasound scan. This motorization, with the addition of control software, will result in a first-generation robotic device, the aim of which is to reduce operation time and irrigant fluid absorption. The frame limits the surgeon to resecting a volume of tissue in the shape of a truncated cone. Before motorization, it was necessary to prove that this resection cavity could objectively relieve outflow obstruction.

The decision to operate on these patients was based on the assessment of symptoms and a flow rate less than 15 mL/sec. Pressure–flow studies were carried out preoperatively, since a persistent low flow postoperatively can be secondary to a poorly contracting detrusor rather than persistent obstruction.[13] Twenty-one patients (75%) who underwent frame

prostatectomy have a flow rate of 15 mL/sec or greater at last follow-up. This compares with 83% of 53 patients who had relief of obstruction in the series of Abrams et al., but those investigators excluded patients who had a poorly functioning detrusor.[13] Of the 7 patients in our series with a postoperative flow rate less than 15 mL/sec, 3 had a detrusor pressure at maximum flow of 70 cm H_2O or less on urodynamic assessment preoperatively.

Neal et al. reported a flow rate of 18 ± 9 (SD) mL/sec at mean follow-up of 11 months.[14] Abrams[15] and Frimodt–Moller et al.[16] reported flow rates at 12 months as a mean of 21.2 (range 5–48) and median 19.6 (range 4.7–42.5), respectively. The mean peak flow rate in the current series is 22.2 mL/sec (9–40.5). The mean follow-up after a frame prostatectomy is shorter, but both Abrams and Frimodt–Moller et al. reported flow rates in their patients at 3 months that were lower than the 12-month figure. We, therefore, suggest that the outcome after a frame prostatectomy is similar to that after conventional transurethral prostatectomy.

The manual frame does not reduce the total operation time. This is partly because of the time taken to set up the device and the fact that the resection is carried out manually by the surgeon. A reduction in operation time and irrigant fluid absorption will occur when the device is motorized and the procedure can be carried out automatically.

ACKNOWLEDGMENTS

We thank Mr. G.F. Abercrombie, consultant urologist, St. Mary's Hospital, Portsmouth, and Mr. P.J.R. Shaw, consultant urologist, Institute of Urology, for permission to include their patients in this study. We are very grateful to the Smith's Charity, the St. Peter's Trust, and the Violet M. Richards Charity for the Aged for their generous financial support.

REFERENCES

1. Holtgrewe HL, Valk WL. Factors influencing the mortality and morbidity of transurethral prostatectomy: a study of 2,015 cases. *J Urol* 1962;87:450
2. Melchior J, Valk WL, Foret JD, Mebust WK. Transurethral prostatectomy: computerized analysis of 2,223 consecutive cases. *J Urol* 1974;112:634
3. Mebust WK, Holtgrewe HE, Cockett ATK, Peters PC. Writing Committee. Transurethral prostatectomy: immediate and postoperative complications: a cooperative study of 13 participating institutions evaluating 3,885 patients. *J Urol* 1989; 141:243
4. Roos NP, Wennberg JE, Malenka DJ, et al. Mortality and reoperation after open and transurethral resection of the prostate for benign prostatic hyperplasia. *N Engl J Med* 1989; 320:1120
5. Coppinger SWV, Hudd C. Risk factors for myocardial infarction in transurethral resection of prostate? (letter) *Lancet* 1989;(ii):859
6. Evans JWH, Chapple CR, Coppinger SWV, Singer M, Milroy

EJG. Transurethral prostatectomy: the acute haemodynamic response. *Eur Urol* 1990;18(suppl 1):Abstract 36

7. Davies BL, Hibberd RD, Timoney AG, Wickham JEA. A surgeon robot for prostatectomies. Proceedings of the 2nd Workshop on Medical and Healthcare Robotics. Newcastle-Upon-Tyne, 1989:91–101

8. Davies BL, Hibberd RD, Ng WS, Timoney AG, Wickham JEA. The development of a surgeon robot for prostatectomies. *J Eng Med* 1991;205:35–38

9. International Continence Society. Third Report on the Standardisation of Terminology of Lower Urinary Tract Function. *Br J Urol* 1980;52:348

10. Davies BL, Hibberd RD, Coptcoat MJ, Wickham JEA. A surgeon robot prostatectomy: a laboratory evaluation. *J Med Eng Tech* 1989;13:273

11. Cinquin P, Laralee S, Demongeot J. Computer-assisted medical intervention. Proceedings of the 2nd Workshop on Medical and Healthcare Robotics. Newcastle-Upon-Tyne, 1989: 63–65

12. Engelberger JF. Parasurgeon. In: Engelberger JF (ed). *Robots in Service*. London: Kogan Page, 1989:130–134

13. Abrams PH, Farrer DJ, Turner-Warwick RT, Whiteside CG, Feneley RCL. The results of prostatectomy: a symptomatic and urodynamic analysis of 152 patients. *J Urol* 1979;121:640

14. Neal DE, Ramsden PD, Sharples L, et al. Outcome of elective prostatectomy. *Br Med J* 1989;299:767

15. Abrams PH. Prostatism and prostatectomy: the value of urine flow rate measurement in the preoperative assessment for operation. *J Urol* 1977;117:70

16. Frimodt–Moller PC, Jensen KME, Iverson P, Madsen PO, Bruskewitz RC. Analysis of presenting symptoms in prostatism. *J Urol* 1984;132:272

Reprinted from *Journal of Endourology* 1991;5:165–168.

28

Video Transurethral Resection of the Prostate

Jerrold Widran

The application of video technology in endoscopy is a natural progression in the advancement of imaging quality. The video camera in combination with the resectoscope is a useful and important new tool for the urologist. Observation of a television (TV) monitor screen for surgical judgments during transurethral resection (TUR) of the prostate gland and bladder neoplasms is a magnificent improvement that adds a new dimension in endoscopic visualization (Fig. 28–1).

Urologists traditionally have been the leaders in the field of endoscopy. Technologic advances in telescope lenses were driven by the desire for improved optical imaging. The skills for performing a TURP have been developed, improved through constant reassessment, and passed on for several generations. Monocular viewing with the resectoscope close to the face has been the conventional operating method (Fig. 28–2). The transition from monovision to television is our goal. There are many advantages to be obtained from this change that will benefit not only the urologic surgeon but ultimately the patients as well.[1,2]

Video TURP, also known as video prostatectomy[3,4] or armchair prostatectomy,[5,6] is the technique, procedure, and method of operating with a video camera attached to the eyepiece of the resectoscope. The video camera offers unique advantages that improve our ability to view the operating field with magnification and clarity. It allows us to stand comfortably and use both eyes to view the high-resolution images transmitted to the TV screen (video monitor) (Fig. 28–3). The video camera replaces having one eye pressed against the scope and projects magnified images of the endoscope field up to 50 times life size on the monitor screen.[7] The entire transurethral resection proceeds by observing the real time visual information pictured on the TV screen (Fig. 28–4) in the course of making judgments about where to resect tissue and fulgurate bleeding vessels.

The video technique initially is perceived as difficult to learn, but with regular use, its potential can be realized and soon appreciated. The motivated urologist will find that his coordination and skills for performing a TUR can be readily transferred and adapted to operating from the TV image. Familiarity with handling the video camera and obtaining confidence with its use during surgery take practice, and it becomes necessary to take the time to learn how to handle this new technology and to gain comfort with its features in order to obtain its maximum benefits.

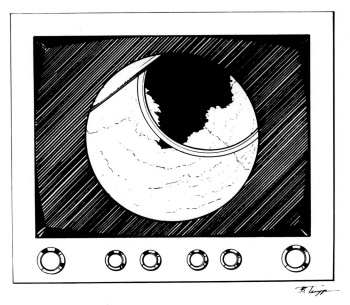

Figure 28–1. Illustration of the endoscope field projected on a television screen.

167

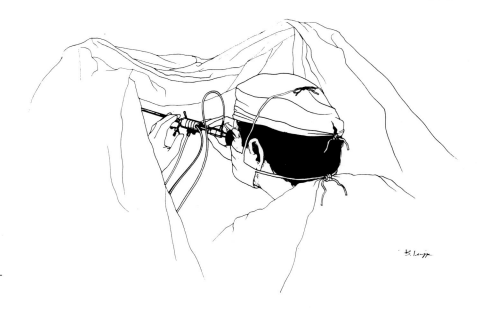

Figure 28–2. Conventional monocular operating method for TUR.

HISTORICAL PERSPECTIVE

In 1984, Aso et al.[8] described the application of closed circuit video equipment for simultaneous viewing of the surgical field during various endourologic procedures. Also during that year, O'Boyle et al. presented their experience with the specific application of a miniature video camera mounted on a resectoscope for operating from a TV screen during TURP.[3,9] Subsequently, several urologists from the United States,[1,10] Israel,[5] and Japan[11,12] have confirmed the successful, safe, and routine use of TV viewing in the performance of TUR.

DEVELOPMENT

The widespread acceptance of color television-assisted surgical endoscopic procedures was dependent on the advance in camera technology from large heavy tube sensor cameras to small, lightweight, sterilizable, high-resolution CCD chip

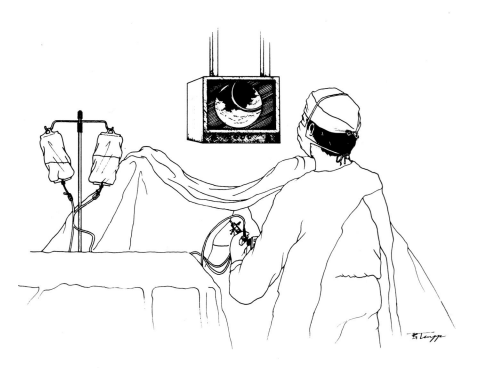

Figure 28–3. Video TURP. Both eyes are used while standing to observe the resectoscope image on a TV monitor.

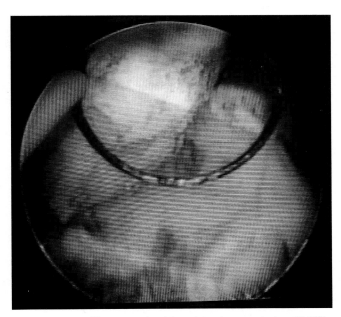

Figure 28–4. Photograph of the video image during TURP.

sensor cameras.[13] During this development period of miniature camera technology, video system prices dropped dramatically, and the equipment became more easily affordable.[10] Improvements in the optical characteristics of endoscopes and the advent of fiberoptics for light source transmission to the surgical field helped popularize the routine use of closed circuit television in the operating room.

Other medical specialties showed the way by using the video camera during relatively bloodless endoscopic procedures, such as arthroscopy,[14] colonoscopy,[15] and laparoscopy.[16] In arthroscopy, a tourniquet is used to stem blood flow to the surgical site so that bleeding is prevented from interfering with visualization. In colonoscopy and laparoscopy, mostly dry surgical environments are encountered where fluid irrigation is unnecessary, blood loss is minimal, and visibility is not a problem.

It seems the urologist may be the last of the endoscopic specialties to take advantage of the video technology on a routine basis. This is probably because the urologist contends with bleeding during the performance of TUR surgery.[7] Vessel bleeding tends to obscure visibility unless it is washed away quickly. Blood loss becomes the limiting factor that makes it difficult to adjust and gain comfort with the video camera. The red color of blood absorbs much of the available light to the camera sensor, causing the picture resolution quality to diminish and the video image to become dark.

There are many subtle difficulties in working with the video camera during TUR that require an adequate flow system to overcome. It is important not to have to pull the instrument apart to drain the irrigation fluids because this disrupts orientation, permits bleeding to go unchecked, and requires extra time to refill the bladder to redistend the bladder and prostate.[4] Since the camera is less sensitive to

light than the human eye, high flow rates are needed to wash blood out quickly, provide fresh, clear irrigant, and maintain proper visibility.

Measurements of the intravesical pressure are important so that high balanced flow rates can be obtained without concern for exposing the patient to high intravesical pressures and associated increases in fluid absorption. Until recently, with the advent of the controlled continuous flow resectoscope, the capability for pressure monitoring with a safety mechanism to prevent high pressures while working from the TV screen was not available, and acceptance of video TURP was delayed.

IDEAL INSTRUMENTATION

In the reality of life, we never quite reach the ideal situation, but we still attempt to approach it as closely as possible. Surgical techniques often change in the pursuit of a better way. Often these changes are only improvements of past methods using newer instrumentation and methods designed to help us reach our goal.

The criteria most likely chosen to evaluate the ideal situation for TUR would be based on ease of surgical performance, safety during the procedure, and a successful surgical outcome. The instrumentation needed to achieve these goals should have features that improve our ability to perform TUR with less difficulty by permitting easier manipulation of the instrument and reduced operative time. Increasing the margin of safety for both the surgeon and the patient is another important requirement. Most importantly, the patient should experience a good functional result, short recovery time, and no complications resulting from the surgery.

The current state of the art in urology for TURP utilizes a TV monitor for direct surgical judgments and a video camera attached to a continuous flow system utilizing two pumps under the control of an intravesical pressure monitor. This combination of instrumentation brings us closest to the ideal situation, and its features help to achieve this goal.[1] The ultimate in optical and video engineering provides a bright, clear, high-resolution image on a TV screen. The surgical field is highly magnified so that all anatomic details and pathologic features can be identified easily. High flow rates are available to help maintain clear visualization for locating difficult bleeders. Intravesical pressures are kept within a safe range and prevented from exceeding a level deemed unsafe so fluid absorption can be minimized. Large glands can be undertaken with confidence.

EQUIPMENT

System Requirements

The basic video system for TUR consists of several components. There is a high-resolution video camera unit, a high-resolution television monitor (Fig. 28–5), a high-intensity video light source, and a high-transmission light cable. A recording device is a useful accessory but is not required. A dedicated video cart for housing all the video components in a single mobile unit is recommended for organizing all the equipment in one location.

The video camera unit is made up of several parts. The video camera head with attached cable plugs into the receptacle of a remote video console. This console houses all the major electronic circuits and controls for the camera, such as white balance button, color contrast, and a possible range of other features. A coupling lens system, mounted on the camera head, joins the camera with the resectoscope.

The coupling lens system focuses the view from the eyepiece of the scope onto the imaging chip inside the camera.[13] Focus adjustment of the endoscope video image is accomplished by manually turning a ring surrounding the middle of the coupler. The coupler should have several air vent holes to help reduce possible condensation buildup on the lens when the camera is attached to the scope. A spring-loaded mechanism manually opens and closes by twisting the end of the coupler to mate the camera firmly with the resectoscope. The scope must be allowed to rotate freely in the seat of the camera coupler.

A choice of two couplers is available in either the split beam or the direct beam lens system. Split beam couplers allow monocular viewing through the resectoscope lens while also transmitting the image to a TV screen. With the direct beam coupler, the eyepiece of the scope is covered completely so the surgeon must view the TV image.

Originally, a split-beam lens was attached to a side scope for help in teaching during TUR.[17] The split beam lens was then coupled with a video camera so multiple observers could view the endoscopic field while the surgeon operated by looking through the resectoscope lens. This capability further improved methods for teaching and communication between instructor and students during TUR.[18] The need for cumbersome articulated arms and fiberoptic attachments was eliminated. Video recordings became possible without interfering with the TUR procedure.

For video TUR, the split beam coupler is no longer needed because during the learning stage with the direct beam coupler, if anxiety arises, the camera can be disconnected easily from the scope to allow conventional viewing through the lens. The direct beam coupler places the camera in-line with the resectoscope and prevents the surgeon from seeing through the lens (Fig. 28–6). The endoscope image is viewed on the TV screen, so that the coordination and skills required for video TUR can be developed.[3] Reducing dependence on the monocular method and developing reliance on the video image enables the urologist to take full advantage of video technology.

Video Cameras

There are many important features needed in a camera for video TUR.[6] Get the highest resolution single-chip camera available. The latest cameras have up to 480 lines of resolution for a sharp video image even on large screen TV. A camera that is sensitive in low light situations is vitally important for obtaining a bright enough image to see well during inspection and treatment inside the prostate and bladder. The camera should have an automatic white balance control and provide good color rendition of the surgical field. The camera should be immersible for cold soaking in gluteraldehyde-based solution prior to surgery. It should be electronically well shielded to prevent radiofrequency (RF) disturbances, generated by cutting and fulgurating currents,

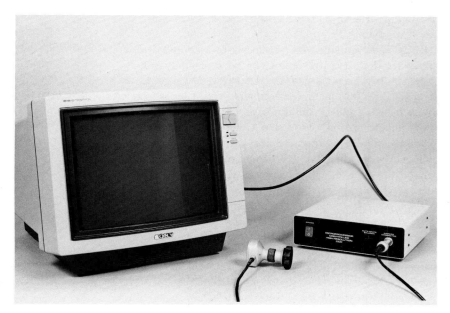

Figure 28–5. Miniature endoscopic video camera (Acufex) attached to high-resolution TV monitor.

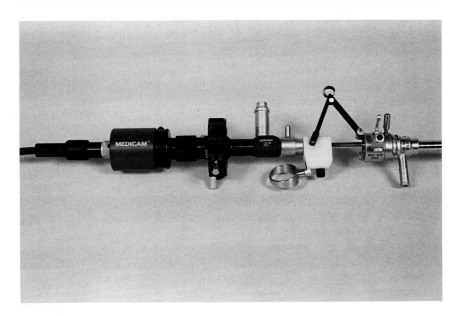

Figure 28–6. A direct beam coupler attaches a video camera (M.P. Video) to the resectoscope.

from interfering with the video image. The video camera head should have a raised reference notch to physically orient the camera on the endoscope and indicate the camera's 12 o'clock position. Also, the camera head with the coupler attached should be as lightweight as possible.

Other video camera features that may be of benefit are as follows. Some cameras have an automatic shutter feature that boosts picture brightness in low light situations and limits excessive brightness to maintain a usable video image under all operating circumstances. Some cameras can be gas sterilized if needed. Some cameras have small buttons on the camera head to activate or deactivate video accessories, such as a recording device. Some camera heads have a removable cable so if the cable breaks down, it can be changed easily without sending the camera out for service. Some cameras generate a color bar so that the colors on the TV monitor can be adjusted properly.

Recently, a three-chip camera has become available providing the highest resolution quality possible for endoscopy.[10] These cameras use red-green-blue (RGB) technology to obtain a superior image transmission of up to 600 lines of resolution. They are terrific for making very high quality recordings. The three-chip cameras are bulkier, somewhat heavier, and more expensive than one-chip cameras, although they provide the ultimate in miniature camera technology.

Couplers

The coupler should lock the camera securely onto the resectoscope. An important feature of the coupler is that it should permit the camera to rotate easily on the eyepiece of the scope with low friction. The resectoscope must be allowed to rotate independently from the video camera.[7] This

capability is necessary for maintaining proper orientation of the camera during the procedure.

Most couplers have a specific focal length that determines the size of the endoscope image on the video monitor. The largest circle on the TV screen possible, without losing the edges of the endoscope field, is best. Some couplers have a zoom lens capability that allows adjustment of the lens focal length. The zoom capability varies the magnification of the endoscope image on the TV monitor so that closeups of interesting pathology can be obtained. This feature makes the coupler more versatile so it can be used for other endourologic procedures with small image scopes, such as ureteroscopes, that require increased magnification.

Television Monitors

The TV monitor should be a professional grade model suitable for hospital use. A 20-inch screen is recommended for video TUR, although a smaller screen TV also can be used. The resolution rating of the monitor should always be of greater or equal value to the video camera to obtain the highest picture resolution possible. Proper shielding and filtering of the video signal input jack on the TV monitor are very important for preventing RF interference from appearing on the TV screen. The video monitor should be RGB capable if a three-chip camera is to be used.

Light Sources

A high-intensity fiberoptic light source is necessary for video use. A 300 W metal halides arc lamp usually is sufficient to provide a bright image for video TURP. Xenon light sources seem to be more popular for video work, although they tend to be more expensive. The video camera manufacturer may be able to recommend the best light source to match your particular camera. Some light sources will tie into the video camera unit and automatically regulate the light intensity provided to the resectoscope. Most illuminators have manual controls for setting the light intensity required. Some units have a standby feature so that once the intensity level has been set, the light output can be dimmed until surgery is ready to begin. This feature helps keep the unit cool and extend the bulb life.

The maximum light intensity of all light sources gradually but imperceptibly diminishes with increasing use. Light source bulbs rarely burn out completely. Many units have a bulb life indicator to measure the length of use. This bulb should be replaced periodically with a new one to maintain adequate light intensity for video TUR.

Light Cables

The most commonly used cables are fiberoptic. These tend to be very flexible for easy maneuvering of the resectoscope. A liquid light cable also can be used in place of a fiberoptic cable. Liquid cables are constructed with a special oil wrapped tightly inside a plastic-coated metal casing. These cables provide brighter light transmission than fiberoptic bundles, but they are very stiff and inhibit rotation of the resectoscope. Liquid cables last longer than fiberoptic cables, but they are more expensive to purchase.

Fiberoptic cables are actually very delicate. The multiple little fibers, compressed to form the bundle, tend to break in increasing numbers during repeated use. As more and more fibers break, the light intensity transmitted to the resectoscope gradually diminishes. Examine the cable periodically and exchange it for a new one if a large number of fibers are broken.

With conventional through-the-lens viewing, a small-diameter bundle usually is sufficient, but for optimal video brightness, a large-diameter fiberoptic bundle is important.[1] The diameter of the fiber bundle should be approximately 4.5 mm, or roughly equivalent to the diameter of the light collector on the resectoscope. The disadvantage of using a thicker cable is that its added weight increases drag on rotation of the resectoscope. In the future, as video cameras improve and require less light, light cables will become thinner, even more flexible, and lighter in weight.

Resectoscope Lenses

The most important factor affecting the video image is the quality and condition of the resectoscope lens.[6] Clarity and brightness of the video image are only as good as the lens permits. Older lenses may appear dark on the video monitor and make it difficult to see well with the video camera. Sometimes, the optic fibers at the distal tip of the scope get burned during the course of resecting tissue, which damages the light output of the lens. Wornout lenses should be replaced.

Newer telescope lenses with improved illumination and imaging capabilities are recommended for video use. Newer lenses increase the brightness of the video image during TUR by including a light-collecting funnel at the connection with the light cable. They add more fiberoptic strands inside the telescope body for greater light transmission to the surgical field, and better optical elements within the scope provide an even brighter endoscopic image.

Electrosurgical Generators

A compatible electrosurgical generator is necessary during video TUR to obtain an image free from RF interference.[6] Tube generator units should not be used because they cause severe interference problems on the video monitor during cutting and fulguration. Most solid-state generators will not cause RF problems, but if problems do occur, they may be the result of improper filtering or shielding on either the video camera or the TV monitor. Sometimes changing electrosurgical generators to a different manufacturer's brand will help solve video interference problems.

Recording Device

Tape recordings of the video TUR procedure can be made and documented for later review. Entire cases can be saved for future showing to referring physicians, consultants, and students.[8,10,12] Tape-recorded procedures may be useful for preoperative and postoperative comparisons and follow-up examinations. A choice of videocassette recording machines is available in VHS, SVHS, U-matic, or 8 mm format.[6] With a color video printer, individual color still images of interesting pathologic conditions can be obtained and placed in the patient's permanent record.

TECHNIQUE

Surgical Adaptations

There are several accommodations required for adapting to the video technique. The surgical field pictured on the TV screen is exactly the same view as normally seen by looking through the resectoscope, although now the view is highly magnified. Landmarks, tissue chips, and blood vessels appear much larger than before and become easier to identify. The surgeon's two eyes both are used for observing the endoscopic field on the TV screen. The resectoscope is displaced from in front of the surgeon's face. Now, the surgery is performed standing while the instrument is manipulated from around waist-high level. Some urologists indicate their preference for sitting upright in a chair and lowering the table to the appropriate height.[5,6]

Preparing for Surgery

When setting up the video system for TUR, the TV monitor normally is elevated high enough so the surgeon can view the screen comfortably while standing. The best location for the TV screen is toward the end of the table by the patient's head so the surgeon can look straight ahead without turning his body. By aligning the TV monitor with the resectoscope, the surgeon easily can glance down occasionally to verify proper orientation of the video camera in relation to the resectoscope. The TV monitor should be tested before surgery begins to verify proper adjustment of picture contrast, picture brightness, color hue, and color intensity. The TV image can be difficult to adjust once the surgery has started.

The video camera head, with attached coupler and cable, is prepared for surgery by cold soaking or gas sterilization, along with the light cable and other instruments needed for TUR. A special cap usually protects the plug end of the camera cable from getting wet during fluid immersion, but, as a precaution, it is best to leave the connector end out of the solution to ensure proper camera functioning and prevent the risk of fluid entering the cap. Before coupling the camera to the resectoscope lens, use a sterile towel to carefully dry all signs of fluid moisture from the inside of the coupler and the surfaces of the telescope eyepiece.

Make sure the camera sits securely on the lens so that it cannot fall off accidentally and be damaged. When turning the video light source on, caution is recommended.[6] Heat generated by the bright light coming from the open end of the light cable or the tip of the resectoscope lens can burn through the sterile patient drapes.

With the light cable attached to the resectoscope, perform a white balance of the video image on the TV monitor.[1] Aim the resectoscope at a group of white sterile gauze towels and have the nurse press and momentarily hold down the white balance button on the remote video console. The white tint on the monitor automatically adjusts for the proper shade of white. The white balance corrects color contrast and color tint so that the entire color spectrum obtained during surgery appears true and natural. A new white balance is needed at the beginning of each case and in the middle of a case when changing lenses or light sources.

During the Procedure

The video camera takes the place of your eye, and it must be maintained in one position regardless of the rotation of the resectoscope.[7] The camera should never be locked tightly to the resectoscope or forced to rotate with it, since rotation of the camera causes disorientation. To obtain proper orientation, the camera must remain at the fixed 12 o'clock position relative to the surgeon's body. The resectoscope is permitted to rotate freely and independent of the camera in the seat of the coupler.

The nondominant hand holds the camera steady while the dominant hand manipulates the resectoscope. Holding the video camera in one hand helps to guide the aim of the instrument and makes it easier to maneuver. A raised notch on top of the camera body indicates the fixed up and down 12 o'clock position. The thumb of the nondominant hand is placed over the notch on the camera, and the palm is wrapped under the camera to support the entire video/resectoscope unit. By maintaining pressure on the raised notch, the surgeon can feel the camera's correct orientation without taking his eyes off the TV monitor.

If the surgeon holds the camera coupler instead of the camera body to maintain orientation, fogging of the video image can occur. The surgeon's gloves usually are wet, and grabbing the back of the coupler blocks venting of moisture. Buildup of condensation inside the coupler obscures the video image and requires interrupting the procedure to eliminate the problem.

During the course of resecting tissue, bleeders should be fulgurated quickly to prevent loss of visualization.[1] If bleeding becomes a problem, causing a red-out of the video image, a dark, red, fuzzy image appears on the TV monitor and completely obscures vision. Increasing the flow rate and placing the lens close to the tissue helps brighten the image and improve visibility. Temporarily close the outflow stopcock valve on the resectoscope to increase the flow of fluids away from the scope until bleeders are found and fulgurated. Bringing the resectoscope behind the bleeders helps in locating them. Search and fulguration are continued until comfortable visibility of the entire field is regained.

Concluding the Procedure

The camera remains coupled to the scope when the working element is removed from the sheath while draining the bladder fluids and evacuating resected tissue. At the TUR conclusion, protect the camera from falling on the floor when it is disconnected from the lens. Immediately detach the cable from the remote video console and replace the protective cap over the plug. Recoil the cable and place the camera head on a stable surface.

PROBLEMS AND LEARNING DIFFICULTIES ENCOUNTERED WITH THE VIDEO TECHNIQUE

Problems and learning difficulties encountered with the video technique include orientation, magnification, light sensitivity, cumbersomeness, and irrigation.

I. Orientation
    Understand where you are operating in relation to the surgical field.
    A. Change of location of instrument away from face.
        1. Initially, it is a strange sensation to stand and not have the resectoscope close to the face while doing loop manipulations.

2. Must alter allegiance and break need to look through the scope.
  B. Learn to trust what is seen on the TV monitor.
    1. The camera is your eye, and similar to your body, it is not permitted to rotate with the scope.
    2. Camera is held in fixed 12 o'clock position, and scope swivels freely on the coupler.
  C. Must adapt to one-handed spring-type resectoscope.
    1. One hand is needed to steady the camera and guide the in and out movement of the scope.
    2. Other hand manipulates resectoscope rotation and moves the loop to resect tissue and fulgurate blood vessels.
II. Magnification
  Learn to judge surgical dimensions.
  A. Blood vessels and tissue chips appear much larger than they are.
    1. The 30–50 times magnification makes everything seem huge.
    2. Use loop diameter for actual size comparisons.
  B. Familiarity with area visualized is determined by using landmarks as your guide.
    1. Maintain proper orientation with verumontanum appearing on TV screen at 6 o'clock.
    2. Know where you are cutting at all times.
  C. Perception of depth of field requires adaptation.
    1. Estimating distances and moving the instrument requires practice.
    2. Develop feel for new hand–eye coordination.
III. Light sensitivity
  Maintain enough light to see well.
  A. Bleeding tends to obscure video image.
    1. Fulgurate arterial bleeders promptly.
    2. Increase irrigation flow to wash blood away.
  B. Fogging of the image makes it difficult to see.
    1. Condensation forms between camera and scope.
    2. Wipe coupler and lens dry before connecting.
  C. Video camera is less sensitive to available light than the human eye.
    1. Need equipment dedicated for video to provide adequate transmission of light to the field.
    2. Light source, fiber bundle, and telescope must be maintained in good condition or replaced.
IV. Cumbersomeness
  Added equipment takes getting used to.
  A. Video camera changes balance point of the resectoscope, making it back-heavy.
  B. Heavy or stiff light cable and attachments add drag to rotation of the scope.
  C. Requires motivation for new routine setup and use.
V. Irrigation
  Continuous flow is mandatory.
  A. Need accessibility to high flow rates.
  B. Maintain continuity of resection and bladder distention.

C. Need safety mechanism to prevent high pressures and bladder overdistention.

FLOW SYSTEMS FOR IRRIGATION

A coordinated continuous flow system with pressure sensor control provides a balanced pump-in and pump-out flow system (Fig. 28–7) that solves many of the problems of gravity-dependent flow systems[19] and addresses the many variables encountered during video TUR.[7] This system, called the controlled continuous flow resectoscope (CCFR) (Fig. 28–8), adds an element of safety and control previously unavailable during TUR.[20] Its features make it ideally suited for video TUR.

The CCFR system uses two pumps for fluid infusion and withdrawal (Fig. 28–9). The resectoscope is designed to allow a 5 F pressure transducer to fit inside the working element (Fig. 28–10) to measure intravesical pressure non-invasively throughout the procedure. High flow rates up to 1000 mL/min are available on demand. Flow rate and flow balance are adjustable electronically by two rheostat dials on the pumping console. The pressure sensor in the resectoscope transmits pressure information along a flexible cable to the pumping console. A meter displays the pressure value on a bar graph scale in centimeters of water. The maximum pressure limit is adjustable on the console.

During the procedure if intravesical pressure reaches the maximum set point limit, the inflow pump automatically shuts off until the pressure is relieved. An audio signal alerts the surgeon when the inflow pump has stopped so he need not pay attention to the actual displayed pressure reading. The outflow pump continues functioning to remove excess fluids. The surgeon advances the resectoscope into the bladder to decompress fluid pressure. When the pressure drops below the maximum set point, the inflow pump automatically resumes functioning, and the procedure continues.

The more typically available flow systems for TUR rely on gravity and the height of the fluid source to determine the rate of irrigation flow. The familiar intermittent flow resectoscope has been available since the first resectoscope was introduced in 1931. With intermittent (reciprocal) flow, cutting and fulguration occur during the inflow of fluids, and the resectoscope must be disconnected from the sheath periodically when the bladder is full to drain the fluids and start again (Fig. 28–11). In 1975, Iglesias et al. developed a flow system with continuous flow potential utilizing outflow suction and eliminating the need to interrupt the procedure[21] (Fig. 28–12). Then, in 1978, Reuter et al. described the use of a trocar placed suprapubically into the bladder as an alternative method for achieving continuous flow[22] (Fig. 28–13).

Using the intermittent flow resectoscope with the video camera can be a frustrating experience. As the bladder reaches maximum filling, the flow rate slows until a pressure equilibrium is obtained between the bladder and the height of

T.U.R. IRRIGATING SYSTEM
CONTROLLED CONTINUOUS FLOW
PUMP IN → PUMP OUT
UNDER CONTROL OF
INTRAVESICAL PRESSURE SENSOR

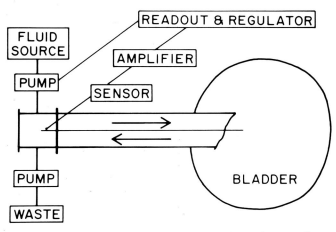

Figure 28–7. Diagram of the controlled continuous flow system for TUR.

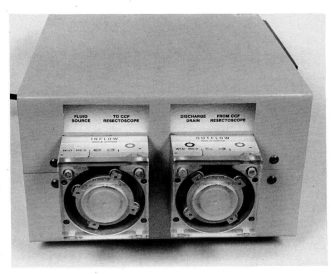

Figure 28–9. The CCFR pumping console uses two pumps for irrigation during TUR.

the fluid source. The TV image becomes increasingly difficult to distinguish as visibility diminishes due to the accumulation of blood mixing with the fluids. Periodic interruption required to remove the working element and drain bladder fluids disrupts orientation and is physically cumbersome with the video camera. Elevating the fluid source to improve

visualization of arterial bleeders frequently is counterproductive because as the bladder fills faster, it reaches capacity sooner, and the instrument must be disconnected more often.[7]

The Iglesias method for continuous flow uses gravity inflow and suction outflow. This system has no means for accurately balancing flow and maintaining the desired level of bladder distention when the flow rate is increased. As with all continuous flow resectoscopes, when the sheath is drawn

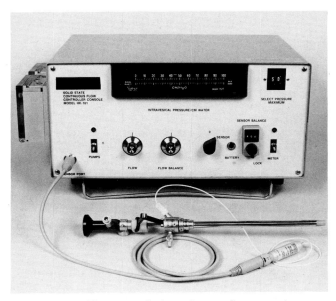

Figure 28–8. The controlled continuous flow resectoscope (CCFR) with pumping console limits the intravesical pressure during TUR.

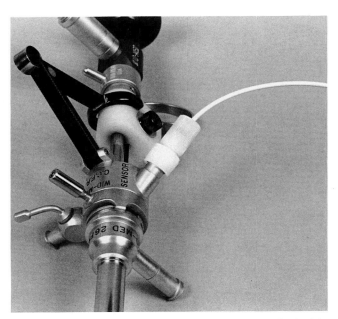

Figure 28–10. An electronic pressure transducer fits inside the CCFR working element for routine measurement of intravesical pressure during TUR.

T.U.R. IRRIGATING SYSTEM
RECIPROCAL
GRAVITY IN → GRAVITY OUT

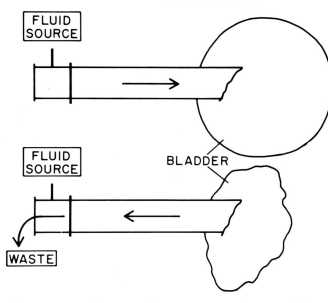

Figure 28–11. Diagram of the intermittent (reciprocal) flow system for TUR.

into the prostatic urethra, unresected prostatic adenoma frequently obstructs the outflow. Also, at times, blood clots or tiny pieces of hypercellular tissue adhere to the outflow openings and completely restrict fluid withdrawal. When this occurs, intravesical pressure rises, and the bladder continues filling under gravity until the intravesical pressure reaches equilibrium with the fluid source.

These gravity-dependent flow systems provide no means for routinely measuring and limiting intravesical pressure.[23]

T.U.R. IRRIGATING SYSTEM
CONTINUOUS FLOW-IGLESIAS TYPE
GRAVITY IN → SUCTION OUT

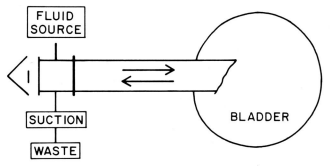

Figure 28–12. Diagram of the Iglesias continuous flow system for TUR.

T.U.R. IRRIGATING SYSTEM
CONTINUOUS FLOW-REUTER TYPE
GRAVITY IN → SUCTION OUT
CYSTOSTOMY

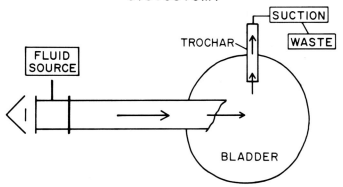

Figure 28–13. Diagram of the Reuter suprapubic continuous flow system for TUR.

A continuous flow system is the best way to accomplish the video procedure accurately and efficiently because it alleviates the need periodically to interrupt the surgery. Without actually measuring the pressure, however, the potential exists for bladder overdistention with the resultant overstretch of the detruser fibers.[24] Vision of the back wall of the bladder is lost with the video camera, and the fine sensation of what is happening there is not perceived.[7] The intravesical pressures commonly are ignored while the surgeon concentrates on the technique of resection and minimizing blood loss. Increasing the height of the fluid source to help maintain visibility on the TV screen also increases the maximum level of intravesical pressure when outflow is obstructed or not available. Repeatedly high intravesical pressures occurring at maximum bladder filling increase the potential risks for hypervolemia and secondary hyponatremia.[25,26] It has been shown that lowering the intravesical pressure by only 10 cm of water (from 70 cm to 60 cm) can reduce total absorption by almost half.[27] Absorption especially can be a problem during the latter part of surgery if numerous venous sinuses are exposed.[28] Judgments of intravesical pressures are based solely on conjecture and the surgeon's prior experience. By the time bladder fullness is actually noticeable by suprapubic feel, the intravesical pressure already may be exceedingly high.

With the Reuter continuous flow method, the surgeon usually works with a collapsed bladder unless a flow controller is used.[29] This recently developed mechanism maintains bladder distention and limits the intravesical pressure regardless of the fluid source height. This system may be suitable for video TUR, but adding the trocar puncture to the patient's abdomen increases surgical invasion and the potential for complications. One advantage of the trocar method is that the flow of blood and fluids is always away from the lens, so visibility should be good with the video camera.[12] The possibility of the trocar being dislodged during the operation, making it very difficult to replace, and leaking of fluids around the trocar and into the perineum add to the patient's surgical risk. Also, the trocar method should not be attempted during bladder tumor resection.

The CCFR system has many advantages that make it recommended and desirable for successful video TUR.[4] Interruptions to disconnect the instrument from the sheath are eliminated except when needed for removing resected tissue fragments. High flow rates are available by simply turning a dial on the pumping console to reestablish clarity of the endoscopic field quickly. The balance of inflow and outflow can be adjusted and fine tuned so the bladder remains distended based on pressure readings. Bladder overdistention is prevented by an automatic safety mechanism that limits intravesical pressure at a predetermined level in order to minimize the potential for absorption of the irrigation fluids.

CASE STUDY

Five hundred patients with prostatic obstruction were operated in three Chicago hospitals between June 1986 and September 1990. TURP was performed in all cases by standing and observing the TV monitor. The video technique, as earlier described, was applied during these cases.

The CCFR with a 30-degree, magnified view lens was attached by a direct beam coupler to a solid-state miniature video camera. Either a 26 F or a 28 F sheath was attached to the resectoscope, and accordingly a 26 F or 28 F cutting loop was used. Intravesical pressure was monitored continuously by a Millar Instruments, Inc., 5 F pressure transducer inserted into the resectoscope working element. On the pumping console, the maximum pressure limit was set at 50 cm of water to deactivate the inflow pump and sound a warning. Irrigation flow rate was adjusted between 300 and 900 mL/min for continuous inflow and outflow during these cases.

An M.P. Video, Inc., model Medicam MC-6 video camera was used during the first 400 cases. This camera provided 330 lines of resolution for a sharp video image with good color reproduction. The last 100 cases were performed using either an M.P. Video, Inc., model Medicam MC-800 video camera or an Acufex Microsurgical, Inc., model AFM-2 video camera. Each of these cameras provided over 400 lines of resolution and had improved light sensitivity over the MC-6 camera.

A 300-W manually adjustable light source with an Osram metal halides arc lamp was utilized with a 4.5-mm fiberoptic cable. A 20-inch screen, professional grade NEC TV monitor with over 400 lines of resolution provided up to 50 times magnification of the surgical field. Either a Valleylab solid-state generator or a Bard solid-state generator was used in conjunction with the resectoscope to energize the loop.

Data were recorded from these 500 TURP cases to examine the safety and efficiency of the video-enhanced procedure. Information regarding the resection rate, blood loss, sodium depletion, and CVP were examined. The mean value and range for each category was determined and averages based on calculations are presented in Table 28–1.

Data obtained from these 500 video TURP cases were comparable with data presented by other researchers examining TURP with conventional vision through the lens operating method.[30-32] Blood loss, resection rate, and sodium change figures appear within an acceptable range.[33,34] These figures corroborate that the video technique is a safe and efficient means for performing TURP.[1,7,9,12]

Experience with the video method shows that there is better control of bleeding during and at the end of the operation than with the conventional method.[7] Postoperative irrigation fluid generally is clearer in the cases where the video camera is used. This is in part due to the continuous flow of fluids and the ability to see better with the magnification created by the TV image. The small bleeders, ordinarily missed by the conventional method, are seen more easily because of the enlarged picture from the scope on the video monitor.

ADVANTAGES OF VIDEO TUR

1. The standing position with both eyes open reduces stress on the surgeon's back, neck, and eyesight.[7,11]
2. High magnification and clarity of the field of view

Table 28–1. Data from 500 Consecutive Video TURP Cases with CCFR

Age of patient (years)	Mean 69
	Range 53–93
Weight of tissue resected (g)	Mean 33
	Range 5–103
Length of surgery (min)	Mean 44
	Range 15–90
Resection rate (g/min)	Mean 0.75
	Range 0.16–3.10
Volume of irrigating fluid (mL)	Mean 19,000
	Range 6000–48,000
Change in hemoglobin (g/100 mL)	Mean 1.3
	Range 0.1–5.0
Change in hematocrit (points)	Mean 3.4
	Range 0.1–11.0
Change in sodium (mmol/L)	Mean 1.5
Estimated blood loss volume (mL)	Average 340
Blood loss per tissue removed (mL/g)	Average 10.3
Blood loss/min of surgery (mL/min)	Average 7.7
Number of blood transfusions	3 patients
Sodium below 130 mEq/L	7 patients
CVP above 20 cm H_2O	0 patients
CVP patients monitored	20%
Postoperative length of stay	Average 4.2 days

improve the visibility of landmarks, capsular tissue, and small, hard-to-find bleeders.

3. The larger angle of mobility and range of motion for movement of the resectoscope make it easier to maneuver and manipulate for more accurate surgery.[2]
4. This remarkable teaching tool facilitates the teaching and learning of TURP by permitting observers in the room to follow and understand the procedure.[12,18]
5. Tape recordings or video snapshots of interesting pathologic conditions can be documented for later review.[6]
6. The surgeon's eyes and mouth are distanced from the resectoscope discharges, providing reduced exposure to possibly contaminated bodily fluids.[1]

LEARNING PERIOD

Cystoscopy is a good procedure for getting acquainted with and practicing the video procedure. Since very little bleeding is encountered, the circumstances are less stressful, and the video technique is easier to learn. All the problems and difficulties encountered during TURP are similar during cystoscopy, although less critical. It provides an excellent opportunity for learning the setup of the video equipment and accommodating the feel of orientation with the video image. All the advantages of the video method are obtained during the cystoscopy procedure as well. Once comfort and skill with video cystoscopy develop, this method can be applied to the confident surgical performance of all TUR cases.

The learning curve for video TUR will vary depending on the individual and the surgeon's prior experience with TUR. It takes approximately between 3 and 10 cases to gain comfort and assume speed of resection with the video camera. With patience and determination, the surgeon will develop a mastery of this technique and gain the benefits of its superior features.

FUTURE DEVELOPMENTS

Once the video technique becomes established in everyday urologic practice, lenses will no longer need an eyepiece, and the camera can be built directly on to the telescope to form a single videolens—camera/coupler/scope combination. Voice-activated switches will be programmed electronically to obey the surgeon's commands for adjusting pump speed and irrigation flow needed during video TUR to help maintain visibility. Soon, even higher quality imaging will become available with the application of high-definition television (HDTV) for endoscopy.

DISCUSSION

Video TUR is a tremendous advance in endoscopic urologic technique. Added to this is the use of a noninvasive continuous flow device that relates to the safety of intravesical pressure monitoring. Magnified endoscopic images and electronic safety allow us to come closer to the ideal instrument for transurethral surgery. Until a better method of removing hypertrophied prostate and noninfiltrating bladder neoplasms than TUR is proven, the video technology must become a part of our armamentarium.

Perhaps the magnitude of appreciation is accelerated by the memories of over 25 years of monocular suffering. With each advancement in technology, a look backward makes us wonder how we did it with such archaic equipment. Each step in the progression from the semidarkness of the battery-activated light bulb to the fiberoptics and magnified view lens seemed adequate for the times. Perhaps the next century will fine tune laser ablation of diseased organs, and the upgrade of video technology for TUR will become another footnote in surgical history.

For now, we should allow ourselves to be liberated and start using this equipment. Once the video TUR is mastered, all endourology becomes video endourology. Not only will the urologist's life be better, but the quality of surgical techniques will be improved. Finally, in any discussion on the merits of video technology and its relationship to urology, it is not how can we do it but how have we done without it for so long.

ACKNOWLEDGMENT

I thank Sanford L. Widran for assistance in preparation of this manuscript.

REFERENCES

1. Widran J. Video transurethral resection: report of 200 cases. *Br J Urol* 1990;65:357–361
2. Tazaki H, Tachibana M. Video-guided TUR using advanced instruments (videotape). *VideoUrology* 1989;1:Program 4
3. O'Boyle PJ, Lumb GN, Appleton GVN. Videoprostatectomy. In: Matouschek E (ed). *Endourology, Proceedings from the Third Congress I.S.U.E. August 1984, Karlsruhe.* Baden-Baden: BuA-Verlag Werner Steinbruck, 1985:323–324
4. Widran J. Videoprostatectomy. *Urology* 1987;29:191–192
5. Yachia D. Videoprostatectomy or armchair prostatectomy (Letter). *Urology* 1987;30:189
6. O'Boyle PJ, Raina S, Holdoway AT. Videoprostatectomy. Guidelines for choosing an effective microvideo operating system. *Br J Urol* 1989;63:624–626
7. Widran J. Video transurethral resection using controlled continuous flow resectoscope. *Urology* 1988;31:382–386
8. Aso Y, Tajima A, Suzuki K, Ohtawara Y. Application of the video-system in urological endoscopy. *Hinyokika Kiyo* 1984;30:13–15
9. Appleton GVN, O'Boyle PJ, Lumb GN. Videoprostatectomy versus conventional TUR. In: Matouschek E (ed). *Endourology, Proceedings from the Third Congress I.S.U.E. August 1984, Karlsruhe.* Baden-Baden: BuA-Verlag Werner Steinbruck, 1985:324–325
10. McDonald HP Jr. Color television endoscopy (abstract). *J Endourol* 1990;4:S45

11. Tazaki H. Video control TURP (abstract). *J Endourol* 1990;4:S46
12. Osawa T, Nakamura S, Kawakami Y, Nishiyama T. Transurethral resection of prostate under TV-monitoring. *Nippon Hinyokiki Gakkai Zasshi* 1989;43:679–682
13. Allhoff E, Bading R, Hoene E, Jonas U. The chip camera: perfect imaging in endourology. *World J Urol* 1988;6:6–7
14. Jackson DW, Ovadia DN. Videoarthroscopy: present and future developments. *Arthroscopy* 1985;1:108
15. Sivak NV Jr, Fleischer DP. Colonoscopy with a videoendoscope: preliminary experience. *Gastrointest Endosc* 1984; 30:1–5
16. Nezhat C, Hood J, Winer W, Nexhat F. Videolaseroscopy and laser laparoscopy in gynaecology. *Br J Hosp Med* 1987; Sept:219–224
17. Iglesias JJ, Kardashian JF, Lanteri VJ, et al. Iglesias articulated endoscopy teaching attachment. *J Urol* 1978;120:465–468
18. Kaplan J, Berci G, Kudish H, et al. New television technique as a teaching aid for transurethral resection of prostate (TURP). In Matouschek E (ed). *Endourology, Proceedings from the Third Congress I.S.U.E. August 1984, Karlsruhe.* Baden-Baden: BuA-Verlag Werner Steinbruck, 1985:629
19. Widran J. Controlled continuous flow (CCF) resectoscope: a report of 200 cases. *Urology* 1985;25:242–247
20. Widran J. Noninvasive transvesical pressure monitoring using controlled continuous flow resectoscope. *Urology* 1987; 29:598–604
21. Iglesias JJ, Sporer A, Gellman AC, Seebode JJ. New Iglesias resectoscope with continuous irrigation, simultaneous suction, and low intravesical pressure. *J Urol* 1975;114:929
22. Reuter HJ, Reuter M, Kleckner N, Gernoth D. Die Nierendruckirrigation-eine neue Technik zur Vermeidring von Kompliakationes wahrend der TUR. *Therapierocke* 1978; 28:2017
23. Madsen PO, Nielsen KT. Devices for monitoring intravesical pressure during transurethral resection of the prostate. *Med Instrument* 1988;22:69–73
24. Bird D, Slade N, Feneley RC. Intravascular complications of transurethral resection of the prostate. *Br J Urol* 1982;54:564
25. Henderson DJ, Middleton RG. Coma from hyponatremia following transurethral resection of prostate. *Urology* 1980; 15:267–271
26. Logie JR, Keenan RA, Whiting PH, et al. Fluid absorption during transurethral prostatectomy. *Br J Urol* 1980;52:526–528
27. Madsen PO, Naber KG. The importance of the pressure in the prostatic fossa and absorption of irrigating fluid during transurethral resection of the prostate. *J Urol* 1973;109:446–452
28. Widran J. The controlled continuous flow (CCF) resectoscope. In: Matouschek E (ed). *Endourology, Proceedings from the Third Congress I.S.U.E. August 1984, Karlsruhe.* Baden-Baden: BuA-Verlag Werner Steinbruck, 1985:321–322
29. Korth K. Suprapubic puncture kit (abstract). *J Endourol* 1990;4:S44
30. Mackenzie AR, Levine N, Scheinman HZ. Operative blood loss in transurethral prostatectomy. *J Urol* 1978;122:47
31. Levin K, Nyren O, Pompeius R. Blood loss, tissue weight and operating time in transurethral prostatectomy. *Scand J Urol Nephrol* 1981;15:197
32. Flechner SM, Williams RD. Continuous flow and conventional resectoscope methods in transurethral prostatectomy: comparative study. *J Urol* 1982;127:257
33. Madsen PO, Frimodt-Moller PC. Transurethral prostatic resection with suprapubic trocar technique. *J Urol* 1984;132:277–279
34. Stephenson TP, et al. Comparison between continuous flow and intermittent flow transurethral resection in 40 patients presenting with acute retention. *Br J Urol* 1980;52:523

29

Urethral Stricture

Maj. José M. Hernandez-Graulau, Richard M. Evans

Urethral stricture can be described as a scar, which usually is the result of tissue injury, caused by urethral trauma, pelvic fracture, inflammatory disease, or neoplasia. As this scar heals, it contracts and creates fibrotic narrowing composed of dense collagen and fibroblast. Fibrosis usually extends into the surrounding corpus spongiosum, causing spongiofibrosis. Urethral strictures also can be congenital.

CLASSIFICATION OF STRICTURES

Congenital Lesions

Congenital lesions are found most commonly at the external urethral meatus, often associated with hypospadiac orifices,[1] but the membranous urethra and the penoscrotal junction frequently are involved. They are seen in both sexes but are more common in males.

Traumatic Lesions

Traumatic lesions are the result of tears or ruptures of the urethra caused by blows to the perineum or pelvic fracture, or they are iatrogenic. They can occur anywhere in the anterior or the membranous urethra, but they probably are most common in the bulbomembranous portion of the urethra. Chemical strictures, which are considered to be traumatic, usually occur in the anterior urethra. Iatrogenic strictures are a common form of traumatic stricture of the urethra in children and adults secondary to instrumentation. Traumatic strictures usually develop much more rapidly than do the inflammatory types. They tend to be dense and longer because of more ischemic necrosis.

Inflammatory Strictures

Inflammatory strictures may be caused by gonorrhea, tuberculosis, syphilis, or nonspecific infections. Although gono-coccal urethritis is seldom a cause of stricture today, infection remains a major cause, particularly infection from long-term use of indwelling urethral catheters. Large catheters and instruments are more likely than small ones to cause ischemia and internal trauma. It has been stated that approximately 75% of inflammatory strictures occur at the bulbomembranous junction. The lesions from infectious causes tend to be more diaphragm-like short strictures. Tuberculosis is a spread from another focus, usually higher up in the urinary tract and most likely from the prostate. The urethra appears to be particularly resistant to tuberculous infection, but when strictures occur, they are intractable and often associated with fistula formation and abscesses. The watering pot perineum results from fistula formation secondary to periurethral abscesses, which are common with inadequately treated *Neisseria gonorrhoreae* infections.

Neoplastic Strictures

Neoplastic strictures are the result of primary urethral carcinoma or are secondary from the bladder or the prostate. They may occur at any place in the urethra but are most common in the bulbomembranous area. Recurrent stricture disease of the urethra, even in the absence of hematuria, demands periodic retrograde urethrography to rule out the possibility of a clinically occult urethral cancer. Transitional cell carcinoma of the urethra may be associated with a bladder cancer. This possibility must be ruled out before the urethral lesion is addressed.

SURGICAL ANATOMY

Male Urethra

The male urethra is a fibroelastic structure that extends from the internal urethral orifice at the vesical neck to the external urethral meatus at the tip of the glans penis. It is divided by the urogenital diaphram into three parts: prostatic, membranous, and penile (Fig. 29–1). The prostatic urethra is the widest and is about 3 cm long in normal adults. The lumen of the urethra is distensible but normally is obliterated by elastic fibers causing apposition of its anterior and posterior walls. In prostatic lateral lobe hyperplasia (BPH), the urethral wall is changed into a wide anteroposterior fissure by encroachment of the enlarged lateral lobes on the urethra.

The urethral crest extends along the posterior floor of the urethra from its origin on the vesical trigone to its bifurcated end. The prostatic sinus is a depressed fossa on each side of the crest and has many orifices from prostatic ducts. The seminal colliculus or verumontanum is the greatest prominence of the urethral crest, and the prostatic utricle opens in its central surface. The finer, slitlike orifices of the ejaculatory ducts open beside the prostatic utricle.

The membranous urethra is the shortest, about 1.5 cm long, and passes through the urogenital diaphragm between its superior and inferior layers of fascia. This part of the urethra has no proper surrounding tissue but contains the circular fibers of the deep transverse perineal muscle, called the external urethral sphincter. This is a voluntary muscle controlled by the perineal branch of the internal pudendal nerve.

Behind the membranous urethra, close to the inferior layer of the urogenital diaphragm, lie the bulbourethral glands of Cowper, which open into the penile urethra at its bulbous part on each side.

The penile urethra is the longest segment of urethra and is surrounded by the spongy body. It is about 15 cm long when the penis is flaccid and has a right-angled curve at the penoscrotal junction. The bulbous urethra is dilated and forms the perineal curve. Openings of the bulbourethral glands of Cowper lie at its posterior wall. On the floor of the penile urethra are numerous small lacunas and mucosa glands, the glands of Littré. The external meatus is the narrowest part. The preterminal urethra next to the meatus has a dilated lumen known as the fossa navicularis. The arterial supply to the urethra is derived from branches of the internal pudendal and inferior vesical arteries. Veins drain into the pudendal or perivesical plexuses. Lymphatic drainage is to the inguinal nodes and lymph glands along the iliac vessels.

Female Urethra

The female urethra is approximately 4–5 cm long and begins at the internal urethral orifice or vesical neck. It follows a slightly curved course downward and forward and terminates at the external urethral meatus on the roof of the vestibule.

The epithelium of the female urethra is squamous in its distal portion and transitional in its proximal segment. Numerous periurethral glands are embedded in the submucosal layer, the largest are the glands of Skene, which open just inside the meatus.

The longitudinal smooth muscle layer of the bladder neck is prolonged to encase the urethra, but at the portion that pierces the urogenital diaphragm, it is surrounded by striated sphincter muscle, as in the male. The urethra also passes through the levator ani muscle before traversing the diaphragm and is supported by bulbocavernous muscle under the diaphragm.

Because the female urethra is short, care must be taken not to damage the urethral wall in operative procedures. A distinct sphincter action is not always demonstrable in the female.

SIGNS AND SYMPTOMS

The patient with urethral stricture usually has symptoms of bladder outlet obstruction. He complains of a slow, halting urinary stream and hesitancy in initiating the stream. Frequency and dysuria often are present. A split stream and terminal dribbling are common complaints. Occasionally, a urinary infection or a chronic urethral discharge prompts a

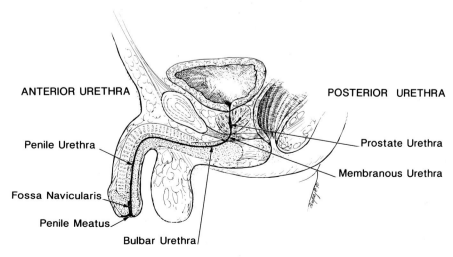

ANTERIOR URETHRA

POSTERIOR URETHRA

Penile Urethra

Prostate Urethra

Membranous Urethra

Fossa Navicularis

Penile Meatus

Bulbar Urethra

Figure 29–1. Normal anatomy of the male urethra.

urologic evaluation, which discloses the presence of urethral stricture as the underlying pathologic condition.

A high index of suspicion should be entertained in those clinical situations in which stricture may occur as a complication of either the treatment or the disease process. The gonorrheal stricture may occur 10–20 years after the original infection. A careful history should be elicited as to any previous urethral instrumentation, including even brief periods of urethral catheterization. A history of a straddle injury or a fractured pelvis may be significant.

Gross observation of the urinary stream may reveal a decrease in the usual force and caliber of the urinary stream. Obstruction from BPH may coexist with a previously undiagnosed stricture, and the effect may be additive. Stricture occasionally may be suggested by a careful palpation of the urethra. Induration may be present, particularly with posttraumatic strictures rather than with strictures from instrumentation or gonococcal urethritis.

LABORATORY FINDINGS

If urethral stricture is suspected, urinary flow rates should be determined. The patient is instructed to accumulate urine until the bladder is full and then begin voiding. A 5-sec collection of urine should be obtained during midstream maximal flow, and its volume should be recorded. With strictures creating significant problems, the flow rate usually is less than 10 mL/sec (normal is approximately 20 mL/sec).

Urine culture should be obtained. The midstream specimen is usually bacteria-free, with some pyuria (80–10 WBC/high power field) in a carefully obtained first aliquot of urine. If the prostate is infected, bacteria will be present in a specimen obtained after prostatic massage. This particular procedure is not usually recommended because of the risk of sepsis. In the presence of cystitis, the urine will be grossly infected.

ROENTOGENOGRAPHIC FINDINGS

Voiding cystourethrograms (VCU) are best to demonstrate dilation behind a stricture, but the retrograde urethrogram (RUG) method best demonstrates the stricture itself. Although strictures may be diagnosed by the insertion of a cystoscope into the urethra, important information, such as length, caliber, location, and multiplicity, cannot be obtained without the use of urethrograms.

Strictures of the urethra appear as narrowed segments, which can vary in length and appearance from valvelike structures to long constrictions. Approximately 10% are multiple. The congenital type is single, usually short and regular in appearance. The inflammatory stricture may be single or, more commonly, multiple, and it may be short or long. It usually appears more irregular than either the congenital or the traumatic stricture. The traumatic stricture

can be single or multiple but more commonly is single. The stricture may be long or short and usually is smooth. Neoplastic strictures are irregular and long and tend to occur with fistulous formation.

FALSE PASSAGES

False passages are produced by internal injuries of the urethra, usually iatrogenic. They usually occur in the region of the bulbous and membranous urethra and are found most commonly on the inferior side of the urethra, appearing as irregular outpocketing extending proximally. False passages can be demonstrated either by VCU or RUG. They must be differentiated from small urethrocavernous refluxes and from the duct of Cowper's gland.

The duct of Cowper's gland usually is smooth and even, and the diameter of its lumen appears to be constant. Small urethrocavernous refluxes usually are more diffuse and do not appear to have a connection with the urethra. False passages are slightly irregular, with narrowing at the terminal point.

CONTRACTURE OF THE BLADDER NECK

Contracture of the bladder neck may be either congenital or acquired. Contracture of the bladder neck is seen in boys and girls in a ratio of about 4:1.[2] In children, contracture of the bladder neck often is seen with strictures of the ureterovesical junction, often bilateral. The obstruction at the bladder neck may involve the entire circumference or only the posterior segment, representing median bar obstruction. Cystoscopically, there often are associated trabeculation and widespread damage to the upper tracts. Contracture of the bladder neck may be seen in adults in the second and third decades and occasionally later in life. Some of these cases may be congenital, but a good percentage are acquired, most likely secondary to infection and often associated with chronic prostatitis in men and chronic urethritis and cystitis in females. Contracture of the bladder neck also can result from prostatectomy. This postoperative contracture, also called iris-type diaphragm, may be the most severe. Contracture may occur after renal transplantation.[3]

DIFFERENTIAL DIAGNOSIS

BPH or malignant prostatic obstruction can cause symptoms similar to those of stricture. After prostatic surgery, bladder neck contracture can develop and must be differentiated from various other obstructions in the urethra, especially valvular obstruction, congenital urethral strictures, hypertrophy of the verumontanum, and sphincterospastic neurogenic disease. The last can be diagnosed by urodynamic studies. Rectal examination and cystourethroscopy will adequately define abnormalities of the prostate. Urethral carcinoma often is associated with stricture. Urethroscopy and biopsy will establish the diagnosis.

COMPLICATIONS

The most common complication of urethral stricture is significant lower urinary tract obstruction decreasing the compliance and elasticity of the surrounding tissues. Intravesicle voiding pressure increases, and urinary flow rate eventually will decrease.

Residual urine frequently accumulates. The integrity of the upper urinary tract may be at risk by the lower tract obstruction.

Long-standing stricture disease may cause urinary extravasation, which frequently becomes infected, and sepsis rapidly develops. The presence of urine within the tissues is an indication for prompt drainage and diversion of the urine at a site proximal to the extravasation.

Periurethral abscess is closely related in its development to that of urinary extravasation. Periurethral abscess may cause multiple urethrocutaneous fistulas in the perineum, the buttocks, and the thighs.

Urinary tract and prostatic calculi are more common in patients with stricture disease and infection than in the normal population. Bladder calculi may develop from chronic urinary stasis and infection. Difficult instrumentation may be followed by hemorrhage, urinary retention, sepsis, and urinary extravasation and abscess.

MANAGEMENT OF URETHRAL STRICTURE

Management of urethral strictures is based on their location and the degree of compromise of the urethral lumen. Anterior urethral strictures with a moderate compromise of the lumen may be managed by gentle dilation using a curved metal Van Buren sound. Experienced hands can treat recurring strictures, but inexperienced ones can result in the formation of false passages and subsequent new scar tissue production. If urethral dilation needs to be performed too frequently, such as more than once every 4 months, alternate treatments are chosen. Urethral sound dilation is uncomfortable, since only local anesthesia is usually utilized, and the complications can make definitive treatment impossible.

Another form of anterior urethral dilation is the use of the filiform and follower catheters. This involves the blind or cystoscope-assisted insertion of a 35 F catheter (filiform) past the stricture region. It is safer to use the cystoscope, flexible or rigid, to direct the filiform to prevent the formation of a false passage. A larger catheter (follower) screws onto the filiform catheter and is advanced gently past the stricture. The size of the follower is advanced gradually until the desired urethral lumen is obtained (16–30 F).

Penile meatal strictures often can be managed with the Van Buren sound. However, recurrent meatal strictures will require a meatotomy. In this instance, a small scissors is used to open the meatus on the ventral aspect of the glans, for a distance of approximately 0.5 cm. Absorbable sutures are placed in the region of the incised meatus and tacked to the lateral border of the glans to promote patent meatal healing. The patient usually is discharged home the same day with or without a temporary Foley catheter.

Most anterior urethral strictures require more definitive treatment than urethral dilation alone. Strictures less than 2 cm are treated initially with an internal urethrotomy. This is a surgical procedure where the strictured urethra is incised from within. The instrument used, a urethrotome, consists of a movable scalpel attached to a cystoscope (Fig. 29–2A). This permits direct vision while incising the stricture at the 12 o'clock location in the urethra. This specific region of the urethra is chosen because the incidence of hemorrhage is lowest.[4,5] The external sphincter must be avoided to prevent urinary incontinence. Other complications of internal urethrotomy are extravasation of cystoscopy irrigation fluid into the corpora and urinary sepsis. Approximately 15% of anterior urethral strictures will recur following internal urethrotomy. A 24 F Foley catheter is inserted postprocedure for an average of 3 days to 2 weeks.

An alternative to internal urethrotomy is balloon dilation of anterior or posterior urethral strictures[6] (Fig. 29–2B). Local intraurethral lidocaine jelly usually is sufficient for anesthesia. Initially, a guidewire (0.035 inch) is inserted past the stricture and into the bladder under direct vision with a flexible or rigid cystoscope. A balloon catheter 10 cm long and 36 F in size is inserted into the urethra over the guidewire and past the stricture. The balloon is inflated with contrast to

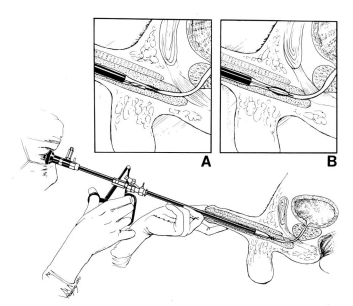

Figure 29–2. **A.** Internal urethrotomy. **B.** Urethral balloon dilation.

12 atm of pressure. Fluoroscopy will reveal the stricture by the waisting appearance. The balloon is deflated after 1 min but usually needs to be reinflated two to three times until sufficient urethral dilation is obtained. Most patients require repeat balloon dilation every 3–4 months, depending on the patient's urinary symptoms. No major complication has been reported, such as impotence, urinary incontinence, or retrograde ejaculation, except for mild hematuria lasting 1–2 days.

Laser therapy has found its way into the treatment of urethral strictures, neodymium:YAG (Nd:YAG) laser can be directed easily with a 600 μm fiber through a cystoscope.[7] The tissue vaporization process is optimized with a sapphire-tipped laser fiber. This special sapphire tip also is preferred because less fibrosis results, since it relies more on tissue vaporization than coagulation to incise scar tissue. Approximately 4–12 W of energy is directed through the laser fiber as it is advanced along the urethral stricture. However, the actual benefit of Nd:YAG laser compared to cold knife internal urethrotomy is in question. The Nd:YAG laser often requires more operative time because it must rely on the slow process of tissue vaporization to open the strictures. Also, urethral stricture recurrence after Nd:YAG laser treatment is quite common. Approximately 50%–60% of strictures will recur after the first year of laser treatment.

Carbon dioxide laser has not been able to be utilized in urethral stricture treatment because of its high absorption in a fluid medium, preventing appropriate delivery. However, KTP (potassium titanyl phosphate) laser is a recent advance of the Nd:YAG laser and is becoming a widely used instrument in urethral stricture management.[8] KTP laser is a double-frequency Nd:YAG laser converted as it passes through a KTP crystal and applied at a 532 nm wavelength. A 400 μm fiber with 5–9 W of energy is inserted through a cystoscope for proper use. KTP has several advantages over Nd:YAG laser in the treatment of urethral strictures. It is more effective in cutting through fibrotic tissue and results in less bleeding. KTP laser has the equivalent success rate to cold knife internal urethrotomy. However, KTP laser may prove to have a lower incidence of stricture recurrence because of less associated tissue injury. Rare complications of KTP laser have been reported, such as a self-limiting bloody urethral discharge and a urethrocutaneous fistula. More commonly, urinary retention can occur when sloughed debris occlude the urethra. This can be prevented by prophylactic insertion of a Foley catheter for 3 days.

The most recent investigational advance in the treatment of urethral strictures is the urethral insertion of a tubular mesh of surgical grade stainless steel wire, known as the Wall-stent.[9] A modified cystoscope allows direct vision implantation of the tightly woven mesh. When the proper urethral location is obtained, the mesh is allowed to expand and mechanically maintain urethral patency. It has been shown that by 4–6 months, the urothelium completely covers the mesh, preventing encrustations, infection, and migration.

Thus far, the stent has been used most often in bulbar urethral strictures, but in the future, it will be applied to all urethral strictures. Ejaculation abnormalities and urinary incontinence have not been reported following Wallstent insertion. The permanent nature of the Wallstent may in the future obviate the need for repeated urethral dilations or surgical reconstruction.

Open surgical management, or urethroplasty, may be required if a urethral stricture cannot be managed successfully with less invasive methods. Usually, urethral strictures measuring more than 2 cm are best managed with initial urethroplasty. The option of different types of urethral reconstruction depends on stricture location, etiology, and length. Bulbomembranous urethral strictures less than 2 cm are best managed with a perineal approach. The strictured region is resected before the two ends can be reanastomosed. This is referred to as a one-stage procedure. If the bulbomembranous urethral stricture is greater than 2 cm, a two-stage procedure is most successful. The first stage involves the opening and marsupialization of the urethral edges to surrounding skin or scrotal skin, as in the popular Turner-Warwick procedure (Fig. 29–3A,B,C). The second stage is performed 4–6 months later, when the neourethra is tubularized to include the adjacent skin from the first stage to form a 26 F lumen (Fig. 29–3D,E). If the neourethra is made too

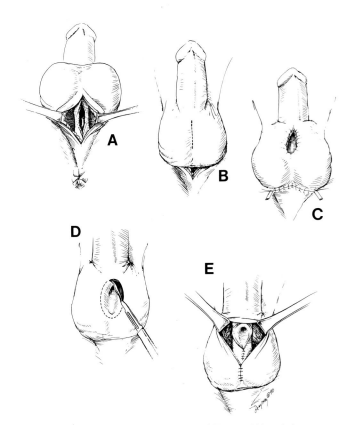

Figure 29–3. A,B,C. First stage of Turner-Warwick procedure. D,E. Second stage of Turner-Warwick procedure.

large, a pseudodiverticulum may result. Thus, careful planning and measurement are essential.[10,11]

Two other types of surgical repair are the use of a free full thickness skin graft and a vascularized island flap. The free full thickness skin graft consists of all layers of the skin, as opposed to a split thickness skin graft, which lacks the dermal support tissue. The full thickness graft has better vascularization and contracts up to 80% less from its original size as compared to the split thickness graft. The most common source for the full thickness graft to be harvested is the preputial or penile skin. Following the excision of the urethral strictures, the full thickness skin graft is sutured into place. If the urethral defect exceeds 1.5 cm, the success rate of repair diminishes. The island flap urethroplasty, as described by Quartey, utilizes penile skin as either a patch or a tube.[12] This one-stage procedure relies on a vascularized pedicle of penile or preputial skin, which can be used to repair a urethral defect of virtually any length.

ACKNOWLEDGMENTS

We wish to express our appreciation to Mrs. Ana Osansky for her help in structuring and refining this manuscript.

REFERENCES

1. Lattimer JK. Similar urogenital anomalies in identical twins. *Am J Dis Child* 1944;67:199–200
2. Campbell MF. *Urology,* 2nd ed. Saunders: Philadelphia, 1963;2:1689–1694
3. Loening SA, Banowsky LH, Braun WE, et al. Bladder neck contracture and urethral stricture as complications of renal transplantation. *J Urol* 1975;114:688–691
4. Sandozi S, Ghazali S. Sachse optical urethrotomy, a modified technique: 6 years of experience. *J Urol* 1988;140:968–969
5. Cohen E. Operative internal urethrotomy. *AUA Update Series* 1982;1:Lesson 24
6. Daughtry J, Rodan B, Bean W. Balloon dilatation of urethral strictures. *Urology* 1988;31:231–233
7. Smith J JR. Treatment of benign urethral strictures using a sapphire tipped neodymium:YAG laser. *J Urol* 1989;142:1221–1222
8. Shanberg A, Baghdassarian R, Tansey L, Sawyer D. KTP 532 laser in treatment of urethral strictures. *Urology* 1988;32:517–520
9. Milroy EJG, Chapple CR, Eldin A, Wallstern H. A new stent for the treatment of urethral strictures. *Br J Urol* 1989;63:392–396
10. Webster GD, Koefoot RB, Sihelnik SA. Urethroplasty management in 100 cases of urethral stricture: a rationale for procedure selection. *J Urol* 1985;134:892–898
11. Webster GD, Sihelnik SA. The management of strictures of the membranous urethra. *J Urol* 1985;134:469–473
12. Quartey JKM. One-stage penile/preputial island flap urethroplasty for urethral stricture. *J Urol* 1985;134:474–475

The opinions or assertions contained herein are the private views of the author and are not to be construed as official or as reflecting the views of the Department of the Army or the Department of Defense.

Index